The Clock and the Mirror

The Clock and the Mirror

GIROLAMO CARDANO AND
RENAISSANCE MEDICINE

Nancy G. Siraisi

PRINCETON UNIVERSITY PRESS
PRINCETON, NEW JERSEY

Library of Congress Cataloging-in-Publication Data

Siraisi, Nancy G.
The clock and the mirror : Girolamo Cardano and
Renaissance medicine / Nancy G. Siraisi.
p.   cm.
Includes bibliographical references and index.
ISBN 0-691-01189-3 (cloth : alk. paper)
1. Cardano, Girolamo, 1501–1576—Contributions
in medicine.   2. Medicine—Italy—History—16th century.
3. Cardano, Girolamo, 1501–1576—Philosophy.
4. Italy—Intellectual life—16th century.   I. Title.
R520.C32S57   1997
610'.92—dc21   96-46354

This book has been composed in Galliard

Printed in the United States of America
by Princeton Academic Press

10 9 8 7 6 5 4 3 2 1

For Nancy Brain

———————

CONTENTS

PREFACE AND ACKNOWLEDGMENTS

THIS BOOK is intended as a contribution to cultural and intellectual history as well as to the history of medicine and science. Where premodern Europe is concerned, it seems to me impossible to separate the history of a large part of medicine not only from social history but also from broad intellectual developments and from the history of learning, reading, and written culture. Accordingly, I began the research that led to this book with the intention of taking a fresh look at areas of Renaissance medicine most closely linked to innovative aspects of contemporary scientific and learned culture. My idea was to complement and move beyond earlier studies that had led me from a group of scholastic physicians in thirteenth- and early-fourteenth-century Bologna to sixteenth-century endeavors to refurbish a medieval textbook. It now seemed time to investigate some of the themes of self-conscious and self-proclaimed renewal in which—as well as in technical accomplishments—sixteenth-century medicine is remarkably rich and to try to see how those themes played out in the actual social context of medical writing, teaching, and practice.

I hope, indeed, that the result goes some way to accomplish those goals. But things never turn out quite as one plans. I did not originally intend to center the book on an individual. Instead, Cardano caught me. My study has ended up being focused on one remarkable person, the diversity of whose interests linked medicine to a much wider world. Whatever the historiographic merits or demerits of this approach, I have enjoyed writing the book. Over the centuries Cardano has been the subject of a large literature, good, bad, and indifferent, and many myths. I hope I do not need to apologize for adding one more book; I have tried not to add to the myths.

I owe thanks to many friends and colleagues for their help at different stages of this work. I am especially grateful to Vivian Nutton and Mary Voss who read the manuscript for Princeton University Press and offered very useful suggestions. At different times Ann Blair, Alfonso Ingegno, Michael McVaugh, Katherine Park, and David Ruderman gave advice and answered queries; Katharine Park also read chapter 1; Andrea Carlino most kindly drew my attention to documents about Cardano in the Archivio di Stato of Rome. Chiara Crisciani shared her learning about medieval medicine in many valuable conversations; I also owe to her kindness much guidance and help in increasing my knowledge of

Milan and Pavia, Cardano's cities. I am also grateful to the various academic audiences who have heard me speak on Cardano; the discussion on such occasions (especially some remarks by Ian Maclean) often helped me to rethink. My deepest thanks go to Anthony Grafton, a fellow Cardanophile who in numerous conversations on the subject gave most generously of his learning and who also read the entire manuscript, much to its benefit. Remaining mistakes are, of course, my own fault.

My research in Rome was aided by a travel grant from the PSC-CUNY Research Foundation. Part of chapter 6 appeared as "Cardano, Hippocrates, and Criticism of Galen," in *Girolamo Cardano: Philosoph Naturforscher Arzt*, ed. Eckhard Kessler (Wiesbaden, 1994), pp. 131–56. I am grateful to the Herzog August Bibliothek, Wolfenbüttel, for permission to reprint this material; part of chapter 9 appeared as "Girolamo Cardano and the Art of Medical Narrrative," *Journal of the History of Ideas* 52 (1991): 581–602. I am grateful to the *Journal of the History of Ideas* for permission to reprint this material.

I should also like to express my thanks to Barbara Welter, Chair of the Department of History, Hunter College, for her continued encouragement of my research during a difficult period for the City University of New York. I am, as always, profoundly grateful to my sons, and above all to my husband, Nobuyuki Siraisi, for their personal encouragement of, and patience with, me over so many years. This book is dedicated to my mother because she was the first to show me, by her example, the pleasure of reading; and because I admire and wish I could emulate her lifelong example of competence and fortitude.

NOTE TO THE READER

IN THE NOTES to this book, citations of Cardano's works are given to the collected edition, Girolamo Cardano, *Opera omnia*, 10 vols. (Lyon, 1663; facsimile edition New York and London, 1967) for the sake of ease of reference. However, in the case of works published during Cardano's lifetime or within five years of his death, all quotations have been checked in such editions (listed in the bibliography) and differences (other than minor variants in spelling and punctuation) noted.

In the passages quoted, the use of *u* and *v* has been modernized. Some punctuation has also been slightly modernized.

ABBREVIATIONS

1. Abbreviations for titles of selected works by Girolamo Cardano frequently cited in this book. In the following list:

a. Except where otherwise indicated, titles are given in the form used in the table of contents in Girolamo Cardano, *Opera omnia*, 10 vols. (Lyon, 1663; facsimile edition New York and London, 1967), vol. 1, fols. IIIr–IVr. In the case of a number of treatises, the title varies slightly from this form either in sixteenth-century editions or in the volume of the collected works where the treatise actually appears.

b. In the case of works published in Cardano's lifetime or within five years of his death, the date of first publication as established by the *Index aureliensis: Catalogus librorum sedecimo saeculo impressorum*, pt. 1, vol. 6 (Orleans, 1976) follows each title in square brackets. For fuller citations of these and/or other early editions of Cardano's works consulted in the preparation of this book, see the bibliography. Some additional information about publication history and, in certain cases, the subsequent appearance of revised, retitled, or recombined works or parts of works is to be found in the notes.

ACP	*Ars curandi parva* [1564]
CA	*De curationibus et praedictionibus admirandis* [1562]. Reissued as MM, sectio 3
comm. AAL	*Commentarii in librum Hippocratis de Aere, Aquis et locis* [1570]
comm. *Aliment.*	*Commentarii in librum Hippocratis de Alimento* [1574]
comm. *Aph.*	*Commentarii in Aphorismos Hippocratis* [1564]
comm. *Epid.*	*Commentarii in duos libros priores Epidemiorum Hippocratis*
comm. Mondino	*Expositio Anatomiae Mundini*
comm. *Prognost.*	*Commentarii in libros Prognosticorum Hippocratis* [1568]
comm. SP	*Commentarii in librum Hippocratis de Septimestri partu* [1568]
comm. *Tetrabiblos*	*Commentarii in Ptolemeum, de Astrorum judiciis* [1554]
comm. VA	*Commentarii in libros Hippocratis de Victu in acutis*

Contradictiones	*Contradicentium medicorum libri duo* [bk. 1, 1545; bks. 1 and 2, 1548] . . . *libri octo posteriores*
De malo usu	*De malo recentiorum medicorum medendi usu libellus* [1536]. The second edition (1545) reissued as MM, sectio 1
Examen	*Examen XXII aegrorum Hippocratis in Epidemiis*
LP 1544	*Ephemerus, de libris propriis* [1544]
LP 1557	*De libris propriis, eorumque usu* [1557]
LP 1562	*De libris propriis et eorum usu* [1562]
MM	*De methodo medendi sectiones tres* [1565]
Opera	*Opera omnia*, 10 vols. (Lyon, 1663; facsimile edition New York and London, 1967)
RV	*De rerum varietate* [1557]
SS	*Somniorum Synesiorum libri* [1562]
ST	*De sanitate tuenda, libri quatuor* [1580]
UC	*De utilitate ex adversis capienda* [1561]
VP	*De vita propria, liber*

2. Other abbreviations

Benivieni	Antonio Benivieni, *De abditis non nullis ac mirandis morborum et sanationum causis*, in A. Costa and G. Weber, *L'inizio dell'anatomia patologica nel Quattrocento fiorentino, sui testi di Antonio Benivieni, Bernardo Torni, Leonardo da Vinci, Archivio "De Vecchi" per l'Anatomia Patologica*, vol. 39, fasc. 2 (Florence, 1963), 429–821 (recently reissued, with revised and abbreviated introductory material, as Antonio Benivieni, *De abditis nonnullis ac mirandis morborum et sanationum causis*, ed. Giorgio Weber [Florence, 1994])
IA	*Index aureliensis: Catalogus librorum sedecimo saeculo impressorum*, pt. 1, vol. 6 (Orleans, 1976)
Ingegno	Alfonso Ingegno, *Saggi sulla filosofia di Cardano* (Florence, 1980)
Kessler	Eckhard Kessler, ed., *Girolamo Cardano: Philosoph Naturforscher Arzt* (Wiesbaden, 1994)
Kühn	Galen, *Opera omnia*, ed. C. G. Kühn, 20 vols. (Leipzig, 1821–33)
Littré	Hippocrates, *Oeuvres complètes d'Hippocrate*, ed. and trans. E. Littré, 10 vols. (Paris 1839–61)

PART ONE

Cardano's Medical World

Chapter 1

INTRODUCTION

"THE studious man," wrote Girolamo Cardano, "should always have at hand a clock and a mirror: a clock since in such a confusion and mass of things it is necessary for him to keep track of time, especially if he is a professor, teaches, or writes"; a mirror to observe the changing condition of his body.[1] The advice seems emblematic of Cardano in more ways than one. At the most literal level, his output of a vast mass of writings on many different subjects while he was simultaneously engaged in medical practice and, at times, teaching might well have left him—as it has left some of his readers over the centuries—with a sense of breathless confusion and difficulty in keeping track of all his projects. More profoundly, the clock recalls Cardano's astrological commitment, which included the belief that the cycles of the heavens influenced entire eras of historic time as well as the phases of individual human lives. The mirror calls to mind not just a favorite Renaissance image of self-knowledge but, specifically, Cardano's preoccupation with his own experience, which led him to reflect endlessly on the chances and changes of his body, circumstances, and fortune and to become the author of a book on his own life.

Cardano proffered the advice just quoted in one of his numerous works on medicine, and it is his medicine that is the subject of this book. But his recommendation about clock and mirror, incorporated into a medical treatise, expresses concerns that recur and are perhaps central to his output in all fields. I use the remark to introduce my own study as a way of emphasizing that his medical ideas, writings, and practice cannot be considered in isolation from his ideas on other subjects and his life experience. More generally, the main purpose of this book is to illustrate some of the ways in which Renaissance medicine was embedded in a cultural and intellectual—as well, of course, as a social—milieu.

By "Renaissance medicine" I mean here simply the medicine of the chronological period from about the late fifteenth to the early seventeenth century. Distinguishing its characteristic features is a more problematic enterprise. For Italy, at any rate, the term "Renaissance medicine" certainly should not be read to imply a complete rupture, either intellectual or organizational, with the preceding period; yet the sixteenth-century practitioner functioned in a very different cultural and social world from that of his fourteenth- or fifteenth-century predecessor. Contemporaries, naturally, took more notice of novelty than continuity. University professors of various branches of medicine were on the whole agreed that their age was one of notable innovation or renovation. Here, for example, is Vesalius on the subject in 1543: "In the great felicity of this age . . . with all studies greatly revitalized, anatomy has begun to raise its head from profound gloom, so that it may be said without contradiction that it seems almost to have recovered its ancient brilliance in some universities."[2] Others saw change in a less positive light. For example, in 1587, Alessandro Massaria, a professor at the University of Padua, sourly alluded to the "infinite and unbridled audacity" of innovators in medical education.[3] In historical hindsight, major sixteenth-century innovations and innovators in medicine and related sciences have long been the subject of intensive study; yet the extent to which and, more important, the manner in which patterns of change permeated medical culture are more difficult to determine and have been less explored. At this point, to attempt a general definition of "Renaissance" scientific culture in medicine and related fields is perhaps not very useful. It appears more profitable to examine how physicians actually deployed the intellectual resources available to them in the context of specific social and professional pressures. This book is intended as such an endeavor, using Cardano's prolific, self-expressive, and eclectic works as one set of examples. They hold up a mirror—sometimes, to be sure, a distorting mirror—to many aspects of a complex medical world.

Girolamo Cardano: Career, Works, Ideas

Cardano's life story has been many times retold and need only be briefly summarized here.[4] Born in Pavia in 1501, he was the illegitimate son of Fazio Cardano and Chiara Micheri. Subsequently he and his mother joined his father in Milan, where his parents eventually married. Although the elder Cardano was a jurist by training, his interests were in mathematics and the occult. Girolamo's relation with his father was ambivalent, but Fazio exercised a strong influence on his son. Pride in the Cardano family (which claimed noble descent), mathematical accomplishments, and much attention—at different times and in different contexts veering between skepticism and credulity—to various types of occultism were all among Girolamo's salient characteristics. He also identifed strongly as a Milanese citizen.

Girolamo's studies in the faculty of arts and medicine at the University[5] of Pavia were interrupted by the outbreak of the war for Milan between France and the emperor Charles V; he transferred to Padua, where he obtained his M.D. in 1526. A few years of medical practice in

Sacco (Saccolongo), a small town near Padua, followed. He married in 1531; he and his wife subsequently became the parents of three children (his wife died in 1546). Beginning in 1529 he made repeated efforts to return to practice medicine in Milan, which were initially frustrated because he was several times refused admission to the Milanese College of Physicians on the grounds of his illegitimacy. After another period of practice in Gallarate, a small town near Milan, he returned to the city in 1534 and obtained a post teaching mathematics. Gradually he built up a medical practice, acquired influential patrons and patients in Milan, and, eventually, in 1539, gained full admission to the College of Physicians. In 1543, he became professor of medicine at the University of Pavia. However, because his academic salary was not paid as promised, his professorship was soon interrupted by another period of several years of medical practice in Milan.

Meanwhile, during the 1540s and 1550s he was acquiring an international reputation outside medicine owing to the publication in northern Europe of his major mathematical, astrological, philosophical, and encyclopedic works. His mathematical works included a treatise on algebra, the *Ars magna* (1545), in which he provided the first printed explanation of a procedure for solving cubic equations, setting off a famous priority dispute with Tartaglia. In astrology, Cardano was the author of the principal commentary on the most important ancient astrological treatise, namely, Ptolemy's *Tetrabiblos* (1554). He also published treatises on moral philosophy, including a once well-known *De consolatione* (1542). But the work that brought him widest fame in his own lifetime was probably an encyclopedic compendium of natural philosophy entitled *De subtilitate* (1550). A second encyclopedic work, *De varietate rerum*, followed in 1557.[6] An invitation to journey to Scotland to treat Archbishop Hamilton of St. Andrews for a complaint that may have been asthma—one of the few aspects of Cardano's medical activity that has entered standard histories of medicine—allowed him to spend most of 1552 taking a prolonged trip through northern Europe. During this visit he traveled through France, England, Switzerland, and parts of Germany and met with several leading northern European intellectuals.

Subsequently, after another period in Milan, Cardano resumed his teaching duties at the University of Pavia. But 1560 marked the beginning of a succession of personal calamities. His greatly loved eldest son, who had followed him into a medical career, was arrested for wife-murder. Cardano's frantic but unsuccessful efforts to save his son from execution only intensified the scandal. This, combined with the hostility of some colleagues and imputations of homosexual activity directed at Cardano himself, ultimately made his position at Pavia untenable. Although emotionally affected for the rest of his life by the loss of his son,

Cardano by this time had social as well as his own considerable psychological resources to call upon. His patrons at Milan included members
of the powerful Borromeo family. The help of the young Cardinal (the
future San Carlo) Borromeo secured his transfer to a professorship of
medical theory at the University of Bologna. Cardano was a professor of
medicine at Bologna from 1562 until 1570. Family troubles did not
cease when he came to Bologna, as his younger son turned violently
against him. In 1570 an accusation of heresy brought his teaching career to an end, but after a brief imprisonment he was released. He spent
the last few years of his life in Rome, where he continued to practice
medicine until shortly before his death. In 1575 he wrote the remarkable account of his own life on which much of his modern fame rests.
He died in 1576.

Although Cardano's autobiography has made his own view of his
medical career well known, his medical works have been little studied in
the centuries since most of them were collected into the edition of his
Opera posthumously published in 1663.[7] He is best known to historians
of Renaissance culture and science as an autobiographer, as an eclectic
natural and moral philosopher who bridged Renaissance occultism and
nascent early modern encyclopedism, as a noted or notorious astrologer,
and as a mathematician whose accomplishments included not only the
work on algebra just mentioned but also a pioneering attempt to develop a theory of probability in a treatise on games of chance. The range
of his interests—which in addition to those already mentioned included
music, history, dreams, physiognomy, and more—presumably reflects an
endeavor to grasp the whole of natural knowledge. Many of his writings,
culminating in the account of his own life composed in old age, are
strikingly self-revelatory and personal; the exploration and recording of
the self was one of Cardano's abiding preoccupations.

His two encyclopedic compilations were popular storehouses of miscellaneous information and as such several times reprinted in his lifetime;
De subtilitate was also translated into French and German. But Cardano's own purpose in writing these works was to present an innovative
philosophy of nature based on his concept of subtlety. Subtlety, according to Cardano, was a special characteristic inherent in things difficult to
grasp by either the senses or the intellect (*Subtilitas est ratio quaedam,
qua sensibilia a sensibus, intelligibilia ab intellectu, difficile compraehen-
duntur*). It was found in all kinds of difficult and obscure things,
whether natural or man-made—the whole "variety of things"—so that
understanding of subtlety was the key to a grasp of all of nature and all
arts.[8] The kinds of understanding he seems to have had in mind ranged
from the relatively pragmatic, such as grasp of the mechanical or mathematical principles involved in various technological devices, to the

magus's insight into occult forces in nature. He also sometimes wrote as if subtlety itself were a quality of mind possessed by specially gifted persons, surely including himself.

Despite the diversity of disciplines on which Cardano wrote and the confusion of some of his works, certain key concepts permeate his thought and underlie his writings on many subjects. His notion of subtlety was undoubtedly one such concept. For example, in medicine, even when not explicitly invoked, it underlies his ideas about medical understanding and the power to cure. Also central to his entire intellectual enterprise was his belief in astral powers and influences. This belief in turn connected him strongly with the world of Renaissance occult sciences, in the sense of ideas about hidden forces in nature, natural magic, and the role to be ascribed or denied to demons. The large role that this complex of ideas played in Renaissance intellectual and scientific culture is now generally recognized.[9] Cardano remains an especially interesting case because he was simultaneously deeply committed to astral beliefs (and convinced of his own mantic powers) and a critic of popular credulity.

Cardano's astral and occult ideas, like his concept of subtlety, appear in many guises throughout his works. They have particular bearing on his medicine because of the medieval and Renaissance commonplace that one of the most indisputably useful functions of astrology was as an adjunct to medicine. The idea usually referred to specific medico-astrological concepts, such as the notions that the planets ruled stages of development of the human fetus or that the course of diseases was determined by the occurrence of "critical days." This type of medical astrology has a place in Cardano's medical writings, but that place is not by sixteenth-century standards unusually large. When he had occasion to discuss such subjects in medical treatises, he did so in a technically well informed manner, but these discussions occupy only a small part of the mass of his medical writings. Over and above the use of specific astrological doctrines traditionally invoked in medicine, however, belief in astral powers and attention to the regularities of the heavenly clock were guiding principles of his thought as a whole that profoundly influenced his medical as well as his other ideas. For example, his interest in investigating relations between regularity and contingency—something he frequently attempted in a medical context—seems to owe much to a habit of pondering the relation between the regularities of the heavens and apparently random terrestrial happenings. The problem of regularity and contingency also connects to the issue of prediction, which in turn is a common thread joining Cardano's interest in prophecy and in the two predictive sciences of astrology and medical prognostication.

Notwithstanding his multiple interests and the multiple aspects of his personality, Cardano practiced only one profession throughout his life. That profession was medicine. He habitually identified himself as a physician in the titles of his works; he practiced medicine for fifty years; and he wrote copiously on medical subjects. Moreover, in his own lifetime and during the century after his death his medical works found appreciative readers, as the numerous copies possessed by physicians in seventeenth-century Paris bear witness.[10] He thus provides one excellent point of entry into two still very incompletely known aspects of the sixteenth century. The first is the interpenetration of the world of medical culture and the larger intellectual universe of natural and moral philosophy, history, encyclopedism, and descriptive, mathematical, and occult sciences. The second is the nature and boundaries of innovation within the medical community itself, boundaries delimited by a complex relation between medieval and classical tradition, scientific innovation, intellectual debate, personal rivalries, social and institutional pressures, and the needs of pedagogy. My claim is not, of course, that Cardano's medical works typify either of these areas. He was much too idiosyncratic to be typical of anything. Rather, he offers the experience and ideas of one exceptionally self-expressive individual. These works are indeed part of his self-presentation and self-image.

Works on medicine constitute almost half Cardano's published output. He produced numerous treatises on various aspects of medical practice, a major series of Hippocratic commentaries, and a vast compilation of debated issues in medicine. His medical career and experiences also informed passages or aspects of his autobiography and accounts of his own writings, some of his philosophical treatises, his encyclopedias, and his works on astrology and dreams. Furthermore, medical sources or ideas influenced some of his fundamental philosophical concepts. His writings on medicine, unlike his works on other topics, were produced in the context of the traditions and expectations of an established profession. For the most part, they fall into the conventional genres of a system of Latin medical learning that had been several hundred years in the making—commentaries on authoritative medical works, treatises on regimen and therapy, *consilia* or advice for individual patients. But Cardano did not treat the medical teaching and practice that provided most of his livelihood—at levels ranging over time from near poverty to modest prosperity—as merely a means to support his other intellectual activities. On the contrary, he was profoundly involved not only in advancing his own medical career but also in intellectual issues specifically pertaining to medicine. Thus he placed his Hippocratic commentaries first in a list of what he considered were his own most important books.[11] To his medical works, moreover, he brought many of the same interests, beliefs, and attitudes that mark his other writings: his boundless curiosity and intellectual avidity; his various philosophical commitments; his aggressive readiness to challenge accepted ideas and traditional authorities; his continuing inquiry into the relation of divine action, natural law (logical, mathematical, astrological, or physiological), and contingent or chance happenings; his tireless reworking, rewriting, and remaking of his material; and his self-expressiveness.

Indeed, even the two branches of his oeuvre that might be thought to be furthest apart from one another—medical treatises written within the conventions of a technical genre and the exploration of personal experience in the *Liber de vita propria*—have more in common than is at first apparent. Cardano's autobiographical enterprise, which seems and indeed is so uniquely his own, was strongly conditioned by social or institutional factors and intellectual precedents. His self-study, far from being confined to the *Liber de vita propria* written when he was over seventy, began by his thirties, or earlier, and continued in multiple versions throughout his life.[12] Initial motivations included the need to establish professional credentials and attract the attention of publishers and patrons.[13] At the same time, as he noted, Galen and Erasmus provided distinguished ancient and modern models of autobiography and autobibliography.[14] Of course, for someone such as Cardano for whom writing was a central activity throughout adult life, a list of his own works, whatever its original purpose, in fact constituted an autobiographical framework. In addition, the structure of his various accounts of himself owes much to astrological conventions, to theories about dreams, and perhaps to traditions of Italian family history. It has further been suggested that his final account of his life may have been required of him by ecclesiastical authority.[15] It was within the cultural framework interwoven by all these factors that Cardano pursued the search for the meaning of his own experience with an intensity and persistence that was peculiarly personal.

Conversely, his medical writings are for the most part highly conventional in format. They are, much of the time, academic and impersonal in tone. But they too frequently bear the unmistakable stamp of his personality and special interests. For example, from time to time he integrated narratives about and analysis of his own experiences into medical and philosophical, as well as autobiographical, writings. One boundary that he breached regularly and persistently was that between impersonal academic or scientific discussion and personal history. The extent to which such a boundary shifted in the sixteenth century and Cardano's contribution to the change await further exploration.

Yet although Cardano was unusually prolific—both as medical author and in the variety of his interests—as well as unusually concerned to record and explain his experience, he was far from unique in combining

medicine with other philosophical and scientific interests. University education in medicine was normally preceded by studies in arts, that is,
chiefly logic and Aristotelian natural philosophy. No doubt the majority
of medical graduates left their obligatory studies in liberal arts and philosophy behind—perhaps with a sigh of relief—when they left the university and began to practice. But some professors of medicine left elo-
quent testimony to their natural philosophical awareness. One example
is Andrea Cesalpino (1519– or 1524–1603), professor successively of
botany and medicine at Pisa for most of his career, one of the most important botanists of the sixteenth century, and author of a set of *Quaestiones peripateticae*. Another is Gianbattista Da Monte, professor first of
medical *theoria* and then of medical *practica* at Padua from 1540 until
his death in 1551, who is famous for teaching clinical medicine to his
students at the bedside of hospital patients. Da Monte devoted many
pages of his commentary on the *Canon* of Avicenna to natural philosophical questions about the four elements and theory of matter.
Equally, the presence of numerous medical examples in Pomponazzi's
treatise *On the Natural Causes of Marvelous Effects* reveals how much
one of the best-known radical Aristotelian philosophers of the early sixteenth century gained from medical studies at Padua.[16] It is, of course,
well known that the remarkable sixteenth-century development of
anatomy and botany was largely an outgrowth of medicine. But other
descriptive sciences, too, benefited from the interest of men trained in
medicine: some notable examples include the work on mineralogy of
Georgius Agricola, who studied medicine in Italy before beginning medical practice in Bohemia and Germany, and Michele Mercati, who grad-
uated M.D. from the University of Pisa before becoming curator of the
Vatican botanic garden and the papal collection of minerals in Rome; on
ichthyology by Guillaume Rondelet, professor of medicine at the University of Montpellier; and on magnetism by William Gilbert, M.D.
Cambridge and London medical practitioner.[17]

Furthermore, Cardano aspired to achieve fame and success in the academic medical milieu according to the normal measure of the age by
combining publication of learned works with a university chair and practice among an aristocratic clientele. Although he actually spent many
fewer years in university teaching than in medical practice, all his medical writings are in one way or another connected with this career path.
In terms of his training—and, of course, intellectual capacity—the goal
was entirely reasonable. Yet although a university degree in medicine was
a necessary prerequisite for entry into medicine's intellectual and professional elite, in the Italy of Cardano's day it was no longer (if it ever had
been) sufficient. In fifteenth- and sixteenth-century Europe only a mi-

nority of medical practitioners were university graduates, but in Italy graduate physicians were more numerous than elsewhere. Some of them spent their entire careers in the kind of inconspicuous small-town medical practice that occupied Cardano for the first eight years after he received his M.D.

In Cardano's case, he was initially hampered by poverty, lack of useful social and professional contacts and patronage, and too evident attachment to interests outside medicine.[18] These problems as well as his illegitimate birth—and perhaps aspects of his personality—help to explain both his repeated rebuffs by the institutionalized medical elite in the shape of the Milan College of Physicians and the length of time it took him to enter the world of university teaching. Not until he acquired the patron who helped him to a post teaching mathematics in the charitable Piattine schools could he even begin to establish himself in Milan. The next year, 1535, the College of Physicians, which licensed medical practice in the city as well as functioning as an exclusive club of leading physicians, grudgingly acknowledged his right to practice medicine. According to his own account, he was first offered a post teaching medicine at the University of Pavia in 1536 but was obliged to turn it down as it was unsalaried. Only after he had spent several more years building up the support of noble patients and patrons was he able to obtain, first, admission to the Milan College of Physicians—which had previously rejected his application for full membership three times—and then the offer of a salaried professorial chair at Pavia (at that time temporarily transferred to Milan). Cardano's early career serves as a reminder that, in sixteenth- as in seventeenth-century northern Italy, the professional and social gulf between the more impoverished products of medical faculties and some of the various medical practitioners without university training could not have been all that wide.[19]

In medicine, Cardano presented himself as reformist and innovative, although, like many of his contemporaries, he tended to express this idea by asserting that he had discovered the way back to ancient truth—in his case to "true" Hippocratic medicine. He claimed improvements in therapeutic method, imitated Galen in criticizing predecessors—most notably Galen himself—and aligned himself with Vesalius and the new anatomy. Above all, he insisted on the cures he had performed and his successes as a practitioner. His claims and autobiographical anecdotes about his therapeutic successes have antecedents in earlier traditions of medical narrative and, especially, in Galen. Nevertheless, both Cardano's self-presentation as a practitioner and his actual career, which interspersed long periods of medical practice with fairly short episodes of university teaching, link him with a world outside academic medicine and with elements in popular medical culture. Somewhat similarly, his encyclopedic philosophical works, though drawing on academic philosophical tradition, are clearly situated outside the academic milieu and appealed to a nonuniversity audience.

Standing in this way simultaneously within and outside the milieu of academic medicine, he bears comparison with two major contemporary medical and scientific innovators, namely, Paracelsus (1493–1541) and Jean Fernel (1497–1558). To be sure, Cardano was far less radical than Paracelsus, whose wholesale repudiation of academic medical tradition and attempt to establish a transformed, alchemical medicine were to have widespread influence and lasting consequences in the later sixteenth and seventeenth centuries. Unlike Paracelsus, Cardano remained to a very large extent integrated into the mental universe and cultural community of Aristotelian natural philosophy and Galenic medicine. Nevertheless, like Paracelsus, he rested his authority largely on personal claims to success as a healer and his own special inspiration, was strongly critical of contemporary academic medical teaching and practitioners, was deeply involved in occult sciences, and was prepared to make radical innovations in metaphysics.

Conversely, Cardano seems less at home in the world of academic medicine than Fernel. Like Cardano, Fernel combined mathematical and occultist interests with medicine. Moreover, he earned a reputation as a neoteric because of unconventional theories about *spiritus* and disease etiology. Nevertheless, Fernel had a highly successful career, not only as as a practitioner but also as the most distinguished professor of medicine at the University of Paris at a time when it was a center of Renaissance Galenism. The difference may be partly due to personal factors: unlike Cardano, Fernel does not appear to have attracted enemies or attacks on his character. But also unlike Cardano, he refrained from explicit attacks on Galen. Indeed Fernel's general survey of medicine—one of the first textbooks of the subject and a hugely successful one, used well into the seventeenth century—came to be valued as a systematic, practical presentation of modern Galenism.

Notwithstanding these differences, Cardano, like Paracelsus and Fernel, belongs to a new type of practitioner in some ways emblematic of the complex interaction—in medicine as in so many other areas of Renaissance culture—of old and new, academic and civic or courtly, elite and popular. In some respects, Cardano invented himself just as much as Paracelsus did; he clearly believed himself to be an original and, indeed, inspired thinker with a new understanding of medicine as of nature in general. But he simultaneously continued to aspire to academic success in the university milieu.

SIXTEENTH-CENTURY MEDICINE: CONSTRAINTS
AND OPPORTUNITIES

Throughout Cardano's lifetime and long thereafter, university faculties of medicine preserved many aspects of their medieval origins. The University of Bologna, where he ended his academic career, had been a famous center of medical teaching since the thirteenth century. Padua, where he studied medicine, came into existence in the thirteenth century, although it emerged as a major center of medical instruction only in the mid-fifteenth; it was also a notable center for Aristotelian philosophy. Pavia, the site of his earliest studies and of his longest professorial appointment, was a younger institution. Nominally founded by a charter of the Holy Roman Emperor Charles IV in 1361, it was actually the creation of the Visconti rulers of Milan during the latter part of the fourteenth century. Nevertheless, it, like other universities founded at the will of a Renaissance prince or municipality, drew on long-established, powerful, and still lively traditions of organization, curriculum, and pedagogy.[20]

Since the thirteenth century, the principal disciplines in the Italian universities were usually law and medicine. Arts (that is, chiefly logic and natural philosophy) and medicine were traditionally linked administratively and, in the careers of many teachers and students, intellectually. The medical curriculum, the content of which was in most respects fundamentally Galenic, was divided into theoretical and practical branches. Medical theory comprised basic physical science common to both Aristotelian natural philosophy and Galenic medicine (for example, the theory of the four elements), philosophy of medicine (for example, definition of medicine's subject matter, goals, and relation to other disciplines), and Galenic physiology. The practical branch of the curriculum consisted of teaching about disease and therapy. In both branches, the main—though not the only—approach to the subject was via exposition of standard texts by ancient and some medieval medical authors, most notably Hippocrates and Galen among the former and Avicenna among the latter. In the thirteenth- to fifteenth-century universities, in the milieu of Arabo-Latin scholastic medicine, an extensive literature of commentaries, compendia, and so on grew up around these authors and texts. Numerous independent treatises on practical aspects of medicine, *consilia* for individual patients, and reference works of various types based on the Hippocratic-Galenic medical system were also produced.

Hence although sixteenth-century medical faculties were, on the whole, remarkably receptive to change, change was much more likely to involve the incorporation of fresh elements than the abandonment of existing ones. Thus in the 1530s and 1540s Padua was among the earliest universities to respond to the rapid development of medicinal botany by establishing first a new professorship and soon after a new site for study—the university botanic garden. But these innovations were simply added to the existing curriculum in *theoria* and *practica*, which continued, for example, to include sections of the *Canon* of Avicenna. Throughout the sixteenth century, leading professors at Padua expounded that venerable medieval text; yet they did so by means of commentaries and editions that took up current as well as traditional issues in medicine and displayed the author's or editor's up-to-date scholarship.[21]

Moreover, medical humanism or Hellenism, a major Renaissance innovation with profound and far-reaching effects, had as its goal the achievement of fuller and more precise knowledge of ancient Greek medicine—that is, fundamentally the same system of medicine as had been taught in the West since the twelfth century (and before). Toward the end of the fifteenth century, medical teaching in the Italian universities began to be penetrated by a humanist ideology. In the medical context, humanism meant a demand for the direct study of a wider range of ancient Greek medical texts and frequent expressions of scorn for the language, translations, and forms of argument of medieval Arabo-Latin scholastic medicine. Although the number of medical humanists actually capable of philological work on Greek manuscripts always remained small, the production of printed editions of medical works in the original Greek, the proliferation of new translations, and the broad diffusion of humanist ideology among physicians strengthened attention to ancient Greek medical texts and, especially, to Galen for most of the sixteenth century. Moreover, Galen himself, in addition to many other accomplishments, had been a scholar who wrote learned commentaries on works attributed to Hippocrates. His Renaissance admirers thus not only valued Galen's physiological and therapeutic doctrines and appreciated his contributions to anatomy (indeed one of the principal achievements of ancient science), but also found in him a model of medical scholarship. The celebrated practical and scientific accomplishments of sixteenth-century university medicine—the expansion of anatomy, the development of medicinal botany, the increased interest in explaining mechanisms of disease transmission—all took place in the intellectual context provided by medical humanism and the intensified study of Greek medicine. The famous critique of Galen's anatomy in Vesalius's *De humani corporis fabrica* (1543) would have been impossible without the recovery, editing, and printing in the original Greek and in Latin translation of a number of Galen's anatomical works for the first time in the preceding decades; probably the most widely read botanical

tific innovation, curricular change, or intellectual debate was probably always small. Certainly much more is known about the ideas and activities of such men than about the way in which their ideas were received and transmitted by others. Furthermore, many aspects of medical life were determined by socioeconomic, religious, or political developments to which individuals obviously had little choice but to adapt. The religious intensification and ecclesiastical pressures associated with the Counter-Reformation affected all aspects of Italian life in the second half of the sixteenth century. Princes and governments took much interest—sometimes benevolent and sometimes oppressive—in regulating universities as a means of ensuring the proper training and political and religious reliability of professional men, clergy, and officials. When the young Cosimo I effectively refounded the University of Pisa in 1543, ducal advisers scoured Europe for distinguished professors. Cosimo's recruiters brought together a teaching faculty of high quality (including the botanist Luca Ghini and, for a time, the celebrated anatomists Realdo Colombo and Gabriele Falloppia)—but the university itself had no control over these appointments. Somewhat analogous situations existed at Padua when Cardano was a student and at Pavia in the early years of his professorship. Both universities had recently been disrupted by warfare; in both, recovery and reorganization brought closer state supervision. Padua had been part of Venetian territory since 1405; in the second half of the fifteenth century the Venetian government began to exercise some control over the various academic corporations that made up the university and to be a source of academic patronage. The temporary loss of Venetian mainland territories during the War of the League of Cambrai (1509–17) produced a complete breakdown of university life. Thereafter, the Venetian government introduced administrative reforms that brought the university under the direct control of a special magistracy of the republic, the Riformatori dello Studio. The University of Pavia suffered badly in the war for the Duchy of Milan between Charles V and Francis I in the 1520s (culminating in the latter's defeat and capture at the battle of Pavia in 1525) and again in campaigns during the early 1540s. But imperial (and hence subsequently Spanish) rule over Milan was established following the death of the last Sforza duke in 1535. In 1541, Charles V issued an edict putting the Senate of Milan in charge of the University of Pavia and giving the same body the power of nominating professors.[23] Notwithstanding these and similar administrative arrangements elsewhere, in scientific or intellectual matters that did not involve religion, university teachers and students were free to accept or reject innovation and to join in controversy. Vigorous polemic was characteristic of Cardano's medical world. But so too was dependence upon the needs and social and intellectual interests of noble patrons and governing circles.

Moreover, academically trained physicians were also obliged to compete as practitioners in a medical marketplace in which they matched their power to heal or reassure not only against each other but also against a universe of empirics, herbalists, mountebanks, and magical practitioners of every kind.[24] Furthermore, medical practice, whatever the practitioner's level of education, undoubtedly always included elements that were empirical, intuitive, or folkloric, as well as those that were systematic. Historical discussion of disease in Renaissance Europe has traditionally focused on epidemics, theories of contagion, and the problem of allegedly "new" diseases. But these were only some aspects of the world of Renaissance medical practitioners. Their practice encompassed all kinds of illnesses and disabilities, some known by traditional names and descriptions, others not.

CARDANO AS WITNESS TO RENAISSANCE MEDICINE

In one sense, Cardano's writings are an exceptionally rich source of information about this complex medical world. Few other authors offer so much detail about a sixteenth-century medical career or so much insight into the mental universe and social world of a physician. But these works also present fundamental problems. In the first place, Cardano himself is almost always his only witness. The diligence of generations of Italian scholars has uncovered and published some basic documentation of his career—principally his wills, some documents relating to his teaching at the University of Bologna, and a small number of his letters. But almost everything that is known about the identity and numbers of his patients, the conditions for which he treated them, his success as a practitioner of internal medicine, and his relations with his patrons comes from his own pen.

Second, most of his medical works exist only in sixteenth-century editions or in the seventeenth-century collected *Opera*. In addition, a small number of manuscripts of such works survive (most of them in the Biblioteca Apostolica Vaticana or the Biblioteca Nazionale Centrale, Rome). Only a small proportion of Cardano's output on any subject and almost none of his work on medicine have appeared in modern editions or translations. Much remains to be learned about the sources, language, and specific intellectual positions of many of his treatises. Moreover, he was an extremely prolific author who made a habit of reusing the same material in different combinations in different treatises and who perpetually revised and rewrote his work. Where autobiographical content is concerned, Cardano's return to the same dreams and the same anecdotes, always in slightly different versions, and his repeated updating of his horoscope and his own bibliography provide valuable clues to his personal development. But in the case of other topics, when one finds

long intervals between his statements about dates of composition and actual dates of publication, the republication of treatises in different combinations or under different titles, or the inclusion of excerpts from one
work in another, there is usually no way to tell whether the cause lies in
external circumstances (for example, the availability or decisions of publishers), in Cardano's desire to extend his bibliography, or in developments in his thought. Indeed, in the absence of modern editions, it is
probably impossible completely to disentangle all the relationships
among different works and among different versions of the same work.

Third, and perhaps most important, Cardano's medical writings, like
all his works, need to be approached with caution because they are the
product of one of the most elusive personalities of the sixteenth century.
His character has baffled and at times infuriated readers from his enemy
Julius Caesar Scaliger (1484–1558) until the present. In his own age of
pervasive supernatural belief in both religious and magical contexts, Cardano's combination of rationalism and occultism may have been less in-
congruous than it appeared to some later commentators. At the end of
the confessional late twentieth century, his emotional intensity and
shameless self-reference probably seem less indecorous and unbalanced
than they did to earlier generations. Nevertheless, variability and eclecticism are salient characteristics of his thought. He was a rational philosopher who simultaneously viewed himself as a magus, in touch with
higher astral forces and gifted with powers of divination. He was a philosophical eclectic, who drew freely on both neo-Platonist and Aristotelian
sources. He was at once a critic and an imitator of Galen. A certain extravagance of personality led him constantly to push his claims and ideas
to extremes. Yet in later years, writing in an increasingly persecuting society in which his own religious orthodoxy came under suspicion, he advocated prudent silence and simulation in professional and civic life.[25]
Even his autobiography, famous for the detail of its self-examination, is
in some respects carefully masked.[26]

Moreover, Cardano was someone for whom the constant production
of written works, and writing itself, constituted a central focus of activity. If his loving description of writing instruments reveals his delight in
the act of writing, his careful instructions as to how to compile a book
by cutting and pasting and rearranging other books suggest one of the
ways in which a very large output could be achieved while the author
was simultaneously pursuing a busy medical career.[27] Furthermore, his
claims about subtlety include the idea that it could not be grasped by
everyone and presumably not by all his readers.[28] His interest in the idea
of contradiction, manifested in the title of one of his principal medical
works, went along with apparent indifference to the idea of consistency
as a value. Labile, freely choosing among ideas, moods, and rhetorical

stances, Cardano challenges us to interpret him correctly even when he is writing sober medical works.

For all these reasons, I am not attempting to provide a systematic or comprehensive account of Cardano's medicine or to trace its development over time. Indeed, I think it would be foolhardy to attempt to do so. Instead, I have chosen topics that, in my view, illustrate Cardano's medical interests and activities while also bearing on larger issues in sixteenth-century medicine and life sciences. But I have also tried to place Cardano in his specific social and political environment. Cardano provides an example of a medical career spent almost entirely in the universities and cities of Milanese territory and the Papal States. The intellectual differences among Italian universities may not always have been as great as has sometimes been supposed; but political and social differences, different patterns of patronage, and different levels of religious pressure surely existed among states and institutions.

Two broad themes weave throughout this book. The first of these is the shifting pattern of the relation of generalization and experience. Cardano's medical writings offer much material for exploration of this theme. His lifelong insistence on the importance of experience and concern with the relation of general law and particular or random instance appear to be linked to his mathematical, astrological, and historical interests as well as to acute sensitivity to personal experience. But this emphasis in his writings also reflects larger developments in Renaissance scientific or natural philosophical culture. On the whole, the scholastic natural philosophy of the thirteenth to fifteenth centuries ascribed higher status to the endeavor to reach general or universal conclusions via syllogistic reasoning than to descriptive information about particulars; but in the sixteenth century, the statements and activities of physicians, anatomists, botanists, and students of natural history in all its branches reveal a notably enhanced status for and attention to the particular.[29] Of course, in examining Renaissance claims about the importance of "experience," or descriptions of phenomena as falling within or outside the regular course of nature (usually by the use of such terms as "natural," "monstrous," or "marvelous"), one needs to be constantly aware that the concepts involved are themselves historically determined.[30] "Experience" could mean many things in the sixteenth century—often, for example, including experiences reported in historical works. Moreover, even the model of regularity offered by sixteenth-century clocks was not that of a later age.

The various causes usually suggested for the enhanced interest in particulars and in experience, although doubtless contributory, are too numerous and too general to have much explanatory force. Furthermore, although some newer factors were obviously relevant (notably, the increased attention to ancient descriptive sciences made possible by humanism or Hellenism), some older traditions of knowlege and practice could equally foster attention to particulars. In medicine, the awkward fit between an Aristotelian definition of certain or scientific knowledge (requiring syllogistic reasoning leading to universally valid conclusions) and the multitude of particulars about diseases and remedies that actually made up much of medical knowledge had been noted since the thirteenth century. Conceivably, no wholly satisfactory synthesis regarding the origins of sixteenth-century interest in particulars of medicine, anatomy, natural history, and curious objects of all kinds will ever be reached. I have preferred simply to follow some of the ways in which some of these interests are manifested in Cardano's writings.

A second major theme is the reception, dissemination, and manipulation of innovation. Cardano imported aspects of his philosophical eclecticism, his highly personal version of beliefs about occult forces in nature, and his reworking of ancient dream theory into his medicine. And, to an even more striking extent, he was an early and enthusiastic proponent of two of the principal innovations in medicine that occurred in his lifetime: greatly enhanced access to the Hippocratic corpus and the work of Vesalius. But like other contemporaries, including Vesalius himself, he incorporated his challenges to Galen's authority in specific areas into a fundamentally Galenist medicine. Cardano's works contain prime examples of the activist approach to the ancients—selecting, rejecting, or adapting material from ancient sources according to current scientific and professional needs—characteristic of sixteenth-century natural philosophy. In other instances, they illuminate the process of reception of new material, suggesting professional or other purposes to which innovations could be put.

Although the arrangement of this book is topical rather than chronological, its five parts are designed as a sequence. The next chapter continues the description of Cardano's medical world, begun in this introduction, with an account of his activities as a practitioner. In it, I consider his self-presentation as a healer, while endeavoring as far as possible to place his own accounts of himself and the men, women, and children he treated in the social and professional context of patients and practitioners in Milan, Bologna, and Rome.

Part Two, "Theory and Practice" turns to Cardano's concepts of medical knowledge and how he applied them. The first of its two chapters examines his treatment of theoretical issues by way of an analysis of one of his major projects in medicine, a huge collection of debated topics—or, as he termed them, "contradictions"—begun early in his career and continued on and off for many years. Cardano's work on medical contradictions both depends on and subverts scholastic medical tradition. It is not easy reading (and no analysis of it can be). But more than any of his other writings, it reveals his ideas about the nature and sources of medical knowledge. It suggests both the extent and the limitations of his program of criticism of medical authority, delineates the relation between his medical ideas and his philosophy of nature, and reveals his roots in the medical tradition in which he had received his early training. In the second chapter of Part Two, rather than attempting to survey all his recommendations for practical medicine, I have decided to present a somewhat more detailed and analytical account of his contribution to one single area. Several considerations suggested the choice of Cardano's views on the regulation of diet for this purpose. The subject is one on which he wrote extensively and in which he evidently took a personal interest. It is also a topic that bridges high and low—or at any rate academic and nonacademic—culture in Renaissance society, linking academic and popular advice, concerns, and images about the body and health.

After the context of theoretical debate and current practice has been established in Part Two, Part Three, "The Old and the New," turns to innovation—in a double sense: the search for a "new" (that is, hitherto unknown or neglected) ancient wisdom; and the reception of new contributions to knowledge. Cardano's vision of a reformed medicine drew simultaneously on the oldest and newest scientific sources available to him, namely, Hippocratism and Vesalian anatomy. The story of his exploitation of his own contacts with anatomists in the rhetoric and reality of medical practice is highly suggestive of ways in which the new anatomy acquired recognition among—and served the professional purposes of—other physicians. At the same time, Cardano's studies of the Hippocratic corpus, which were extensive and in some respects pioneering, pressed Vesalius into service to interpret Hippocrates.

The remaining parts investigate the way in which two of Cardano's central preoccupations, which also represent distinctive elements in Renaissance culture, enter his medicine. Part Four, "Medical Wonders," considers his ideas about occult forces in nature in the context of disease and cure. It examines the relation between his medical rationalism and his belief in his own special powers of grasp of subtlety, divination, and prophetic dreaming in the light of earlier and contemporary discussions of the marvelous in medicine. Part Five, "Medical Narratives," looks at Cardano's stories of patients in relation both to earlier narrative traditions in medicine and to his own interest in collecting and studying exemplary narratives about particular events from history, historical astrology, and his own life story (including his own health history). Thus the book moves from the subversion of scholastic arguments at the beginning of Part Two to narratives of experience in Part Five. The arrangement does, to my mind, mirror one kind of development in Renaissance medicine, but that development certainly did not take the form of a straightforward chronological progression. As for Cardano, he intermixed stories and personal narratives with other material from the beginning of his career to its end.

With some exceptions—notably Jackie Pigeaud's study of his Hippocratism—Cardano's medical writings have attracted little attention from recent historians.[31] But I have been greatly helped by some of the valuable studies that have appeared in recent years on other aspects of his thought. Only a few of these can be named here (more are listed in the bibliography), but mention should be made at least of Alfonso Ingegno's comprehensive and penetrating book on Cardano's philosophy and introduction to the *Vita*, of the various studies of Ian Maclean, and, most recently, of the volume of conference proceedings edited by Eckhard Kessler.[32] New work on Cardano, now recognized as a key figure in sixteenth-century culture, continues to appear. His astrology is now the subject of much-needed scholarly attention.[33] Recently, a group of scholars associated with the Centro Studi del Pensiero Filosofico del Cinquecento e del Seicento at the University of Milan has taken the ambitious step of proposing a critical edition of all Cardano's works.

More generally, the writing of this book has been greatly illuminated by the rich literature on the social and cultural history of medicine and a broad penumbra of related fields and of health and disease in late medieval, Renaissance, and early modern Europe that is now available. Newer trends have variously stimulated research into a social history of medicine that includes the experience of patients and nonelite practitioners; fostered a cultural history of the life sciences that takes full account of the role of Renaissance courts, patrons, and collecting, of religion (both in terms of institutional power and as a belief system) and magic, and of the contexts of the classroom, the printer's shop, and the marketplace; called attention to the material culture, the iconography, and the performative aspects of natural history, anatomy, and other sciences; and enhanced comprehension of the very large role of writing and compiling as itself a form of medieval and Renaissance scientific activity. In attempting to come to terms with such a compulsive reader, writer, and would-be masterer of disciplines as Cardano, I have found approaches via the history of the book and of reading, the uses of narrative and self-expression, and the formation of disciplines to be especially useful ways of taking a fresh look at Renaissance scientific culture. But whatever approaches are adopted, for the understanding of a system of knowledge and practice as highly textual as Renaissance medicine, the content of texts remains of primary importance. The task of struggling with the texts and endeavoring as far as possible to explain the ideas they transmit remains inescapable.

To a considerable extent, of course, recent contributions reflect developments in historical studies in general over the last twenty years, developments that have included a focus on social and cultural history and the influence of insights from such fields as sociology, anthropology, gender studies, and literary criticism. The history of medicine now intersects with a broader history of health, disease, and the human body in society. The history of science now routinely includes attention to social and cultural context, institutional factors, economic issues, and the material culture of science, and is more attentive to the life sciences than was always the case in the past. Historians of science and medicine as well as political and intellectual historians pay attention to rhetoric and to the uses of rhetoric in the service of power relations. A fortunate conjunction—to use a Cardanian metaphor—of historical trends has, I think, made this a favorable time for an appreciation of the place of medicine in Renaissance scientific and philosophical culture and society.

One man, especially one as sui generis as Cardano, provides only one reflection of a world. I hope the reader will find, as I have done, that Cardano's mirror is worth looking into.

Chapter 2

PRACTITIONER AND PATIENTS

CARDANO'S self-presentation as a physician emphasized above all his success as a practitioner who effected cures. In a work entitled *On Wisdom* published in 1544, he announced: "Since in this city [Milan] I bore the burden of others' ill will and did not make enough to cover my expenses, I tried many things in the art of medicine so that I might find something new. . . . At length I thought out a cure for phthisis (which they call phthoe), which for many centuries was considered incurable, and I healed many people, who are still alive; nor was it more difficult than curing *morbus gallicus*."[1] Over the next two decades, he published lists of his successfully treated patients on three separate occasions.[2] And at the very end of his life, in 1575, he was still insisting on the number and remarkable nature of the cures he had effected: "You should not be amazed, O reader, nor suspect that I am lying; all these things happened, and things like them, and even greater ones and many more: I do not remember the exact number but I think it reached 180 and even more; nor should you think I am vainly boasting or that I want or hope to be thought better than Hippocrates."[3]

Cardano's medical practice is necessarily seen through his own eyes, since his copious autobiographical comments on his medical activities and successes (and occasional failures) and his relations with colleagues and patients constitute the principal source of information about it. The relation of these accounts to his actual practice is as ambiguous as that of his prescriptive treatises on aspects of medicine subsumed under *practica* (diseases, prognosis, therapy, regimen).[4] Although his various works yield the names and illnesses of considerably more than a hundred of his patients, as well as passing references to "many" others, the full extent of his practice and its size and significance relative to that of other north Italian physicians of the period are unknown.[5] The valuable studies of health, disease, and mortality and of practitioners and patients in early modern northern Italy that have appeared over the last twenty years make possible a greatly enhanced appreciation of the general context of Cardano's medical practice.[6] Nevertheless, there is no possibility of placing his stories about his patients and their illnesses in any but the broadest social and demographic, let alone epidemiological, context. It is only occasionally possible to relate sixteenth-century descriptions of disease to modern understanding. Moreover, his accounts of his experiences with patients and colleagues show many traces of imitation of ancient models, both in the shape of the influence of Galen as medical autobiographer and in that of parallels drawn between himself and both Galen and Hippocrates.[7] In addition, medical practice seems to have been for Cardano a theater of sometimes conflicting needs and ambitions: for immediate economic survival, for lasting fame, and for mastery of true knowledge.

Furthermore, any evaluation of his standing as a practitioner can only be tentative, because the criteria by which the sixteenth century measured success in a medical career are by no means self-evident. For one thing, these criteria were not necessarily in all respects the same inside and outside the medical profession. Within the medical profession, there was a hierarchy even among university-educated practitioners. Senior professors of medicine in the universities, authors of learned medical books, and members of civic medical colleges constituted the often overlapping categories of an elite superior to other university-trained and licensed physicians. By the sixteenth century, as Carlo Cipolla has pointed out, in Italy as elsewhere university-educated physicians as a group held themselves sharply apart from and above licensed surgeons and apothecaries. All categories of licensed practitioners expressed nothing but scorn for the efforts of empirics, who, however, continued to flourish in the marketplace. Although it is impossible to estimate their numbers, empirics attracted much attention in sixteenth- and early-seventeenth-century Italy and played an important role in popular culture. The term most often appears to refer to unlicensed and informally trained, but otherwise unremarkable, practitioners, but sixteenth-century cities also swarmed with flamboyant "professors of secrets," charlatans, mountebanks, snake-handlers, and herb-sellers, all peddling natural and magical remedies, hope, and entertainment.[8]

Patients, too, clearly valued the learning, formal training, and prestige of physicians at the upper end of the professional hierarchy. Yet instances in which empirics as well as physicians were summoned to attend noble or royal invalids suggest that sometimes ranking within the medical hierarchy mattered less than a reputation for performing cures.[9] Evidence for a similar attitude also comes, as Gianna Pomata has pointed out, from contracts between patient and practitioner specifying that the practitioner would cure the patient of a certain ailment for a given sum of money. Such contracts placed buyer and seller in an equal commercial relationship and made the buyer the judge of the service purchased. The criteria of success or failure were presumably the patient's own perceptions of change in his or her state of health. By the time Cardano was practicing medicine, such contracts were usually entered into only by barber surgeons and empirics, not by university-educated physicians; such is the case with the few that survive from late-sixteenth-century Bologna. But the fundamental patient attitude expressed in them probably remained widespread. That attitude contrasted strongly with the ideals of "correct" treatment, legal or educational qualification, and "true" doctrine espoused by medical professionalism and institutionalization in their various early modern forms.[10]

No doubt the differences within the hierarchy and the different attitudes of practitioners and patients had existed ever since the thirteenth century when the medical hierarchy took shape. But, in addition, in Renaissance Italy, the upper hierarchy itself underwent disruption and reshuffling. The relative status of professors of theory and professors of *practica* seems to have shifted in favor of the latter;[11] and anatomists for the first time took the role of leading figures within the orthodox medical profession. The same period saw the emergence of a few figures who did not fit into any of the ordinary categories of the medical hierarchy: they resembled empirics in their insistence on their power to cure; but, at the same time, and completely unlike empirics, they aligned themselves with new philosophies of nature, drew on learned forms of occultism, and presented themselves as reformers of medical knowledge. The prototypical such personage is, of course, Paracelsus. Although, as noted in the previous chapter, Cardano was much more steeped in Galenic orthodoxy and scholastic and humanistic medical learning than was Paracelsus, he too in some respects fits this last model.

Cardano's assertive insistence on the record of his successes in practice makes success as a practitioner into both test and authentication of medical knowledge and skill. His practice guarantees the validity of his medical learning and his suitability to teach medical theory in an academic context, not the other way round. The emphasis was clearly a matter of choice, since in reality, his dedication to writing (including the writing of learned medical works) and to the mastery of other disciplines besides medicine must have limited the time available for practice. Moreover, in a medical environment in which medical scholarship and learned authorship were very highly valued, Cardano could easily have rested his claim to a place within the academic medical community primarily on these attributes.

But ambiguity lurks in his claims of power to cure. His language sometimes appears to refer to a uniquely personal and occult gift, sometimes to discovery or mastery of techniques of prognosis and therapy that could be passed on. For example, he was inspired to write his *Ars curandi parva*, subtitled "a most perfect method of healing," in a dream. He thought that its contents were partially responsible for his own, surely unique, success in curing more patients than "Galen or any of his successors."[12] Yet he revised and rewrote the work many times in order to ensure that the final product would be a little handbook that would teach any reader how to attain the same kind of certainty in medicine as his *Ars magna* did in mathematics.[13] But whatever stages *Ars curandi parva* went through, it ended up as a manual of conventionally Galenic medical practice. Occult or philosophical content is more or less confined to the explanation that "the *anima Mundi* fights against nature" and is responsible for illness.[14] The work's chief distinguishing feature is the use of an exemplary series of likely combinations of symptoms or conditions (e.g., interior abscess accompanied by acute fever, fever with diarrhea, pp. 188–89) to teach proper treatment of different kinds of illnesses and injuries. By the time Cardano finally published this handbook in 1564, he claimed that it demonstrated his medical orthodoxy, and he used it in direct rebuttal of an attack launched by a fellow professor of medicine at Pavia, the philosopher and physician Andrea Camuzio. The preface contains an indignant repudiation of Camuzio's accusation that he was a "heresiarch of medicine" and anxious protestations of both Galenic and—significantly—religious orthodoxy.[15] The work's lasting usefulness as a handy practical manual of medicine is perhaps demonstrated by its presence among the books that John Winthrop Jr., alchemist, physician, and first governor of Connecticut, brought to New England.[16]

Cardano, like so many of his contemporaries, saw himself as both engaged in and teaching a reformed or renovated medical practice. His version of renovation called for the application of rules of prognosis that he believed could be learned from Hippocrates, and for increased attention to anatomy in diagnosis and therapy and to autopsy as a postmortem diagnostic tool, aspects of his medicine that will be the subject of subsequent chapters. Other reforms of medical practice were the result of his own *inventio*, a gift that consisted in his knowing how to combine reason and *experimentum*: "reason will be the leader of *inventio*, but *experimentum* the master."[17] As is well known, Cardano greatly prized *inventio*, by which he meant both the finding of new things and the recovery of lost ones, such as true Hippocratic medicine. In a famous passage of the *Vita*, he proudly stressed his appellation as "a man of inventions."[18] In medicine, the idea is yet another way for him to associate himself with Hippocrates, since Hippocrates was considered the finder or discover of medical science.[19] He included his new exposition—that is, his recovery—of Hippocrates, one of his major projects (see chapter 6), among the medical findings listed in the same passage. Two others are improvements in method: an astronomically correct method of reckoning of critical days to which he attached much importance (see chapter 6); and a method of extrapolating appropriate treatment for a disease by studying accounts of other diseases resembling it in some respects. Presumably the sample combinations of conditions in the *Ars curandi parva*, referred to above, constitute an example of the second, which is also adumbrated in one of his manuscript collections of *Experimenta*.[20] Another item was improvement in food preparation—dietary regimen was one of his major areas of interest, as will appear in chapter 4. He also claimed to have found cures for several diseases (other than phthisis/phthoe, terms he seems to have used indifferently) and to have improved some types of medication, without describing either therapy or ingredients in detail; for example, among the medications were purgatives made from nonpurgative ingredients and horrible medicines made into ones that were easy to take.[21]

Whatever the level of innovation in these therapies and pharmaceutical preparations, the content of his treatises on practice, like his *consilia* for individual patients, suggests that he easily accommodated both his medical reformism and his possession of special personal gifts of healing and *inventio* within the framework of the usual procedures of sixteenth-century Galenic medicine. Indeed, it seems unlikely that he could have held his own in the medical marketplace as well as he evidently did, had his actual practice not been fairly conventional. In addition to one reputed diagnostic insight[22] and a defense of anatomy,[23] the critique in *On the Bad Practice of Recent Physicians* contains a major structural criticism of the medical profession. Cardano lamented the exclusion of obstetrics, infant care, dentistry, care of the eyes, and surgery—anything where failure would be obvious, as he acidly remarked—from the purview of physicians.[24] (In his old age, he made a personal attempt to extend the scope of medical subject matter by writing on dental problems and diseases of the joints, treatises that were not published in his lifetime.)[25] Otherwise, the great majority of the specific examples of bad practice consist of failure to follow one or another ancient or medieval authority in details of therapy. What is most unusual about this treatise is not the content of the individual criticisms but the range of their targets. Cardano's model may have been the similarly named *Sixty Errors of Recent Physicians* by the medical humanist Leonhart Fuchs.[26] But whereas Fuchs had blamed the sorry state of medicine exclusively on the Arabs and medical scholasticism, Cardano leveled his attacks indifferently at Aristotelianism and scholastic disputation, Hellenizing medical philology, ancient Greek and medieval Arab medical authors, and readiness to take practical advice from surgeons.[27]

More significant than the content of some of the individual criticisms may be the uses to which Cardano put the work. Protesting his embarrassment about mistakes in the first edition (1536—his first medical publication), he reissued it in expanded and corrected form in 1545. The publisher, as for the first edition of the theoretical *Contradicentium medicorum liber*, which appeared in the same year, was Octavianus Scotus in Venice. Thus the *Contradictiones* (as he sometimes called the work)[28] and *De malo usu* presented Cardano's ideas about medical theory and medical practice, respectively, to an Italian readership at the time when his career as a practitioner and professor of medicine at Milan and Pavia was finally becoming established, but his fame as a philosopher and mathematician was only just beginning to penetrate to a wider European audience through his northern publishers. Twenty years later, however, *De malo usu* was transformed into part of a much more ambitious project. The little treatise was conjoined with a revised version of Cardano's account of his own "remarkable" cures (now severed from the bibliography of his writings in which it had first appeared) and some other short pieces to form his *De methodo medendi*.[29] The juxtaposition was appropriate, since criticism of medical predecessors was, of course, a very Galenic activity and Galen was an acknowledged model for Cardano's autobiographical account of the cures he had performed.[30] In the Galenically named *De methodo medendi* Cardano—so often in particular respects a critic of Galen—himself appears as almost a new Galen.

Cardano was in medical practice for almost fifty years in Venice, Sacco, Gallarate, Milan, Pavia, Lyons, England, Scotland, Bologna, and Rome. Ever quick to draw a Hippocratic parallel, he noted that Hippocrates too had practiced in many regions, and opined that such experience contributed to success in medicine.[31] But at a number of these places, Cardano's practice was severely limited in either duration, extent, or fame, and sometimes in all three. Any practice at Venice must have been while he was still a student. Sacco and Gallarate were obscure country towns. For several years after his return to Milan, his efforts to establish himself in medical practice there ran into formidable difficulties, which have been many times rehearsed by his various biographers. According to both his own account and that of hostile investigators from Bologna, he did not practice much at Pavia while he was teaching there.[32] His experiences of practice outside northern and central Italy redounded to his fame but they were very brief, for his entire trip when he went through France and England to Scotland to treat the archbishop of St. Andrews and back through England, Germany, and Switzerland occupied only ten months of 1552.[33] He continued to practice in his later years at Bologna and Rome, but although he had some distinguished patients, they do not by this time seem to have been very numerous.

The one time and place in which he evidently built up a fairly extensive medical practice over a period of decades was Milan between the mid-1530s and the late 1550s (with some intermissions for teaching at Pavia and travel). Most of his more dramatic accounts of his own successes in therapy and in developing a circle of patrons and patients come from this context; so too do the two treatises dedicated to attacking the therapeutic preferences of medical colleagues. Yet in the same period, as already noted, he was deeply involved in writing major works on subjects other than medicine and publishing them outside Italy for a European scholarly audience. Furthermore, he included his local and particular experiences as a practitioner in his grand project of reaching audiences outside Italy and beyond academic medical circles. As a result, his accounts of his patients cannot be read simply as a record of his efforts to build up a local reputation for therapeutic successes and acquire local patronage, informative though they are on that score. They are productions consciously composed as part of his presentation of himself to a European public as a philosopher, mathematician, astronomer, and physician endowed with special gifts. Thus the great majority of the patients named in the three treatises listing his medical successes that Cardano published in his lifetime were Milanese or resident in Milan. But the treatises were printed in Lyon, Paris, and Basel; only one was included in a medical work, the other two being, respectively, part of his autobibliography and an appendix to his treatise on dreams.[34]

But he also took steps evidently intended to build up his practice at Milan. The most striking feature of Cardano's position within the medical profession at Milan and Pavia is its persistently anomalous character. He clearly both sought and ultimately achieved a place in the upper ranks of a tightly organized and exclusive local professional and social hierarchy, and subsequently in the academic circles to which that hierarchy was closely linked. His long campaign to gain admission to the College of Physicians (whose members were required to be of noble as well as legitimate birth and to have studied logic, philosophy, and medicine for seven years in a university),[35] the publication of the erudite *Contradictiones*, and his acquisition of a professorship in medical theory all fall into this pattern. Nor was it necessarily particularly unusual to move to a professorial position after years spent exclusively in medical or surgical practice. The appointments of Berengario da Carpi as professor of surgery at Bologna (1502) and of Giovanni Argenterio as professor of medical theory at Pisa (1543) were both of this type.[36] Yet Cardano's own actions also show that he never wholly defined himself in terms of this standard path to an elite medical career. The complaints of colleagues that he devoted a great deal of his time to subjects other than medicine in these same years were, after all, justified.[37] The aggressive rhetoric of *On the Bad Practice of Recent Physicians* fell well within the limits of learned medical debate in a combative age, but the initial publication of the work in 1536, when he was still seeking entry to the college, could hardly have helped to win support from its members.

Furthermore, whatever the reality of his relations with established local medical colleagues in Milan, the attitude to them expressed in his writings is consistently hostile. On the one hand, he portrayed himself as an underdog, repeatedly obliged to overcome their enmity, suspicion, and attempts to exclude him. A reference to "certain of our well-born physicians . . . by conspiracy snatching [a patient] from my hands" is only one of many similar anecdotes or allusions.[38] On the other, he judged them by the standards of the most advanced medical and philosophical learning and found them wanting. His attitude is made very clear in one of his few surviving contributions to the then popular genre of the medical epistle, a letter written from Milan in August 1551 to his former pupil Taddeo Duno in Switzerland. Duno had become involved in a controversy with both another university-educated physician and an empiric over the proper treatment of pleurisy and was looking for his former teacher's backing. Instead, he received an unsympathetic reply that left him thoroughly dissatisfied. In addition to criticizing Duno's specific views on therapy, Cardano informed him that whatever he had to put up with was certainly no worse than his, Cardano's, own experience with the medical practitioners of Milan, who "do not know how to speak Latin correctly, nor attain to any part of philosophy, nor understand reasoning about the art of medicine or the precepts of healing. They feign for themselves certain comments, by which they deceive the populace."[39] (Cardano's own command of Latin came in for a good deal of criticism from more philologically minded contemporaries, notably Julius Caesar Scaliger.)[40]

Conversely, he was very respectful of physicians of European fame—especially perhaps those from outside Italy—whom he knew via their writings. In the same letter, he ranked leading contemporaries. Leonhart Fuchs, Janus Cornarius, and Antonio Musa Brasavola were all undoubtedly distinguished, on the basis of their numerous and widely read works. He was considerably less appreciative of Matteo Corti, one of the most famous Italian physicians of his generation, whom "I would not have dared to put in the same category if I had not heard him lecture [*nisi audisse non auderem his adnumerare*]."[41] The judgment on Corti, an enthusiastic proponent of Renaissance Galenism, undoubtedly had personal as well as scientific elements. Corti, who came from Pavia, had been Cardano's teacher at Padua. He thought well enough of the young Cardano to recommend him for a professorship of medicine at the University of Pisa, even though the two had quarreled over a debt. When Cardano looked back on the episode at the end of his life, he took pride in remembering that it had never caused him to deny Corti's erudition ("*non eruditioni eius invidi*"). In a horoscope for Corti published in 1547 (after the latter's death), Cardano characterized him as a famous medical practitioner and professor of medicine, with great knowledge of things, but envious and full of suspicion. He also expressed the opinion that Corti's mistaken dietary recommendations had hastened the death of Pope Clement VII.[42] Envy and suspicion seem to have been the hallmarks of this professional relationship, perhaps on both sides but certainly on Cardano's.

Despite his insistence on practice and cures as crucial elements in his own reputation, his favorable judgments of other physicians really depended on successful scientific authorship. His tepid remarks about Gianbattista Da Monte (1489–1551), another famous Italian physician among his older contemporaries (who was well known to Cardano by repute, though apparently not in person), are explained by the fact that most of Da Monte's writings had not yet been published when Cardano's letter to Duno was written. Although he acknowledged that Da Monte had a high reputation, he based his opinion on one pamphlet (*opusculum*) of Da Monte's that he had read, which he thought showed *ingenium* and judgment, but no erudition. He reserved his highest praise for Sylvius, Fernel, and Vesalius; these were "the most famous [*famosissimi*]." As usual, Cardano was up-to-date with his reading. This early appreciation of the Paris professor of medicine Jean Fernel (whom Cardano was to meet in the following year) must refer not to his comprehensive textbook of medicine—first published in 1554—but to Fernel's treatise on physiology (*De naturali parte medicinae*, 1542) and/or his work "on the hidden causes of things" (*De abditis rerum causis*, 1548). From these works the reader could gather both Fernel's insistence on the importance of anatomy and his theories about innate heat, celestial spirits, and occult influences in physiology and pathology.[43]

Cardano further urged Duno, who was planning to publish a pamphlet attacking Leonhart Fuchs's views on the treatment of pleurisy, to avoid pointless controversies and instead imitate Galen by concentrating on solid erudition, especially—since Duno had already progressed far in medicine—in languages and mathematics (no doubt including astrology).[44] Even though Fuchs himself had engaged in controversy, one should imitate not the vices of outstanding men but their virtues; in any case, "we ought to be very grateful to Fuchs who added grace and brevity to erudition so that the writings of living authors could begin to be read with pleasure."[45] Fuchs, moreover, "commands fairly polished Latin, is skilled in Greek, writes briefly and with minimal confusion, and is clear and well organized, knows the works of Galen well, knows a great deal about simples, has written a lot, freely teaches what he knows, and is certainly a hardworking and erudite man."[46] This succinct description of a model medical scholar by the standards of the most advanced medicine of the mid–sixteenth century shows Cardano as both just and generous when it came to evaluating a contemporary physician on the basis of his learning.

Yet in his descriptions of his own successful cures, the power to heal, not academic medical learning or professional authorization, emerges as the primary test or justification of his eminence as a physician. These descriptions in some respects recall the world of empirics and professors of secrets recently and vividly described by William Eamon. As will become apparent in a later chapter, in their most developed form Cardano's Latin narratives about his cures have learned, literary antecedents; they derive from older traditions of Latin medical narrative and incorporate ideas that he drew from his reading of the Hippocratic *Epidemics*, as well as involving the direct imitation of Galen as autobiographer that has already been noted. Nevertheless, the claims quoted at the beginning of this chapter do not seem totally remote in spirit from the vernacular boasts of his contemporary, the famous empiric surgeon Leonardo Fioravanti.[47] Indeed, Cardano's claimed cure for phthisis, which apparently included incision of the chest, was itself a medical secret, although like many "secrets" of the period it was published in a printed book.[48] Moreover, Cardano's insistence on his cures was by no means merely a strategy adopted to assist his rise from obscurity but continued to the end of his life.

Thus although by the 1540s Cardano was indeed, as he has recently been described, "a controversial member of the medical elite,"[49] the description does not encompass every aspect of his practice. Acceptance by local medical colleagues confirmed Cardano's professional status and legitimized his practice, but that practice nevertheless also had links both to elements in popular culture and to Cardano's broader philosophical reputation and goals and his vision of himself as a reformer of medicine, as of other disciplines. Its basis was the dissemination of claims to cure among networks of patients, patrons, and readers. All these aspects of his practice are exemplified in the famous, and subsequently rescinded, claim to be able to cure phthisis quoted at the beginning of this chapter. In particular, this claim provides a notable instance of the way in which his fame as a philosopher of nature disseminated his medical reputation across Europe. Cardano linked his initial claim firmly to his experience in Milan—"this city"—and dedicated *De sapientia*, in which the claim appears, to Francesco Sfondrati who had been one of the principal patrons and employers of his medical services there. But *De sapientia* is a philosophical, not a medical, treatise and was published in Nuremberg. Cardano's summons to distant Scotland to treat Archbishop Hamilton of St. Andrews came about because the archbishop's physician, who was impressed by the first of Cardano's autobibliographies and admired *De subtilitate*, came across the claim while reading *De sapientia*.[50]

But at the local level Cardano's reference to his economic straits as a motivation to "find something new" in medicine suggests competition to cure in Milan's medical marketplace. His attention may have fallen on phthisis because he perceived it as a particularly pressing local problem. *Phthisis* (or *phthoe*) was conceived of as a disease marked by wasting, coughing, and fever, sometimes accompanied by bloody sputum;[51] it was therefore a construct that encompassed what would now be diagnosed as pulmonary tuberculosis, but also other conditions. The exceptionally complete Milan death registers, which run in an uninterrupted series from 1452 until 1806, include the cause of death for adults, the determination of cause of death being made by members of the College of Physicians or other approved medical practitioners. No complete analysis of this vast body of data has so far been published. However, a recent study of about 18,000 entries in the registers for nonepidemic years between 1452 and 1503 has concluded that it is extremely likely that tuberculosis was a major cause of both mortality and long-term morbidity, with large numbers of pulmonary cases; another study suggests that respiratory problems were similarly prevalent a century later.[52] The universe of disease in Cardano's accounts of his patients and *consilia* seems to have consisted mostly of fevers, *morbus gallicus*, and various chronic or endemic ailments. With the exception of one outbreak in 1545, which, according to him, attacked chiefly young girls, he left little record of any practice during epidemics.[53] Among the endemic diseases that he treated, phthisis, phthoe (again, he seems to use both terms indifferently), difficulty in breathing, wasting (*tabes*), and catarrh recur continually. In some families, one person after another died of phthoe: Cesare Bozio and Francisco Serio had each lost two brothers to it when they consulted Cardano; in the family of Lorenzo Gadi, two children had already died and a third was moribund when the father and four other children were stricken. Phthisical patients evidently sought out Cardano because word spread that he had a cure; thus. sometime in the late 1530s, Donato Lanza, a pharmacist who shared Cardano's interest in music, overheard him discussing his cure. Soon after, Cardano was hearing about Lanza's own wasting, fever, and bloody sputum.[54]

Cardano's comparison of the cure of phthisis with the cure of *morbus gallicus*, which by the 1530s had become endemic in Europe, suggests how easily claims to cure could be made sincerely and believed in the case of diseases of long duration in which periods of complete remission or temporary improvement might take place. *Morbus gallicus* was regarded as curable because the tertiary stage of syphilis was not recognized, because syphilis was not clearly distinguished from other diseases affecting the genitals, and because, above all, its recognized symptoms disappeared after a time.

The most remarkable thing about Cardano's claim to be able to cure phthisis is therefore his willingness to give it up in the face of evidence to the contrary. By 1554, nine years after publishing the claim that he had discovered a cure for phthisis, he realized his mistake; his disavowal was published in 1557. With the passage of time, he came to realize that phthisical patients who seemed to recover under his treatment survived for only a few years. Such was the fate of a patient whom he had apparently cured so completely that Cardano's enemies in the medical community were driven to allege that the man had never had "true phthisis [*vera phthoe*]" in the first place. Five years later the patient died, "coughing up his lungs like other phthisis victims." Subsequently, Cardano questioned the man's widow and learned that his cough had in reality never completely gone away. Thus, as Cardano summarized the episode, "since I dared to write that I had cured patients with phthisis . . . the physicians and I had both lied, but I had written these things in good faith, and I was deceived by my hope."[55] Despite Gabriel Naudé's strictures, there seems to be no reason to disbelieve the last assertion.[56] However, Cardano continued to have faith that he had cured patients suffering from simple wasting (*tabes simplex*), difficulty in breathing, and other similar conditions, some of whom, to be sure, may indeed have recovered completely.[57]

On the part of both Cardano and his critics, the episode is illustrative of Renaissance interest in identifying specific diseases and clarifying the application of classical disease nomenclature to conditions currently encountered in clinical practice. It is also suggestive of the indeterminacy of the concept of cure and its dependence on professional or community consensus. But as far as Cardano himself is concerned, the most striking feature of the entire episode is his readiness to make a public reassessment of his own claims in the light of further experience. In medicine as in astrology, this trait sharply distinguishes him from other Renaissance practitioners, whether popular or erudite. But it remains difficult to evaluate his willingness to reverse his opinion, given both the ambiguity of sixteenth-century standards of evidence in disease and cure and the indifference to consistency as a value frequently manifested throughout Cardano's nonmathematical writings.

Cardano's claims to cure may have owed something to the idea of public competition or challenge. As is well known, he was certainly familiar with such challenges among mathematical practitioners, even though he refused to participate personally in a viva voce contest with Tartaglia, apparently on grounds that to do so did not befit his position as a professor of medicine.[58] Yet in medicine he issued such challenges, which were more commonly associated with empirics, even when he was an elderly professor of medical theory *supraordinarius*. But Cardano's principal challenge, unlike that of the empiric Fioravanti some ten years later, was limited by considerations derived from medical doctrine as well as by caution learned from experience. Thus whereas Fioravanti proclaimed his conviction that he would win a competition with "all the physicians of Milan" to see who could cure "twenty or twenty-five sick people with diverse ailments . . . faster and better," Cardano promised "publicly at Bologna, that I would cure every sick person under the age of seventy and over seven who came into my hands," provided he or she were not suffering from a long list of excluded preexisting conditions (the language of modern American medical insurance springs irresistibly to mind). The excluded conditions fell into the categories of mental illnesses, traumatic injuries, and incurable diseases—among them phthisis.[59]

Whether or not this challenge was ever taken up, there is no reason to doubt that at times Cardano did encounter the kind of patient population that it implies—random individuals of any social origin, classified only by age and medical condition. But his accounts of his named patients suggest a practice heavily dependent on particular social and family networks and structures. Although the roster includes the sons of a carpenter and an innkeeper, most patients are described as belonging to the middle and upper ranks of society: the families of merchants, members of the learned professions, and the urban patriciate. A substantial proportion of those named are women. There is also a numerically small but highly significant representation of Milan's Spanish rulers, of noble Milanese families of the first rank, and of the higher clergy. At Milan, in the absence of a local princely court after 1535, these three groups were the major sources of cultural patronage. Patients or their relatives from these groups were potentially and often actually also patrons of Cardano's erudition in fields other than medicine. A striking example is provided by Francesco Sfondrati (1493–1550), who served both Francesco Sforza, the last duke of Milan, and the subsequent Spanish regime until shortly after his (Sfondrati's) wife's death. He then entered the church, was rapidly elevated to the rank of cardinal, and was considered a possible candidate for the papacy on the death of Paul III.[60] After his departure for Rome in the early 1540s, Sfondrati could do no more for Cardano at Milan; however, Cardano subsequently owed a great deal to ecclesiastical patrons at Bologna and Rome.[61]

Patients came to Cardano in two principal and overlapping ways: through what amounted to a system of informal referrals among the patients themselves; and as a result of his own social and professional strategies. Some people, as we have just seen, appear to have been attracted by his reputation for curing particular conditions. In other instances, word about him seems to have spread among members of an extended family or lineage: Lorenzo Gadi and his sons were presumably related to Gianfrancesco Gadi, prior of the Augustinian Canons, who had been one of Cardano's first patients in Milan; Cardano treated both a child of Count Camillo Borromeo's and the wife of his cousin Giberto Borromeo.[62] What might be described as vertical social contacts were also important. Treating a nobleman's client might lead to practice among the noble family itself and to patronage by its head: thus the pharmacist Donato Lanza, a grateful patient in the service of Sfondrati, first drew Cardano to Sfondrati's attention when the latter's infant son fell ill.[63] The fact that among the families of two of his principal noble patrons, the Borromei and Sfondrati, Cardano seems frequently to have treated the women and children as well as or instead of the master of the household is probably significant evidence of his ability to inspire confidence in patients; as recent studies have pointed out, the health and medical attendance of the women and children who transmitted the lineage to the next generation was something noble families took extremely seriously.[64] Thus even though the terms of the challenge quoted above may suggest that Cardano would have liked to exclude pediatric and geriatric cases, he was often called on to treat infants and young children. He also devoted much of his attention—at any rate in his didactic works on health care—to problems of old age (see further below).

Insofar as one can judge, therefore, it appears that Cardano joined a fairly broad practice among Milan's middling and prosperous classes with access to a few households whose heads enjoyed sufficient wealth and power to be true patrons. His native state, no longer an autonomous dukedom, did not offer him the possibility—or the hazards—of becoming the physician of a prince.[65] However, Cardano achieved what was presumably the next best thing, since he enjoyed the patronage of three successive Spanish governors of Milan.[66] But the extent to which he acquired patronage specifically as a result of his activities as a medical practitioner as distinct from his other accomplishments is as ambiguous as most other aspects of his medical practice. Cardano several times dedicated works to important patients: in addition to *De sapientia*, two other examples are the *Practica aritmeticae* to Gianfrancesco Gadi and later editions of *De subtilitate* to Gonsalvo Ferrante (Gonzalo Fernandez), governor of Milan, whom Cardano treated sometime between 1558 and 1562.[67] It is impossible to determine the relative importance attached by these men to Cardano's medical services, and in particular to his claims to cure, and to his mathematics or philosophy. Cardano himself stated that with one exception—the comte de Brissac who was looking for an engineer—various nobles and rulers throughout Europe who had sought his services had all wanted him as a physician.[68] Nevertheless, it seems likely that for his patrons, clients, and patients his various roles appeared mutually enhancing. Cardano's own view of his relations with the powerful varied according to the individual: he took one hundred gold crowns for treating Ferrante but did not ask for a fee from Cardinal Morone "since I thought I owed him more than he owed me." Instead, Morone as patron/patient sent an unsolicited gift.[69]

Yet the situation of a medical attendant on the powerful was very different from that of someone who was purely a literary or scientific client. Cardano expressed his lively awareness of the potential hazards of practice among the nobility in terms that recall his feeling remarks about the precarious situation of a court astrologer (with reference to his unfortunate prediction of long life for Edward VI of England, he described his terror that an unfavorable prediction might arouse suspicions of conspiracy and his fear that, if so, he might never get home safely).[70] Among "perilous" medical situations (for the physician, not the patient) he listed "if the sick person is a prince, or if he is the only son of his father or mother, or if his relatives are violent, or if the sick person himself is a wrathful man."[71] He was no doubt justified in regarding medical treatment of the male children of irascible noble fathers as a particularly risky business (for an example, see chapter 8).[72] Notwithstanding these anxieties, however, he evidently cultivated patients of elevated status with some care and considerable success. Moreover, in at least one instance he used connections forged through medical practice to secure patronage, quasi-official endorsement, and fame for his nonmedical writings. Before 1552 he had successfully treated Giovanni Paolo Negroli, a prosperous merchant, for headache and his sister for fever. In 1554 they referred their relative Niccolo Sicco, a military commander, to him for treatment for fever, arthritis, jaundice, and dropsy. Sicco, in turn, was a relative of another Niccolo Sicco, this one prefect of criminal justice in Milan, to whom Cardano dedicated two successive editions of his autobibliography.[73]

Throughout his career, a series of distinguished Milanese patients or their relatives came to Cardano's aid as patrons in times of crisis. Their helpfulness presumably indicates satisfaction with Cardano as a family or personal physician, as well as appreciation of his intellectual accomplishments. However, when powerful ecclesiastics of Milanese origin came to his aid in Bologna and Rome, they may also have been motivated by a wish to assert influence on behalf of a fellow countryman. In the late 1530s and early 1540s Sfondrati played a part in securing Cardano's admission to the College of Physicians of Milan and his professorship at Pavia.[74] In the next generation, the young Carlo Borromeo, whose mother Cardano had attended, proposed his appointment to a professorship at Bologna and overrode local opposition.[75] Giovanni, Cardinal Morone, for whom he provided a dietary regimen, was a patron and in some sense, surely, friend for nearly thirty years. In 1570, when Cardano fell under suspicion of heresy at Bologna, Morone advised him to stop teaching voluntarily, presumably in the hope of demonstrating his sincere intention not to offend. Cardano came to believe that Morone had been too ready to credit the accusations of his enemies, but the strategy suggested may well have helped to ensure the relative mildness of Cardano's treatment by the Inquisition. Moreover, the cardinal worked to obtain papal protection and a pension for Cardano after the latter's arrest, private abjuration, and release. Morone certainly knew from personal experience the difficulties accusations of religious unorthodoxy could bring. Despite long service as an ecclesiastical statesman and trusted papal adviser—he was the chief papal representative at the first session of the Council of Trent—in the reign of Paul IV he had endured a lengthy trial and two years' imprisonment on charges of crypto-Lutheranism before being totally absolved in 1560.[76]

One expression of dissatisfaction with Cardano as a medical practitioner came from Bolognese civic and university authorities. Their initial resistance to his appointment was due to a number of factors: rumors about his troubles at Pavia, resentment at the way powerful ecclesiastics in Rome overrode local autonomy, and desire to get value for money (there was much haggling over Cardano's stipend) evidently all played a part. Stated grounds for objection were, however, lack of confidence in him as a practitioner "into whose hands no serious person in the city, either noble or popular, would entrust his or her life or health." Since Cardano had not previously practiced in Bologna, this judgment could have been based only on rumor or secondhand reports. In 1563, after the Bolognese authorities had had a year's firsthand experience of his teaching and practice, they renewed his contract for a longer term, adding words of praise and a raise in salary; they also granted him Bolognese citizenship. But once he had been accused of heresy, the officials of the university again began to grumble that he had not attracted enough patients to justify his large salary. Cardano's insistent claims to cure now appear in a different light, as both stimulating and responding to the demands and expectations of his employers. What attracted patients was a reputation for performing cures; and at this point in Cardano's career the administrators of a bastion of medical learning seem to be complaining (however speciously and however much really motivated by financial, prudential, or religious considerations) that their professor of medical *theoria* has not cured enough people.[77] Yet it is no easier to evaluate their dissatisfaction than the evident satisfaction of Cardano's noble patrons. Medical reputations among the lay public depended (depend) to a large extent on consensus, which may be achieved in a variety of ways.

Ultimately, Cardano's medical practice remains in many respects elusive. Even though his descriptions of his patients and their illnesses, treatment, and outcome constitute an exceptionally rich source of information about the practice of medicine as he and, to some extent, his patients experienced it, his accounts resist easy analysis. Interpretative strategies that pay exclusive attention to any single factor, however apparently promising—such as, for example, the social and professional aspects of his medical career—are likely to be as unsatisfactory as the earlier attempts of various biographers and historians of medicine to isolate specific medical insights or innovations for which he was responsible.[78] Rather, both his accounts of himself as a medical practitioner and his prescriptive writings on aspects of medicine subsumed under *practica* invite multiple levels of interpretation that acknowledge his self-appointed role as a prophetic reformer of all knowledge, his classicizing imitations of Hippocrates and Galen, his responses to a professional, social, and religious context, and the influence of the epidemiological and demographic environment.

PART TWO

Theory and Practice

Chapter 3

ARGUMENT AND EXPERIENCE

MANY of Cardano's ideas about the nature and sources of medical knowledge and the construction of medical theory, the subject of this chapter, were a product of his early academic training in Aristotelian natural philosophy and Hippocratic-Galenic medicine. But in important respects his response to intellectual assumptions built in to the philosophical and medical system in which he was educated was also subversive. His medicine was in most respects Galenic, but he was strongly critical of particular doctrines of Galen. He worked in standard genres of medical writing but used some of them in idiosyncratic ways. As reader and writer of medical books he was a collector and producer of texts and profoundly respectful of textual authority—but the textual authority was sometimes his own, and he also constantly claimed a privileged role for "experience." His characteristic attitudes appeared early: "In the year 1526, when I was at Sacco . . . I wrote out for myself a pretty big collection of passages from different authors, which was of almost no use to me"; "I wrote a work on the epidemics that occurred between 1526 and 1533, which begins, 'On September 24, 1526, which was my birthday, I went to Sacco.' " [1] His practice of periodically sorting through his constant flow of writings, destroying some and incorporating others into different treatises, has ensured that neither of the two works mentioned has survived as an independent publication or recognizable entity. But these reminiscences, written down many years later, of his activities as a young practitioner capture enduring features of his medical science. They show him diligently forming two collections: one of authoritative but also strongly criticized texts; the other of "experiences."

One project that he began in the Sacco years or even earlier and that occupied him, on and off, for much of the rest of his life was the *Contradicentium medicorum libri*, a collection of citations and arguments about issues on which standard medical authorities differed. As noted in the previous chapter, the first octavo volume of *Contradictiones* appeared in print in 1545; a second edition, doubled in length, appeared in 1548. The dates of publication of the first two editions, both within five years of Cardano's receiving his chair at the University of Pavia, probably reflect his determination to publish a work appropriate to a professor of medical theory as soon as possible after his appointment. The dedication of the work to the Senate of Milan, which controlled professorial appointments to the University of Pavia, is further evidence that the timing of the publication was not coincidental. The *Contradictiones* is also one of very few medical works of any kind that he actually published during the 1540s and 1550s when, simultaneously, his medical career at Milan and Pavia was at its height and he was at his most productive in disciplines other than medicine.[2] But Cardano continued to enlarge the collection long thereafter. By the end of his life it had grown almost as long as both his encyclopedic works combined.[3] In the amount of effort the author devoted to it, this must be rated one of his major works. And although plenty of controversies are incorporated into his medical writings in other genres (most of them treatises on practice or Hippocratic commentaries), the *Contradictiones* is the only work in which he focused exclusively on the analysis of controversies in medicine.

The *Contradictiones* is at once a key text for Cardano's ideas about medical knowledge and a prime example of the multiple and often confusing strands in his thought. Alfonso Ingegno has rightly drawn attention to the presence in it of essential aspects of Cardano's philosophy of nature and a strongly revisionist approach to medicine.[4] Other features are consonant with traditions in Latin medicine extending back to the thirteenth century. Not all the ambiguities can be resolved; the project was not necessarily in every respect a coherent one. Yet the work casts much light on Cardano's agenda as a medical reader, teacher, and writer. In this chapter, I shall draw on it to explore, first, the process of assembling the collection; then, in turn, his ambivalent relation to Latin scholastic medicine; the functions that he may have envisaged for the *Contradictiones* in aiding reading, memory, and debate; his understanding of the roles of textual authority and experience in the construction of medical theory; and, finally, the extent to which he was prepared to allow his general (and in some instances radical) philosophical ideas to drive his medical theory.

COLLECTING TEXTS, COLLECTING EVENTS

As his remarks quoted above indicate, in the same period in which he was beginning to amass the texts for the *Contradictiones* Cardano was also collecting events that he had personally experienced in his capacity as a practitioner. The diseases that occurred at Sacco between 1526 and 1533 were also to be sources of medical knowledge. No doubt his fascination with the analysis of all aspects of his personal experience had already led him to begin what would presumably be a lifelong practice of keeping notes or some form of journal. His accounts of his illnesses, his year-by-year chronicle of his literary activities, and his lists of those who had written well and ill of him were evidently all, like the record of his dreams, the result of a habit of note taking (see chapter 8).

In principle, the combination of attention to experience and bookish compilation from authors was fully congruent with the existing system of medical knowledge. Medicine was held to include both general and universally applicable theory and innumerable disparate pieces of information about diseases, remedies, and patients. Theory was supposedly arrived at by a combination of reason, reliance on textual authority, and experience but in actuality mostly by arguing about texts; many of the details of recommended practice were allegedly the fruit of "experience" (without distinction between ancient and contemporary or between personal and reported experience). What remained unclear, despite much scholastic discussion, was the relation between the two categories of knowledge.[5] But in thirteenth- to fifteenth-century Latin medicine accounts that claimed to be related to some form of experience had a well-established place and took various forms. They included *experimenta* (in most instances, allegedly proven medicinal recipes), *exempla* (occasional illustrative anecdotes, not necessarily based on the writer's own experience), and *consilia* (advice given to individual patients, often preserved in standardized and edited collections). By the fifteenth century, moreover, a good deal of evidence points to growing interest among medical practitioners in details of practice, in the individual and the particular, and in a few cases in the record of personal experience.[6] Nevertheless, Cardano's desire to record the diseases that afflicted Sacco in the years when he lived there was novel, and indeed radical, because it reflected three concerns peculiarly his own that would remain with him for the rest of his life: endeavors to analyze the significance of contingent events; the autobiographical and astrological commitment that led him to introduce his own birthday into a town's medical record; and pioneering interest in the Hippocratic *Epidemics.*[7]

Thus Cardano's interest in the epistemological status of particulars in medicine and in framing rules for practice on the basis of analysis of experience cannot be divorced, either chronologically or conceptually, from his approach to textual authority. His interest, in medicine as in various other disciplines, in the problem of the relation between particular instances and general theory seldom or never involved repudiation of reliance on texts or ancient authority. Rather, he selected, manipulated, and juxtaposed texts according to his own preferences or substituted one authority for another. Cardano's mathematical ability, interest in technology, and endeavors to restructure knowledge set him apart from most other humanistically educated intellectuals of the period. Nevertheless, he as much as any of them was the product of a bookish and verbal philosophical, natural scientific, and medical culture in which ancient texts provided much of the currency for intellectual exchange.

The enterprise of collecting points on which authorities disagreed began in a logical or philosophical, not a medical, context during his student years. While he was a student at Padua, he compiled a set of 100 points of difference between the teaching on dialectic of Aristotle and Averroes.[8] About the same time he started to collect differences among medical authorities or between Galenic physicians and Aristotelian philosophers. By 1531, he had accumulated almost 400 such differences, and by 1543 he had in hand the material for a work in twelve books.[9] The volume containing one book of 108 differences published in 1545 therefore comprised only a fraction of what he had amassed by that point. But parts of the published Book 2, added in the edition of 1548, were evidently written, or rewritten, after the publication of Book 1.[10] Eight more books survive in a version that includes additions or revisions made in the 1550s or early 1560s; with the exception of a short excerpt from Book 3, these books were printed for the first and last time as part of Cardano's collected *Opera* long after his death.[11]

In the form in which Cardano published it, the work incorporates elements of several different genres and conveys several different messages. Most strikingly, it presents scholastic and verbal analysis, as exemplified by the *Conciliator differentiarum philosophorum et medicorum* of Pietro d'Abano (d. 1316), and the brand-new tool of Vesalian anatomy as two equally effective and in some sense parallel methods for a critique of authoritative medical texts. Thus the preface to the first edition of 1545 declares, "There is no need for me to list those who came before us, who treated these things lightly and listlessly, except one, the Conciliator, and in dissection Vesalius."[12] At the same time, the format of a collection of discrete short treatments of controversial topics gave Cardano scope to intersperse long essays on his own philosophical views as they related to medicine, or on aspects of medicine of particular interest to him, among many shorter routine summaries.

CONTRADICENTES AND CONCILIATOR

Pietro d'Abano was the most celebrated professor of the medieval *studium* of Padua, equally famous for his medical, philosophical, and astrological learning. The *Conciliator*, his principal work, is a collection of scholastic *quaestiones*. Most of them concern debated issues within medicine, many of them of a practical variety ("should one give wine to fever patients?"); some, as the title indicates, concern issues equally pertinent to philosophy and medicine—both specific problems arising from the differences in the physiological teaching of Aristotle and Galen and more abstract issues concerning, for example, the proper understanding of terms such as "substance," "accident," and "form" in relation to the human body. As the title also indicates, the method is the normal scholastic one of laying out views of authorities, with the goal of harmonization. But Pietro also devoted lengthy passages to the exposition of an all-encompassing astrological worldview. He was, for example, one of the most explicit proponents of the idea—which originally reached the West from works of the ninth-century Arabic astrologer Albumasar (Abu ʿMashar) translated into Latin during the twelfth century—that conjunctions of the planets determined the times in history at which great religious leaders appeared.[13]

In choosing a title emphasizing contradictions, Cardano seems both to allude to the *Conciliator* and to signal an intention to subvert it. Yet his remark about his predecessors suggests that one legitimate reading of the title of the *Contradicentium medicorum libri* is as an homage to, not repudiation of, Pietro d'Abano. The idea of emulating or surpassing Pietro emerges in his statement that the collection of contradictions that he had accumulated by 1531 was "almost as big as the *Conciliator.*"[14] Moreover, since Cardano initiated his project as early as the 1520s, the relation to the *Conciliator* long antedates his acquaintance with the work of Vesalius.

Obviously, Cardano was drawn to the *Conciliator* by its author's reputation as an astrologer and as an extreme exponent of occult but naturalistic and astrological determinants in human affairs. These were areas of inquiry to which Cardano himself was profoundly committed. Pietro d'Abano was in fact one of his chief predecessors in exploring such potentially hazardous topics as the horoscope of religions. But whereas Pietro had confined himself to general statements about the responsibility of conjunctions of the planets for the rise of religious leaders, Cardano went so far as to cast the horoscope of Christ.[15] More generally, both authors shared an interest in astrological history.

But although Cardano's own astrological and related interests gave him special reason to appreciate Pietro d'Abano, his familiarity with a major work of scholastic medicine was scarcely unusual among the generation of physicians educated in Italian universities in the 1520s. By that time the advent of, and vogue for, medical Hellenism had led in advanced medical circles to a great deal of loudly expressed contempt for Arabo-Latin scholastic medicine. The printing history of works in the last category tells a different story. Among Arabic authors, Rasis and, especially, Avicenna continued to be read. Scholastic medical commentaries by authors who flourished in the fourteenth- and fifteenth-century Italian faculties of medicine were available in numerous printed editions and frequently reissued until at least about the 1520s.[16] Moreover, as

the most famous—and in some respects notorious—philosopher, astrologer, and physician of the early history of the University of Padua,
Pietro d'Abano seems to have held his place in the canon of medical literature for longer than most scholastic authors, since several editions of
the *Conciliator* were published after 1540.[17]

But Cardano drew a sharp distinction between Pietro d'Abano and
later-fourteenth- and fifteenth-century scholastic medical authors. In
part, this distinction was connected with his desire to counter the knee-
jerk anti-Arabism that so often accompanied medical Hellenism. He
thought that the way to do this was to distinguish the important contributions of the Arabs and Pietro d'Abano from the inanities of later
medical scholasticism. In 1548, he wrote: "I have not despised the opinion, reasonings, and *experimenta* of the Arabs. Was it fitting for very
learned men and excellent philosophers to be scorned solely on account
of roughness in language or poor translators? . . . I admit Jacobus [Gia-
como da Forlì] and Ugo [Benzi] and the crowd full of chimerical apparitions that Gentile [da Foligno] stirred up contributed little to medicine. But what do you have in the Conciliator, Avicenna, and Rasis
besides language—which was the calamity of the region or the age—that
is unequal to your own outstanding findings? What can be compared
with the subtlety of Averroes, with the judgment of Avicenna, with the
gravity of Rasis, with the doctrine of the Conciliator?"[18]

One medical topic explored by Pietro d'Abano that was also of great
interest to Cardano was that of the perfect temperament (that is, combination of elementary qualities). Ingegno has drawn attention to the
central significance of this aspect of the medical concept of temperament
for Cardano's understanding of subtlety and the attributes of specially
gifted people.[19] Galenic theory held that mankind is the most temperate
of all animals. This idea was problematic in itself, since it could be argued that the mixture of qualities most suited for human function was
not a perfectly temperate balance among hot and cold, wet and dry. The
Aristotelian view was that animals were characterized by heat and moisture and mankind more so than any others. But the question also arose
as to whether perfect temperament, however defined, was a purely no-
tional standard from which every individual human being deviated to a
greater or lesser extent, or whether an individual with perfect temperament could ever actually exist.[20] The discussion of the issue in the *Conciliator* threads its way through the intricacies of the late medieval theory
of temperament (in medieval Latin, *complexio*)—the subject of endless
scholastic discussions—to make two striking contributions to the development of the theme of human perfection. Pietro drew attention to
Galen's use of the story of the statue of Polykleitos, so well propor-
tioned that it served as a standard, or canon, of human perfection, a pas-

sage of Galen that later interested Vesalius as well as Cardano. In addition Pietro noted that those rare prophets and founders of religions whose occasional appearance was made possible by extremely unusual celestial conditions were also endowed with perfection of temperament, adding that "some people" cited as examples Moses and Christ.[21]

Cardano's own fascination with the idea of a human being with perfect temperament led him to devote two long *contradictiones* to the subject.[22] In the first of these, he reproached Pietro d'Abano—and Pomponazzi—for discussing Christ in terms of naturalistic physiological theory, a reproof that may seem somewhat odd coming from someone who would later publish a horoscope of Christ.[23] Perhaps his restraint in this instance was due to the link between the publication of the *Contradictiones* and his appointment to a university teaching position. Although Cardano questioned the idea that the proper or ideal human temperament was a perfectly temperate balance of qualities on the grounds that heat and moisture predominate in all animals, he asserted both that it approached such a balance and that certain rare individuals could actually possess it.

He next sought to establish that a temperamentally perfect human body would actually be perfect in all its operations. In order to do so, he disposed—at any rate to his own satisfaction—of some fairly powerful pragmatic and theoretical objections: the superior speed and ability, as compared to human beings, of some animals; the Galenic teaching that a warm and hot, not a perfectly balanced, temperament was most conducive to longevity; and the universal susceptibility of even the best-tempered human bodies to disease. His conclusion, again calling upon Galen's analogy of the statue of Polykleitos, was that the presence of numerous superior human qualities in one individual were signs of temperamental perfection. These qualities were both physical and intellectual. In a temperamentally perfect person unusual ability to overcome disease, exceptionally acute senses, and longevity would be allied to inborn skill (*ingenium*) exceeding that of Archimedes, oratorical gifts greater than those of Cicero, and the ability to "do many other innumerable things all of which would be taken for miracles."[24] As Ingegno has pointed out, the Galenic idea of balanced temperament as a mean (according to which mankind was at a midpoint as regards other animals, all of which were supposedly either hotter, wetter, colder, or drier, and the palm of the hand was similarly at a midpoint as compared to the other parts of the human body) has here given way to the idea of perfect temperament as the summit of human perfection. Of course, the image of the canon of Polykleitos—also supplied by Galen—lent itself to the latter interpretation. Perhaps, as Ingegno further suggests, Cardano did after all have the qualities of Christ in mind—and may well also have seen himself among the rare and exceptionally privileged group of the temperamentally perfect.[25]

In addition to praising Pietro d'Abano in the preface and sharing his astrological and related interests, Cardano also repeatedly cited the *Conciliator* throughout the *Contradictiones*. For all that, the *Conciliator* served him as a model only in a very limited sense. He did not imitate its organization and often had goals other than reconciliation of authorities in mind. A telling example is provided by his positioning and treatment of some of the same questions that open the *Conciliator*. Pietro d'Abano began his work with a series of ten lengthy questions about the nature of medical knowledge and the place of medicine in the scheme of the arts and sciences. The practice, which became standard, of discussing these topics at the beginning of commentaries or general works on medicine reflects their fundamental importance to scholastic medical theory. The issues addressed in such questions included whether or not medicine, or any part of it, could be considered a science (*scientia*) in the Aristotelian sense of offering certain knowledge of universal truths arrived at by rational demonstration from generally accepted premises; whether, instead, medicine or some part of it should be considered an art with a practical goal; whether the subject of medicine was the study of the human body or the achievement of health; what was the relation of medical theory and medical practice; and whether medicine should make use of logic, the tool par excellence of medieval natural philosophy. Thirteenth- to fifteenth-century medical writers often ended up by claiming that medicine was both *ars* and *scientia*, but that medical theory, which overlapped with natural philosophy, was the part closest to *scientia* (Pietro d'Abano thought the latter was true only in a loose sense, and that much in medical theory rested on conjecture).[26] These and similar questions were usually dealt with in highly abstract philosophical terms, but they were not of purely philosophical significance. They had broad implications not only for the epistemological status of the discipline, but also for the social and intellectual status of its practitioners in the academic milieu.

Three of the same questions discussed in the opening pages of the *Conciliator* also appear in the *Contradictiones*, namely, "Whether a physician should know logic"; "Whether medicine is a science"; and "Whether the human body is the subject of medicine."[27] Both authors use some of the same citations on each side of the various issues; moreover, Cardano's citations of the *Conciliator* make it clear that he had attentively studied the corresponding sections. Yet in Cardano's hands, these topics have completely lost their privileged position. They are scattered at random, rather than grouped at the beginning; and, as compared with the treatment in the *Conciliator*, they are greatly abbreviated. Formal exposition of medicine's place among the disciplines was evidently simply not of much interest (it was, after all, a very well worn subject). Instead, Cardano used these brief questions to bring in some of his own concerns. He declared that medicine was a science; he likened it, however, not to natural philosophy but to mathematical disciplines, which were simultaneously sciences directed toward action and arts: "I say therefore that a science directed toward *opus* is really an art whenever logical demonstration is not involved, as is the case with medicine and music [*Dico igitur, quod scientia quae ad opus tendit sublata demonstratione est vere ars, ut medicina et musica*]." He ended the question on the subject of medicine by comparing music, geometry, astrology, and medicine. His remarks reflect both contemporary interest in the question of the certitude of mathematics and his own persistent interest in parallels between the epistemology of astrology and that of medicine.[28] He asserted that practitioners in all these fields were simultaneously experts in a science (*scientes*) and artificers; but the *scientia* of music, geometry, or astrology involved knowledge of an unchanging and essential reality— that is, musical harmonies and mathematical relationships—that remained unaffected by the practitioners' activities or operations. But "since a *medicus* is a man of science and not a pure artificer and [yet] has to have an effect on his subject by his work, and the subject does not stay constant in one condition on account of matter: the *medicus* alone among all experts in a science is compelled to judge from sense, not from the truth of the thing." Something of the same idea emerges from his statement in another *contradictio* that medicine was certain in and of itself, although conjectural in actual practice. Elsewhere, he opined that as far as knowledge obtainable by human beings in this world was concerned, medicine was more certain than natural philosophy, astrology, and theology—in that order.[29]

Again, Pietro d'Abano's handling of the question about the use of logic in medicine turned on the distinction between instrumental logic and logic as a speculative discipline in its own right, and justified the use of the former. In Cardano's version medicine is said to have its own *ratio inquirendi*, which, unlike that of philosophy, is not directed toward universal conclusions. The same question also provided him with the opportunity to counter humanist critics who objected to the continued use of *quaestiones dialecticae*, or disputed questions, in medicine (that is, precisely, the format of the *Contradictiones*), citing Galen's objections to useless dialectic in support of their argument. According to Cardano, Galen's criticism had actually been directed at inquiry based on medical principles but not directed toward medical purposes; such inquiry, while valid in itself, should indeed be excluded from medicine. With a touch that seems typical of him, he chose as an example of this category Book 3 of the Aristotelian *Problemata*, which is devoted to problems connected with wine drinking and drunkenness.[30]

Reading, Memory, and Debate

Considered as a collection of disputed questions, the *Contradictiones* belongs to a tradition of question literature that extends far beyond the *Conciliator*. Furthermore, many of the individual topics are well-worn favorites discussed by a long series of earlier authors. The presence of *quaestiones* embedded in commentaries, the circulation of independent *quaestiones*, and the compilation of collections all became standard features of Latin medical literature in the fourteenth and fifteenth centuries. The origins of the genre lay in the coming together of the tradition of "natural questions," with antecedents stretching back to antiquity, and practices of scholastic disputation first developed in other faculties of the thirteenth-century universities.[31] Of course, some *quaestiones* reflected local and particular controversies. But when standard topics were discussed—for example, "Whether the heart is the only principal member?"[32]—they also served the purpose of familiarizing the reader with a specific set of issues considered to be of importance and with the positions of the main authorities (in this case, the different views of Aristotle and Galen on the role of the heart). Cardano described another work of his, which does not appear to survive but which was evidently connected in goals and perhaps content with the *Contradictiones*, as follows: "[In 1536], I wrote two *Libri floridorum*, that is, of medical disputations. . . . The special and very great use of the book is that it teaches very difficult medical questions with simple exposition. We also followed an easy order, as is very necessary if you have regard to the subject matter, as without knowledge of these things it is not possible to be a physician."[33]

As this remark suggests, the usefulness of *quaestiones* in medicine was in part simply as a device for organizing knowledge. As Cardano put it, referring to the *Contradictiones*, "These books were necessary, indeed useful, so that memory of many authors could be gathered together at once."[34] The acquisition of medical as of most other learning in the sixteenth century consisted chiefly of gaining control of a large body of reading. Whatever the ambiguities of the *Contradictiones*, one thing the work reveals with striking clarity is the extent of Cardano's mastery of ancient, medieval, and contemporary medical literature and his continuous and assiduous efforts to update his medical reading. He was, as one might expect, thoroughly familiar with the Renaissance Latin editions of Galen, Celsus, and other ancient medical writers. He also knew the literature of medieval medicine very well: not only the Arabs and Pietro d'Abano, but such luminaries of the thirteenth- and early-fourteenth-century Bologna school as Taddeo Alderotti, Turisanus, and Dino del Garbo, as well as the more recent scholastics—Gentile da Foligno, Giacomo da Forlì, and Ugo Benzi—whom he sometimes professed to despise.[35] Some of his remarks seem to imply that he seized on Fabio Calvo's translation of the Hippocratic corpus, which made a number of important works ascribed to Hippocrates readily available in Latin for the first time, almost immediately after it was published in 1525.[36] Cardano's Greek was acquired in middle age. He began to study the language in 1535 but only took it up intensively in 1541 (when he was warned in a dream to do so); by the time Book 1 of the *Contradictiones* was ready for publication, it showed evidence of his reading of Greek medical texts.[37] The remarkable rapidity with which he absorbed the central message of Vesalius's *Fabrica* within a year of its first publication has already been noted.

His reading in ancient and modern authors on topics other than medicine was dauntingly wide, much wider, no doubt, than that of most of his medical colleagues. Thorough knowledge of Aristotelian philosophy and of Aristotelian commentators from Alexander of Aphrodisias to Pomponazzi was perhaps to be expected from anyone educated at Padua in the 1520s. But Cardano also read on an extensive array of other subjects, ranging from mathematics to dream theory to descriptions of the New World. He prided himself on his ability to read rapidly and seize the essential content of a volume. In pursuit of this goal, he devised his own system of marking "useless" passages that could safely be skipped and obscure ones that could be postponed for later consideration.[38] This confident approach to speed-reading is pure Cardano, but its fundamental motivation—to enable him to isolate and remember key passages that were neither useless nor obscure—was by no means idiosyncratic. Instead, his reading practices, which doubtless also included much excerpting, belong to the world of sixteenth-century erudition. They were part of an intellectual environment in which treatises on the art of memory offered help in controlling vast amounts of reading and the use of commonplace books served to process information into brief, easily manageable, and easily retrievable chunks for use as needed.[39] As far as medicine in particular was concerned, *quaestiones* were only one of several ways of organizing texts and authorities for use in study, teaching, and practice. For this purpose they were not necessarily much less useful than some of the others recommended, such as, for example, the suggestion of Martin Stainpeis, writing in 1520, that medical neophytes should copy all the chapters on a particular disease from an array of authorities into a single notebook.[40]

But questions functioned specifically as a guide to *debated* issues and the literature on them. Nor were they only a written genre. The "medical disputations" Cardano had in mind included two spheres of activity. The first was formal debate in an academic setting, a practice that traced its origins to the quodlibetal debates of the medieval universities and survived in various university exercises in medicine. Thus, for example, in 1561, Cardano was called upon to defend his views in a debate with his fellow professor of medical theory at Pavia, the philosopher and physician Andrea Camuzio, "on the customary day for disputing."[41] As will become apparent, Camuzio and Cardano were in vehement disagreement on issues of considerable intellectual significance; moreover, this particular debate was part of an orchestrated and successful campaign to end Cardano's career at Pavia. However, *quaestiones* could also serve more mundane purposes in the academic setting. The discussion of standard *quaestiones* in lectures on medical theory was at once a form of routine pedagogy and a confirmation of medicine's claimed links with philosophy and of the intellectual prestige of medical professors.

Second, urban or court medical practice often demanded that physicians be able to marshal textual arguments and authorities in debates about disease, diagnosis, and treatment. Such debates came about as a result of the custom of summoning several medical attendants at once to the bedside of important patients. Practitioners were obliged to discuss and defend their recommendations in consultations that, though nominally collegial, were potentially highly competitive and fraught with professional risks—risks that increased in severity with the social status of the patient. A centuries-old tradition of medical deontology advised practitioners to avoid disputing with one another about the causes and proper treatment of cases of illness in the presence of people outside the medical profession, especially the patient and the patient's relatives; as the thirteenth-century surgeon Guglielmo da Saliceto put it, "the laity always denigrate the wise."[42] But in sixteenth-century reality, members of the patient's household seem often to have been on hand when a group of practitioners discussed a case with one another and made their separate recommendations in each other's presence. In particular, if the patient was a noble woman or child, the head of the household—the primary patron of its medical attendants—was likely to be present. In such a situation a physician needed ready command of appropriate citations in support of his own recommendations and of countercitations to deflect criticism. The fifty formal consultations, fourteen of them in the presence of King Philip II, held by the physicians and surgeons who attended the head injury of Don Carlos in 1562 were doubtless unusual, evidence of the special care due the heir of the most powerful monarch in Europe. On those occasions, the physicians and surgeons sat in a semicircle in front of the king and were called on in turn to speak: "the physician thus addressed gave his opinion, supporting his statements by authorities and reasons."[43] At a more modest and probably usual level, when Cardano was summoned to attend the infant son of Francesco Sfondrati—one of his principal noble patrons, as noted in the previous chapter—he was obliged to consult with two colleagues, both of whom he thought regarded him critically and with suspicion, in the presence of the anxious father.[44]

Probably the most successful collection of medical *quaestiones* to be produced in the sixteenth century was the *Controversiae medicae* of Francisco Valles. Originally published in Alcalá, it was subsequently reissued in Germany, France, and Italy (one edition was revised, without the author's knowledge and much to his annoyance, by two leading German physicians, Crato von Krafftheim and Peter Monau). The work's contents dealt sequentially with philosophical and physiological issues, pathology, regimen, cures, prognosis, and anatomy. The author's goal was chiefly to defend the superiority of Galen against medieval Arabo-Latin medicine on the one hand and Galen's modern critics on the other. He acknowledged Pietro d'Abano as a predecessor, but much less prominently than Cardano had done and in considerably more reserved terms, doubtless because Valles' commitment to both religious orthodoxy and Galen was considerably more wholehearted than Cardano's.[45] Valles promised his readers that all traces of scholastic methods of argumentation and "barbarous" discourse had been eliminated from his own questions, which were not only well organized and useful but also a pleasure to read.[46] His readers seem to have found them so, for the substantial volume went into ten editions between its first publication in 1556 and 1625.[47]

Cardano, too, claimed—and may originally have envisaged—the *Contradictiones* as a systematically arranged guide to controversies and debated issues in every area of medicine. The preface to the reader, first included in the 1545 edition of Book 1, explained the design of all twelve books, each supposedly devoted to questions arising from works on a different branch of medicine. The context is unambiguously academic: Books 1–3 are described as pertaining to the rotation of three lectures customarily given in the morning hours, that is, to the courses on medical theory, and Books 4 and 5 to alternating courses on fevers and diseases of the whole body given in the evening hours. Seven other books purportedly cover, respectively, anatomy, surgery, prognosis, regimen, simple and composite medications, and a miscellaneous category.[48]

Thus described, the work seems intended to present a programmatic statement of his approach to medicine considered as an academic discipline and perhaps also an ideal curriculum. Judging by the texts listed in conjunction with each branch of medicine, the idea was to encompass all three categories of current medical debate: long standard *quaestiones*, issues raised by Renaissance Galenist critics of medieval Arabo-Latin medicine, and the Vesalian critique of Galenic anatomy. Thus portions of the *Canon* of Avicenna were to be read in the light of Galen's works on physiology, while for anatomy Vesalius's *Fabrica* was set alongside Galen's *De usu partium*, the survey of physiological anatomy that was at once Vesalius's chief textual source and his main object of criticism. The list of books and topics seems likely to have fitted in fairly well with current interests of the medical faculty at Pavia. There, as at other Italian universities, a traditional medical curriculum of lectures on medical *theoria* and *practica* using Arabo-Latin texts was supplemented by participation in recent trends in medical teaching. Lecturers on simples, medical texts in Greek, and anatomy were appointed in the 1530s and 1540s; in 1552 there was a proposal to build an anatomy theater.[49]

But the pedagogical arrangement promised in the preface is handled in very arbitrary fashion in the text. According to the announced scheme, Books 1 and 2 were supposed to relate to courses in medical theory taught from the Hippocratic *Aphorisms* and Galen's *Ars*. Many of the individual questions bear some relation to the texts named, although that relation is not always easy to discern. However, the sequence of topics neither follows the texts in the manner of *quaestiones* embedded in a commentary nor constitutes a systematic survey of medical theory in the manner of a forerunner of early modern textbooks of the type known as the "institutes of medicine."[50] Instead, the questions move haphazardly and apparently at random from subject to subject and between the highly specific and the general and abstract. "Can there be several definitions of medicine?" follows directly on "Is bread more digestible than meat?"[51] Individual items vary greatly in length, depending on the degree of Cardano's interest in the topic. He devoted twenty folio pages to considering "Whether incantations can have any effect in medical treatment,"[52] but dealt with three questions directly related to the text of the *Ars* in a page and a half.[53] Just as Aristotelian natural philosophy is subverted, but not discarded, in Cardano's *De subtilitate*, so the methods of scholastic medicine survive transformed in his medical *Contradictiones*.[54] It would be hard to imagine a greater contrast to Books 1 and 2 of Valles's *Controversiae*, which plod methodically through a survey of medical theory by way of *quaestiones* of approximately equal length on topics pertaining to the elements, temperaments, humors, parts of the body, faculties, and senses.

The apparently unsystematic character of the *Contradictiones* as Cardano published it cannot, presumably, be attributed either to his haste to issue a medical work after receiving a chair in medicine or to the defects of the publisher of the first edition, since subsequent editions published in his lifetime, although otherwise revised—and issued by publishers in whom he had more confidence—were unchanged in this respect.[55] Rather, the adherence to organization by texts or disciplinary subdivision claimed in the preface dissolves in the body of the work into a medicine of innumerable separate topics, priority among which is determined by the tastes and interests of an individual. The humanistic pleasure in free selection, miscellany, and randomness also evident in some other areas of Renaissance scholarship seems here to have found its way into an academic medical compilation.[56]

AUTHORITY, PARTICULARS, AND THE METHOD OF CONTRADICTIONS

Cardano had no hesitation in calling attention to the association of the *Contradictiones* with Pietro d'Abano and to its usefulness as a memory guide to medical literature and debate. But he also claimed it as "almost" belonging to the genre of "scholia and castigations," that is, as a work of criticism.[57] In his letter of dedication to the Senate of Milan, he set out what amounted to a program for a reformed use of the question method. Redirected toward particulars, it could be used to build up an effective critique of Galen by the method of "the study of contradictions." Attention to particulars was crucial because of the practical and urgent nature of the task of medicine: "because we are engaged in a serious matter and one in which human lives are exposed to danger, we require not confusions of philosophers or oratorical precepts but more diligent clear reasoning about each single thing [*in singulis*] when the matter [*res*] demands it."[58] What was necessary was to lay out dubious or self-contradictory statements clearly so that the reader could see where the problem lay: "I have tried to submit things that seem dubious to reasoning. . . . in all I have been led by reason as well as authority, so that if the opinion of both agrees, the judgment will be the firmer: if reason and authority disagree, having given my own opinion, I shall leave to the readers the whole power of choosing what is more pleasing."[59]

Galen was the appropriate object of such a critique precisely because he was generally regarded as the best representative of the entire ancient medical tradition. The Hippocratic writings were difficult to understand, Celsus was useful only for interpreting vocabulary, the Greek writers who came after Galen were inferior to him, and the Arabs had misinterpreted him on many points, "so that Galen's judgment was the only

hope left." But those of Galen's works that survived contained numerous inconsistencies. Hence "by the study of contradiction it would be
possible for me to be a willing judge of every disagreement, even if it
had not clearly appeared in dissections that he constantly affirmed that
he had seen things which he had not seen at all and which were not true:
so that already I, believing not Vesalius but rather my own eyes, have
doubts not about his [Galen's] judgment, as often happens, but about
his good faith."[60] In this formulation, the arguing of *quaestiones* has
metamorphosed into "the study of contradiction." The title of the *Contradicentium medicorum libri* is now to be read simultaneously as
homage to the author of *Conciliator differentiarum medicorum et
philosophorum* and as a declaration of intent to abandon that work's goal
of reconciliation. Moreover, "the study of contradiction," which reveals
inconsistencies in Galen's texts, is presented as just as effective as—and
indeed as exactly parallel to—the confrontation of Galen's statements
with the dissected human body. The idea of a parallel enterprise emerges
again in Cardano's remark "I certainly have in common with [Vesalius]
that for the sake of truth itself I have sometimes set myself against
Galen."[61]

   The insistence that close attention to particulars provided the most effective tool for a general critique of Galen is reiterated in a second letter
to the reader added at the end of the expanded edition of the *Contradictiones*. Noting that medications unknown to Galen and Hippocrates,
such as sugar and rhubarb, were cheap and in common use—even by
practitioners who prided themselves on their Galenism—Cardano continued, "But if Galen was ignorant even of these obvious things, why
should one not suppose that he was much more ignorant about more
hidden things? But you will say that he might have been ignorant about
single species of things [*singulares rerum species*], but the art of medicine
is established with general principles. . . . [I]f by general reason you
mean that rule which teaches contraries are cured by contraries, then indeed I think Galen handed down everything, but [so did] also Hippocrates before him. . . . But if we mean the signs, modes, causes,
symptoms, and remedies for particular diseases and the number, site,
usefulness, and quality of the parts of the body, then necessarily many
things are lacking in Galen's writings, just as many and extremely necessary things are lacking in his medications."[62]

   There is no doubt that this program represented a genuine set of priorities for Cardano. Exposure of internal inconsistencies within or
among Galen's works is a recurrent theme throughout the *Contradictiones*. The 659 separate questions that make up the ten surviving books
of the work, most of them relating to physiology, diseases, remedies, and
treatment, can reasonably be regarded as a huge collection of particulars,
of "single things," about which medical authorities were in disagree-

ment. Nevertheless, the actual content of the work fulfills the promised program only very partially. For one thing, scholastic conciliation has by no means disappeared; plenty of questions are resolved by purely verbal reconciliation.[63]

A more fundamental problem, as with many Renaissance calls for attention to particulars or to things, not words, is to determine what the concepts of *singuli*, *singulares*, or *res* meant to Cardano.[64] Clearly, his insistence on the importance of particulars as distinct from speculative philosophizing or broad generalization is a demand for attention to specific, medically useful ("lives are in danger") details. Furthermore, the parallel that he drew between "the study of contradictions" and Vesalian anatomy evidently rests on the notion that both proceed by close and critical study of detail. In a sense, this is true enough. But whereas the *Fabrica* confronts statements in texts with a mass of directly observed descriptive detail about objects in nature, the *Contradictiones* essentially proceeds by setting details of texts against one another (even when one of the texts is the *Fabrica*). Moreover, although many of the individual *contradictiones* examine statements about limited and specific aspects of Galenic medicine (for example, the attributes ascribed to individual plant remedies), others take up broad aspects of physiological function, such as reproduction. And although Cardano was never committed to medical philology as a method and often expressed his contempt for those who were, yet other *contradictiones* concern the meaning of words. For instance, his inquiry whether *staphyloma* was a disease of the uvea or the cornea traced inconsistencies in the use of this term by Paul of Aegina, Celsus, and Aetius.[65] Such inquiries had value in the period of the remaking of medical vocabulary that was a major consequence of medical Hellenism. But in the *Contradictiones* no real distinctions are made among collecting information about words, collecting views of authors on specific points ("Is ginger humid?" "Is rhubarb hot?" "Is lily bad for the stomach?" "Is pain in the joints always cured by bloodletting?"), and collecting other forms of data.[66]

Of course, Cardano's insistence on the importance of particulars is connected to the intensive interest in collecting data that marked all his intellectual activities. He referred to his own life as a "collection of events" to some of which his students were witnesses.[67] In medicine, he collected *experimenta* (that is, mostly remedies, not necessarily all his own or even all tried out by him), his own *consilia*, and accounts of cases he had treated.[68] There seems little reason to suppose that he regarded data collected as a result of direct personal experience or observation as essentially different in character from his store of historical anecdote, evidently gathered by diligent excerpting, or from the innumerable descriptions of minerals, plants, and animals that fill long sections of his encyclopedic works, many of which were clearly accumulated in the same way. Substantial mathematical and technological content, as well as the author's self-expressiveness and his views on subtlety and other matters, distinguish *De subtilitate* and *De rerum varietate*; their sections on natural history have much in common with other sixteenth-century encyclopedic treatments of nature.[69]

In the *Contradictiones*, the importance that he attached to *experimenta* found in texts emerges strongly from his recurrent praise of medieval Arab medical writers, in which their superior knowledge of *experimenta* in medicine is a principal theme. Thus, for example, an exposé, of the inconsistency of the temperaments ascribed to poppy and water lily by Galen and various other authors turns into an attack on medical humanists (especially Giovanni Manardi and Leonhart Fuchs) "who now care not a straw about the opinions of all the Arabs, even in *experimenta*, as they do not wish to attribute anything to them," and who "desert Avicenna, Rasis, Avenzoar, and so many physicians and philosophers of the most outstanding gifts [*ingenium*]. . . . Therefore let the grammarians follow the grammarians, when we will be with the physicians. . . . They certainly want to err with Galen, but it is not given to them to act rightly with Galen. We see every day that those who imitate Galen allow in serious error and are inferior in *experimentum* to the Arabs."[70]

Cardano's own experiences in medical practice, although brought to bear upon the assertions of authorities from time to time, are less prominent in the *Contradictiones* than in some of his other medical works. Almost the only section where *exempla* from his practice or personally known to him appear to be systematically deployed is in a long discussion of poisons.[71] There, a series of such cases illustrate discussion of different types of poisons and their actions. One way of looking at this collection of stories is simply as an attempt to gather at first hand descriptive particulars about cases of poisoning. In some instances, moreover, empirical evidence is used to substantiate conclusions contrary to common assumptions, asserted fact, or learned opinion. Thus Cardano presented two cases known to him that disproved the opinion that powdered steel was poisonous: one of his patients had admitted having fed powder or scrapings of steel to someone (Cardano thought the intended victim was probably the man's adulterous wife) without doing her any harm; and Francesco Todeschini, who ate powdered steel while insane, had also survived unscathed. The story of the crazy nun who, "released from her chains [*vinculis soluta*]," put ground glass in the convent's chickpeas, killing two of the sisters but leaving most of them unhurt, implies that poisonous substances are not always lethal to everyone who ingests them. A realistic appraisal of the difficulty involved in distinguishing symptoms of poisoning from symptoms of disease is suggested by the story of the blood that looked like milk, sent to Cardano from one of the patients of his friend Tommaso Iseo: this was either the result of poison ingested when the man was already ill or the result of long-standing disease of the liver.[72]

But taken as a whole, this discussion suggests that the selection of examples may have been determined by priorities other than—or in addition to—an intention to test textual authority or common belief by confrontation with empirically collected evidence. The exposition seems both to reflect a generalized social anxiety about poisons and to be specifically connected with the genre of treatises on poison written for princes.[73] One of the main issues addressed is whether there are poisons that, having been administered on a single occasion, act imperceptibly over a series of months, eventually altering the body to produce illness of which the victim dies. (The model for this idea of a type of poisonous action was the bite of a rabid dog.) As an example, Cardano recounted the story of an episode from his time at Gallarate, when a cleric, who wanted to get the parish priest out of the way so that he could succeed to his position, mixed poison in a cake. Nine guests at a dinner died as a result, but not until between one and six months later and from conditions mimicking natural illness (this was a very special poison made by priests at Rome [*"Attulerat ex Roma id veneni genus, ubi Christi sacerdotes ei clarissimae industriae operam dant"*]).[74] The extent to which anxiety about poisons was focused upon the persons of princes emerges from Cardano's description of how he had seen the chair, table, and even dais that were to be used by Charles V at dinner carefully cleaned so as to remove any poisons that might be absorbed through the imperial skin, clothing, or shoes. As he remarked, citing the example of plague spreaders, "the perfidy of our times invented this great subtlety, which the ancients did not know."[75]

Cardano apparently at one time intended some of the material in this section of the *Contradictiones* for a treatise on poisons for a prince, since it includes the remark, obviously anomalous in a *quaestio*, "And you should know, most illustrious prince, that of ten people who drink poisons scarcely one dies, unless the dose is repeated."[76] The reassuring nature of this remark perhaps suggests that the anecdotes about ingestion of supposed poisons that turned out to be harmless, recovery from attempted poisoning, and the possibility that some supposed cases of poisoning might be disease were also chosen for their reassuring quality. The prince Cardano originally had in mind was presumably a secular one, given the remark about the Roman clergy quoted above. However, the independent treatise on poisons that he finally published is dedicated to Pope Pius IV and contains very little personal or anecdotal material.[77] It appeared in 1564; that, of course, was after the younger Cardano had been executed for murdering his wife with a poisoned cake.

Another kind of use of personal experience to evaluate Galenic theory occurs in a discussion of inherited characteristics, in which Cardano used himself as a test case. If, as Galen claimed, the rule was that if the paternal semen was stronger the offspring would resemble the father, but if the female semen and menstrual blood were stronger it would resemble the mother, how could one explain the characteristics of a person who had his father's nose and his mother's eyes or who, like Cardano himself, was very like his maternal grandfather in inborn skill (*ingenium*) and physique? Really, he thought, just as the soul possessed distinct powers of imagination, reason, and memory, so too in the body there must be many forms, each transmitted from one of the parents, distinct in location as well as nature. In his own case, his heart resembled that of his father, Fazio Cardano, and his paternal grandfather, Antonio Cardano, and his great-grandfather, another Fazio Cardano, and the ancestor of the family, Aldo, and all the intermediate ancestors who had lived since his day 220 years earlier, "for they were all extremely vital [*vivacissimi*] but not, as I have heard, similar in form."[78] Thus when it came to the ruling organ of the body according to Aristotle and the source of heat and vital power (*virtus vitalis*) in Galenic physiology, Cardano insisted on his strictly paternal inheritance. In this way he found physiological and philosophical support for his strong identification with even remote ancestors of his paternal family in preference to a close maternal relative—the grandfather whom he actually resembled.

If the concept of particulars in the *Contradictiones* is in some respects problematic, its anti-Galenism is not nearly as sweeping as Cardano's programmatic statements suggest. The criticisms of particular details of Galen's writings, numerous and frequently cogent though these criticisms are, certainly do not constitute a wholesale rejection of Galenic medicine. Notwithstanding his philosophical eclecticism and intellectual adventurousness, Cardano remained relatively close to academic medical tradition. The strongly Galenist system (to some extent synthesized with Aristotelianism) in which he had been trained provided most of his basic medical ideas. He also expressed admiration for aspects of Galen's character and treated him as an important literary model.[79] One respect in which Cardano did indeed resemble Vesalius was in combining criticisms of Galen on specific issues with an understanding of physiology, pathology, and therapy that remained fundamentally Galenic. Moreover, although Cardano's critique of Galen led him to endorse specific views or achievements of other authors, he by no means always preferred their views to Galen's. Throughout the *Contradictiones* he often demonstrated a preference for Aristotelian over Galenic positions and continually cited Averroes. But he was equally ready to repudiate Aristotle when it suited him; it would be highly misleading to describe the *Contradictiones* simply as an Aristotelian work.[80]

On occasion, too, he was willing to conciliate Aristotle and Galen in traditional scholastic fashion, as he did when handling the two main physiological issues on which Aristotle and Galen disagreed: whether or not the heart was the only ruling organ of the body and the respective roles of the male and female parent in conception. These differences of opinion had long been standard subjects of medical debate.[81] Their treatment in the *Contradictiones* reveals an impressive command of every conceivably relevant passage of both Aristotle and Averroes, as well as of Galen, but in neither case is the main Galenic idea repudiated either on Aristotelian or any other grounds. On the role of the heart, Cardano adopted a conciliation of the Aristotelian and Galenic positions going back to Avicenna: the heart was in some ultimate, philosophically truer, sense the ruling organ, but for medical purposes three principal organs, heart, brain, and liver, had to be taken into account—"and thus the middle way between the philosophers and physicians is embraced, which in my judgment is also the truer."[82] On generation, he favored the Aristotelian position that the male parent alone contributed generative virtue over the Galenic idea of an active female role in conception, but nevertheless conceded that female semen might contribute "some light formative power [*aliquam levem vim ad formationem habeat*]," adding with regard to a cluster of subsidiary problems about generation, "neither Galen, nor Aristotle, nor Hippocrates spoke badly, only imperfectly."[83]

Yet both these lengthy *quaestiones* also include brief appeals to anatomical evidence to correct or amplify Galen on points of detail. In one, the reader is referred to Book 5 of the *Fabrica* for a clearer discussion of the fetal coverings than that provided by Galen. In the other, in the course of considering Galen's belief that the liver provides the "origin" of the blood and the venous system, Cardano cited and endorsed Vesalius's denial that the circumference of the vena cava is greater in the liver than the heart, and described the difference of opinion between Galen and Vesalius as to whether or not the portal and caval systems are joined by capillaries in the liver as "a question of fact, as the jurists say [*Quaestio est de facto ut iurisconsulti dicunt*]."[84]

Even more revealing is his handling of the relation between his version of element theory and the medical theory of temperament. His repudiation of central aspects of Aristotelian teaching on the elements was one of the most notoriously unconventional aspects of his philosophy of nature. Cardano removed fire from the number of the elements. In *De subtilitate* he denied the existence of the elementary sphere of fire and stated that there were only three terrestrial elements. The heavenly bodies were the source of heat in mixed bodies (i.e., all actually existing bodies), and this celestial heat was responsible for their formation from the elements. He further added that coldness and dryness were only absence of heat and moisture, not positive qualities.[85] Moreover, he did not relegate these ideas to a context remote from medicine. He claimed a Hippocratic source for the idea that there were only three elements and used medical analogies in support of his arguments.[86]

One might expect, therefore, that Cardano's element theory would have equally radical consequences for the theory of temperament, since the four qualities that composed temperament were, according to standard Galenist teaching, elementary qualities. In its various ramifications, the theory of temperament, or *complexio*, constituted an extremely intricate and far-reaching system of explanation that underpinned much of physiology, pathology, and therapy. The ideas about the temperaments of human beings and animals discussed above were only one aspect of a much larger scheme. Pairs of elementary qualities were supposed to inhere in each of the four humors. Each part of the body had its own temperament, and the temperaments of the different parts affected one another (as in the originally Aristotelian idea that the brain cooled the heart). In addition, in human beings temperament was assigned to individuals as well as to the species; each person had his or her individual temperament, linked to psychological as well as physical traits. Temperament was also supposed to differ according to age, sex, region, and condition of health. Furthermore, most internal disease was explained as the result of imbalance of temperament or of humoral qualities. Since medicinal substances were also characterized in terms of elementary qualities and cure was held to be by contraries, "rational" therapy involved finding appropriate simple or composite medicines with qualities to counterbalance those of the disease. Hence a significantly revised theory of temperament would have had serious consequences for the entire system of medical thought.

But Cardano adopted positions that guarded medicine from the extreme consequences of his element theory. In *De subtilitate*, he took care to divorce the number of humors from the number of elements—even though he also toyed with the idea of reducing the number of humors to three: "There are four humors in animals; but what has this to do with the elements? What if I were to say that there were only three, together with Turisanus, the commentator on Galen's *Ars medica*?"[87] In the *Contradictiones*, he made a conscious decision to play down his own views on the number of the elements. His ideas appear briefly and rather obscurely in Book 1 in a passage in which he rejected Galen's analogy between the heat in the human body and the heat of a furnace and cited Aristotle (*Generation of Animals* 2.3.737a1–7) in support of the celestial rather than fiery origin of animal heat.[88]

Further, he preserved every aspect of the medical theory of temperament. At the beginning of Book 2 he took up the much discussed topic of the manner in which the elements or their forms remained in composite bodies. Having rejected the theory that the temperament, or *complexio*, was itself the form of a composite body, Cardano asserted that in animate things the soul was the only form; in inanimate ones the form was that of the predominating element ("*Ut vero declaravimus, unam tantum esse formam animatorum animam, inanimatorum autem elementi praedominantis*").[89] But he then went on to allow that in animals the "form of the temperament" was inseparable from the soul and to note that Galen had extended this idea to include human beings.[90] He qualified the idea that the properties of medicines were those of their dominant element by explaining how, in the case of simple medicines that seemed to have qualities associated with more than one element (for example, to be of earthy, hence cold, substance and have an astringent, hence hot, power), the temperament supplied by the plant's vegetative soul when it was alive somehow remained after it was cut and dried.[91] The result of these formulations—a result to which the *Contradictiones* bears abundant witness—was that, despite the genuine radicalism of his view of the elements, Cardano's understanding of physiology, pathology, and therapy, much like that of his less philosophically adventurous medical colleagues, remained wedded to the theory of temperament. It functioned at too fundamental a level of medical explanation to be critically examined as a whole or subjected to any wholesale modification, much less abandoned.

But on theory of temperament as on so many other aspects of Galenic medicine, he was as usual able bring cogent criticisms to bear on details. One example will suffice. Returning to the Galenic idea that the temperament of mankind is at a midpoint among animal temperaments, he examined Galen's claim that fish were colder in temperament than man, noting that what led Galen to believe this was their cold skin. But cold skin is no evidence that an animal is cold internally; if fish were completely cold throughout, they would not be alive; moreover, even if some animals do have a colder temperament than man, this is no evidence that man has the mean temperament among all animals ("*non valet dantur animalia frigida in cute, ergo sunt frigida intus. . . . Et concesso quod possent esse frigidiora temperamento, nihil hoc facit ad demonstrandum hominem esse medium temperamento in actu inter omnia animalia*").[92]

PRIORITIES

Notwithstanding the qualifications just indicated, the analysis of particulars and the critique of Galen are substantial themes that run all through the *Contradictiones.* In Book 1, moreover, Cardano more or less kept to his announced intention to avoid philosophical topics of only tangential relevance to medicine. Most questions, it deserves to be emphasized once again, inquire about particular remedies or particular disease conditions. The longest and most passionately argued segment in Book 1, amounting to a small treatise on the subject and fortified with a dense web of citations, addresses the vehement controversy over the proper method of bleeding for "pain in the side" that divided the medical world in two in the 1520s and 1530s.[93]

The remaining books have a notably higher proportion of material reflecting his other personal and philosophical preoccupations in a medical context. The long question about the usefulness of incantations in medicine addresses his interest in remarkable happenings outside the ordinary course of nature; a cluster of questions on anatomical topics shows him endeavoring to incorporate details of Vesalian anatomy into medical discussion.[94] He also turned the question of whether God knows singulars—meaning in this instance individual human beings and their actions (as distinct from mankind in general)—into an opportunity to discuss his favorite subjects of prophetic or warning dreams and the personal genii or guides who assisted specially favored individuals.[95] But some striking examples of the way in which Cardano's beliefs and philosophical commitments in areas apparently remote from medicine could sometimes drive his medical exposition are provided by questions on whether the human soul is immortal according to the physicians, and whether there is resurrection of the dead. Neither of these questions was included in the *Contradictiones* published in Cardano's lifetime; but since in Book 2 he advertised for a patron to support the publication of the remainder, they were presumably not deliberately withheld by him.[96]

In the years in which he was putting the *Contradictiones* into final form, Cardano was much preoccupied with the immortality of the soul. He published a treatise on the subject in 1545, the same year in which Book 1 of the *Contradictiones* appeared.[97] In the late 1550s and early 1560s, when he was working on Books 3–10, he was also engaged by his *Theonoston*, two books of which are dedicated to, respectively, the immortality of the soul and the life and felicity of souls after death.[98] The nature of the human soul was, of course, the subject of a major controversy in Italian academic philosophy in the first half of the sixteenth century; two of the principal participants were Pomponazzi, who in a famous treatise maintained that the authentic Aristotelian view was that the human soul was mortal, and Agostino Nifo, who adopted a syncretistic position and held that the teaching of all ancient philosophers could be reconciled to endorse the immortality and individuality of the human soul.[99] Cardano's discussions of the subject allied a thorough knowledge of various Aristotelianisms with a syncretizing and Neoplatonic tendency, with religious awareness, and with his own strong interest in dreams, apparitions, and spirit guides. According to Cardano, the teaching of all ancient philosophers, including the Aristotelians, endorsed the immortality of the soul; but they had understood it imperfectly, since they had not reached knowledge of the Christian doctrines of individual immortality and resurrection of the body, as distinct from reincarnation.[100]

The discussion of immortality of the soul "according to the opinion of the physicians" in the *Contradictiones* brings the subject into a medical setting and endows it with medical consequences. It provided Cardano with the opportunity to insist, pace Galen, both that the soul was something other than temperament and that the nature of the soul was a practical medical concern. Given that the body was the instrument of the soul, it followed that if one of two similar human bodies functioned better than the other, this superior functioning might be due to superiority of soul, "just as we see with barbers, one barber shaves better than another with the same razor, and one copyist writes better than another with the same pen, ink, and paper." Furthermore, "it would help in many diseases to cure the soul."[101] The exposition also reveals the intimate connection between a tight cluster of Cardano's central philosophical ideas and his Hippocratism. The main thrust of the argument was to add the chief medical writers, and especially Hippocrates, to the list of authorities testifying to the immortality of the soul *naturaliter loquentes*. According to Cardano, Hippocrates and Avicenna taught the soul's immortality; Galen, although undecided on the subject, never definitely asserted that the soul was mortal. Hence the consensus of the physicians could be said to be that the soul was immortal.[102] Cardano demonstrated Hippocratic endorsement for the immortality of the human soul by quoting the same two passages that he also used to provide textual foundation for his element theory and his equally unconventional ideas about generation and corruption. The first of these, in *On Fleshes*, describes the hot as immortal and heat as a component of human beings as of all bodies. The second is the statement in *Regimen* that "No body perishes entirely, nor is anything made that was not before; but mixed and separated things are changed about."[103]

The appeal to Hippocrates—almost always a figure of irrefutable authority for Cardano—and the significance of the quoted passages for his entire philosophy of nature are fairly unambiguous indications that his own understanding of the immortality of the soul, *loquens naturaliter*, drew on these passages. (On religious grounds, as we have seen, he proclaimed his allegiance to orthodox Christian teaching.) He returned to the same cluster of ideas in the question "Whether generation takes place? And whether there is resurrection of the dead?"[104] There he discussed at length the idea that there is no real generation or corruption, but only a process of mixing and separating and adding and taking away, once again citing the key passage from *Regimen* and contrasting this view with that of Aristotle. Despite a remark distancing himself from the opinion he ascribed to Hippocrates, Cardano seems to have endorsed something like this naturalistic version of immortality.[105] His medical Hippocratism requires a chapter to itself. But the extent to which Hippocratic sources provided important concepts in his philosophy of nature, which, in turn, underpinned his medical ideas, also deserves to be emphasized.

Twenty-five years before the first edition of the *Contradictiones* was published, Gianfrancesco Pico had included a chapter reviewing conflicting authoritative statements about human physiology in his *Examen vanitatis doctrinae gentium* (1520). He thereby demonstrated that the study of medical or medical and philosophical contradictions could be turned to skeptical—in his case fideistic—ends. When Cardano's attacks on Galen and his unconventional element theory led his colleague and enemy Camuzio to accuse him of overturning the foundations of the whole of natural philosophy, Camuzio invoked the name of Gianfrancesco Pico.[106] But Cardano's accumulation and study of contradictions cannot be construed as the work of a skeptic. His essentially reformist enterprise proceeded piecemeal within an existing medical system. His moves toward a new epistemology were tentative and frequently ambiguous. Indeed, even Camuzio's rhetorical denunciation recognized that Cardano wanted to change medicine, not destroy it. Using metaphors that were acquiring ever more menacing overtones by the time his attack was published in 1563, Camuzio described his opponent as a heresiarch who had almost founded a new sect in medicine. What especially distressed Camuzio was that not only students but also medical graduates were responsive to Cardano's self-styled "Hippocratic" medicine.[107]

Cardano's eclecticism makes it as difficult to evaluate his medical ideas as to assess his philosophy of nature or his writings on moral or political subjects. The same paradoxical combinations of Aristotelianism and criticisms of Aristotle, of insistence on particulars of experience and dependence on texts, of Neoplatonist or occultist metaphysics and attacks on credulity that have struck interpreters of his output in these fields are also characteristics of his medicine.[108] To them his medicine added other special features of its own: simultaneous dependence on and hostility to Galen; the endeavor to substitute Hippocrates for Galen as the primary medical authority; appreciation of the methodology and results of Vesalian anatomy; and, above all, the technical, social, and personal realities of medical practice. Thus the presentation of medical knowledge in the *Contradictiones* brings together aspects of Renaissance thought that to a twentieth-century reader are likely to appear opposed, or at any rate distinct: traditional Arabo-Latin medical erudition with Renaissance Galenism; Aristotelian natural philosophy with new eclectic philosophy of nature; Galenism with the critique of Galen; philosophical or philological critique of ancient scientific writers with critique based on empirical data obtained at first hand; scholastic method with self-expression; philosophical abstraction with interest in particulars; Aristotelian rationalism with occultism.

Although Cardano was an extreme example of eclecticism in Renaissance medicine, he was by no means unique. If one novel feature of sixteenth-century scientific culture was intensified attention to describing and collecting, another was the availability of a wider range of methodological and philosophical options. These options were seldom treated as mutually exclusive. The notion of a single correct scientific—or, for that matter, philosophical—method that rigorously excluded other approaches was not part of the sixteenth-century mental universe. Cardano freely selected from and combined a variety of approaches to nature and the art of medicine, just as he selected and combined ancient texts, as the topic, situation, or context demanded. The resulting mixture of genres, content, and ideologies in the *Contradictiones* reveals much conflict, ambivalence, and revisionism in medicine but also suggests the still vast capacity of the traditional system of medical knowledge to absorb new material without wholesale change. But medicine, as the commonplace ran, was distinguished from natural philosophy by its practical goal. Cardano's medical knowledge was intended for use, not only in the classroom and the study, but primarily in practice. It is now time to turn to some of his practical recommendations.

Chapter 4

TIME, BODY, FOOD:
THE PARAMETERS OF HEALTH

CARDANO'S views on diet will serve here to exemplify his prescriptive recommendations on practical aspects of medicine, among which he gave a large place to conservation of health. Yet, perhaps more than any other aspect of his work, his writings on nourishment of the body cross and recross—in both genre and content—the boundaries between academic medicine and the culture of cities and courts, between natural history and medicine, between medicine and moral or political philosophy, between the care of others and the examination of the self. Marked, like so much of his output, by eclecticism and internal contradictions, these writings simultaneously suggest an attempt to grasp the entirety of natural knowledge and a willingness, learned in the course of a difficult career, to try out different traditions and forms of practice and to adapt readily to changing situations.

Although passages on diet in illness are scattered through his medical works, beginning with *On the Bad Practice of Modern Physicians* in 1536, diet in health became a major focus of his attention in the early 1570s, shortly after he had given courses of lectures on two Hippocratic treatises on diet.[1] In those years, he completed three major works largely devoted to this subject. One was his treatise on regimen, to which he gave the Galenic title *De sanitate tuenda* and which was seen through the press by a pupil in 1580, four years after the author's death.[2] In this work, arranged according to the conventional scheme of the six non-naturals, about half the total contents are taken up with discussion of diet and foodstuffs (nominally only one item of the six). He wrote another shorter medical tract, *On the Usefulness of Foods*, and diet is also the subject of Book 2 of his philosophical dialogue *Theonoston*.[3]

His dietary concepts reflect several of the main interests or clusters of ideas that recur through many of his works. One of these was his self-conscious Hippocratism. In his writings on food, this specific commitment appears alongside the more general influence of the long tradition of medical advice about regimen based on Hippocratic-Galenic humoral physiology, on which, as was to be expected, he also drew heavily. Second, some of his principal discussions of diet occur in the context of writing about old age, a subject with which he was profoundly concerned, especially—since with Cardano the political was always personal—toward the end of his life. From yet another standpoint, Cardano the political and moral philosopher showed his concern for the civic, social, moral, and religious implications and consequences of various aspects of diet. In addition, when he came to describe particular species of plants and animals used for food, his encyclopedic natural philosophy, most fully displayed in *De subtilitate* and *De varietate rerum*, easily spilled over into his writings on diet. Finally, where diet was concerned too, he followed his habitual practice of informing his readers of his personal experiences over a span of time. Cardano recorded his diet at different ages and his efforts to put his own dietary theories into personal practice. In the last endeavor, like most of us, he had only limited success.

Eclectic and idiosyncratic as Cardano's writings on food and diet are, they nevertheless have many features in common with other Renaissance works on the subject. His decision to include extended discussion of dietary theory in a philosophical dialogue was unusual, but in writing a treatise on regimen largely devoted to diet he joined a minor Renaissance literary industry. Since antiquity, diet had had a significant place in medical literature. All Hippocratic-Galenic humoral physiology taught that health was the result of a proper balance of the elementary qualities, a balance that was responsive to substances ingested by the body, all of which were themselves endowed with elementary qualities. Several Hippocratic and Galenic treatises provided instructions for selecting foods with the appropriate qualities for different ages, conditions of life, and states of health. Hellenistic—especially Galenic—and Arabic medicine laid more stress on the medication of illness than the Hippocratics had done, but the regulation of diet in both illness and health, ideally on an individual basis, remained fundamental in the medical system transmitted to and further elaborated in the Latin West. Diet usually took pride of place in medical discussions of the so-called nonnaturals, that is, states of the body and environmental and external factors that influence it.[4]

The social conditions of the late Middle Ages and Renaissance ensured that treatises on conservation of health in general and diet in particular increasingly emerged as a separate genre. The context and intended audience of these works was not purely medical—although many of the authors were physicians—but was rather the world of princely courts and urban intellectuals. The multiplication of manuals on diet (or of health manuals in which diet played the leading role) in the fifteenth and sixteenth centuries was doubtless connected with a growing elaboration of meals, dishes, and rituals of eating among the prosperous classes. As recent cultural historians have noted, in the Renaissance and early modern period the various sectors of society were increasingly differentiated by different styles of eating and choices of foodstuffs. Certainly, the literature of dietary theory needs to be considered in conjunction with culinary literature and the life of noble households, although I shall not attempt to do so here. Nor shall I make any attempt to evaluate actual nutritional conditions in Italian cities: throughout Europe, however, the diet of the rich involved the consumption of a great deal of meat protein and alcohol, and that of the poor was mainly based on grain. In Italy, all classes presumably consumed more fruit and salad greens than in northern Europe. The principal health problem of the rich in connection with diet was likely to be excess; that of the poor, actual shortage of food—or of money to buy it, which comes to the same thing—both at vulnerable stages of life (notably old age) and in periods of general dearth.[5]

In fifteenth- and sixteenth-century Italy, the content of dietary advice was largely rooted in Hippocratic-Galenic medicine (even when revisionist or critical of some medical doctrines). Thus cultural beliefs and practices, as well as economic realities, that associated different foodstuffs with different social groups coexisted with a medical dietetics that was in principle based on the theory of individual temperament. Broadly speaking, most authors taught that health was maintained by a diet of foods of complexion similar to the healthy individual's own, and restored by a diet of foods with contrary complexional qualities to the weak, ill, or elderly individual's own. It deserves to be emphasized that the actual advice about particular foods in most of these works therefore comes from an extremely conservative literary tradition. Generally stable conventions attributed particular complexional qualities to individual foodstuffs (cold and moist lettuce, hot and moist pork), recommended certain foods as beneficial (temperate chicken and veal), and excoriated others as harmful (dangerous melons). But the theory of temperament could also take social factors into account, as when certain vegetables were characterized as suitable only for peasants.[6] The extent to which this literature either reflected or influenced what anyone actually ate is a matter for speculation, but it certainly both reflected and influenced ways of thinking about food.

Notwithstanding their common elements, diet books came in a diversity of forms and addressed a diversity of special interests. A very few examples must suffice to give an idea of the scope of the genre. Physicians who wrote handbooks for individual princely patients/patrons tailored their work to the noble mentality: for example, about 1450 the learned Michele Savonarola wrote his advice book for Duke Borso d'Este of Ferrara in the vernacular; while in late-fourteenth-century Lombardy wealthy patrons could gain an idea of the contents of the *Tacuinum sa-*

nitatis, a dry little Arabo-Latin manual about the complexional qualities of different foodstuffs, by leafing through luxuriously illustrated but simplified picture-book versions.[7] Other works responded to current intellectual as well as social trends. Platina's *De honesta voluptate*—the work of a literary humanist, not a physician—combined historical and philological inquiry into the food and culinary practices of the ancient Romans, advice on the health properties of foods, and recipes, and served the useful and courtly purpose of providing intellectual and, as its title suggests, moral justification for an interest in food preparation, food nomenclature, and, indeed, eating.[8] A proliferation of treatises on diet and hygiene for two particular groups, intellectuals and the aged, has been attributed, at least in part, to humanistic interest in classical writings on these topics and, in the latter case, perhaps also to the actual social influence of the elderly in the upper ranks of society.[9] Marsilio Ficino's *De vita*, published in 1489 and famous for its Platonizing astral magic, combines these categories since, taken in conjunction, its three parts constitute a health regime for elderly scholars.[10] Another early example is Gabriele Zerbi's *Gerontocomia*, published in the same year.[11] But works on regimen largely devoted to diet did not appeal only to the elderly: among the few books actually in circulation at the court of Duke Galeazzo Maria Sforza of Milan, a young man whose tastes were lavish but not bookish, were several on health, including one on weight control.[12] In the course of the sixteenth century, many new items on health and or diet were added and older ones were reissued or translated into Italian.[13] As Jean Céard has pointed out, however, celebrated learned physicians generally paid much more attention to therapy than to conservation of health, presumably because, as Cardano himself complained, they regarded the latter as a somewhat peripheral aspect of medicine.[14] His willingness to accord the subject full-scale learned treatment in Latin in the almost three hundred folio-size pages of his *De sanitate tuenda* is perhaps yet another measure of his ambiguous position in the world of erudite academic medicine and his openness to other disciplines and forms of practice.

Turning to themes especially characteristic of Cardano's approach to diet, one may begin with his self-conscious Hippocratism. In his writings on diet as elsewhere, Hippocrates came to serve two broad general functions for him: the first was as a support for specific criticisms of medical colleagues and traditional school authorities; the second, as a source and endorsement of philosophical ideas. Cardano's views on diet were very much part of his combative stance toward other members of the medical profession; this attitude appears with particular clarity in his teaching about invalid diet, of which, although the main subject here is diet in health, one particularly salient example may be cited. A number of his one hundred examples of "the bad practice of modern physicians" concern deficiencies in prescribing diet for the sick. In several of these instances what is being vehemently criticized is either failure to follow Hippocratic advice (for instance, by giving heavy food to invalids) or modern innovation (allowing melons, which Cardano, following much ancient and more recent precedent, declared were so dangerous that they should be forbidden by law).[15] As usual with Cardano, occasional remarks imply a much more radical, if intermittent, skepticism. A case in point is his comment on the practice of prescribing rice or almond flour, chicken, sugar, and lemon juice for invalids—a practice confirmed by Terence Scully's analysis of ingredients in dishes for the sick in early recipe collections. As Scully has pointed out, such a diet could be and probably was justified in terms of complexional characteristics ascribed to these foods. Cardano suggested that the real reason for their popularity as items of invalid diet was simply that they were all white.[16]

From the standpoint of underlying philosophy of diet, one Hippocratic treatise in particular seems likely to have been particularly important. The previous chapter has already called attention to Ingegno's exposition of the significance of Cardano's use of the Hippocratic *De diaeta* (*Regimen*) as a philosophical source. The same work could also be read to imply an endorsement of astrology and thus accorded with another of his major commitments.[17] Moreover, at any rate in its Renaissance Latin versions, it associated medicine and prophecy, and Cardano at times believed himself to have a gift of prophecy.[18] In addition, this treatise expounded a dietary theory that fitted well with some of his ideas about subtlety.

The Hippocratic author insisted on a connection between the blending of heat and moisture in the body and the condition of the soul, mental faculties, and powers of perception. The body's economy is presented in terms of a balance between the intake of nutrition and the expenditure of effort in exercise. The goal of regimen is to regulate this balance between them so as to achieve good proportions of heat and moisture. Consequently, according to this author, an improved regimen can improve the soul as well as the body: less food and more exercise will make "slow" people both healthier and more prudent or perceptive. But people already endowed by nature with a perceptive soul can make it even better by correct regimen; they should eat fish rather than meat, avoid violent exercise, and "reduce their flesh."[19] It may be noted that ancient and Renaissance beliefs about higher astral influences or dream inspiration often included the idea that the state of the body affected receptivity. One well-known example is provided by Marsilio Ficino's advice regarding the food, physical environment, and clothing of the adept in Book 3 of *De vita*. Book 4 of *De diaeta* is in fact a treatise on dreams which makes it clear that while most dreams indicate physical states of health, others are of divine origin.[20] I think it may be assumed that these ideas about the connections between diet and faculties of the soul are implicitly present in Cardano's discussions of the appropriate balance of food and exercise, even when the overt subject is purely physical regimen, as in his De sanitate tuenda.

Cardano's discussions of the regimen of old age in the first and last books of De sanitate tuenda and in Theonoston 2 draw on but also criticize three main bodies of theory. The first is medical dietetics based on Galenic physiology; the second, ideas about the prolongation of life by alchemical, astrological, or magical means. The third is a kind of secular asceticism practiced with the goal of prolonging life and physical health for the vita activa civile advocated by Cardano's contemporary, the Venetian patrician Alvise Cornaro.

Medical Dietetics

In most respects, Cardano's understanding of the physiology of aging, dietary theory, and the relation between them was the conventional one of Galenic medicine as reworked by Galen's Arab interpreters, notably Avicenna. According to this view, aging was a process of dessication and decline in heat. Life involved a continuous consumption of the body's "innate heat" and "radical moisture," of which the latter served as fuel for the former (like the oil of a lamp, in a continually invoked metaphor). Natural death inevitably supervened when all that was left of the radical moisture was a watery, excrementitious substance no longer capable of being transformed into fuel for the innate heat. As Luke Demaitre has pointed out, depending where the emphasis was placed, support could be found in this complex of ideas either for the idea that natural death was the result of physical developments that could not be postponed (apparently Galen's own position) or for the theories about ways of prolonging life artificially that attracted many medieval Arab and Latin writers. Cardano himself believed that completely natural deaths—that is, not involving trauma, disease, or poor regimen—occurred, but not very often. Much more commonly, he believed, death occurred as a result of a mixture of natural causes and disease; moreover, some deaths were the effect of injudicious diet on the weakened bodies of the elderly.[21] This was a view that left considerable scope for medical (or astrological) explanation and advice.

Similarly, his explanation of dietary theory was firmly based on the physiology of temperament. It divided the human population into nine gradations of health, moving down from a top category of strong young men with temperate bodies and no diseases or injuries who resembled the canon of Polykleitos, pressed into service once again as the image of human physical perfection. The next two categories contained people in good to fairly good health, whereas the remaining six classified people who were ill or disabled by various chronic conditions, among them old age. Those in categories 1 and 2 should eat foods similar to their temperaments, those in category 3, whose health was only slightly defective, could benefit from moderate use of some foods with contrary qualities to their own, but those in categories 4–9 stood in need of corrective "contrary" diets. Thus for Cardano as for many other Renaissance writers old age was to be treated as an illness, at any rate where diet was concerned.[22] Consequently, he too included palliatives for the disabilities of age, among them a diet for those who had lost their teeth (he lost most of his own teeth as he aged and was interested in problems of dentistry; his treatise on the subject has already been noted).[23]

But he also emphasized two ideas that he presented as revisionist, Hippocratic, and anti-Galenic. The first insisted on a distinction between robust physical health and the best life: "*Sanitas ergo et optima vita, non idem sunt.*" The physical constitution, and consequently regimen, most conducive to robust good health was not the same as, but different from, the constitution and regimen most conducive to the best life. Cardano made his point by drawing a vivid word picture contrasting a strong, sanguine, sweaty soldier, eating and drinking heartily, and ready for all kinds of physical exertion, but completely lacking in good sense ("*consilii nullus*"), with an intellectual ("*studiosus*") or citizen who ate little, shunned physical exertion, had clear senses, and was strong in mind ("*mente valens*").[24] Moreover, although in principle the best temperament for longevity should be one with much natural heat and "fat" radical moisture of high quality that would make good fuel for the innate heat, such was not the case in practice. People so endowed would live long if they followed a good regimen, but in reality they often shortened their lives by overexertion, drunkenness, and sexual excess.[25] Thus the regimen of abundant nourishment and vigorous exercise that Galen had recommended for optimum health was doubly unsatisfactory: not only was it quite unsuited for citizens and scholars, but the soldiers and athletes who flourished on it were seldom long-lived and often became prematurely deaf, blind, and senile.[26] On the theory that with a low level of innate heat and abundant moisture, the radical moisture would last a long time, Cardano maintained that, on the contrary, the best endowment for long life was a cold and humid complexion; he proposed nuns, in addition to scholars, as another example of thin, pale people who were likely to live long.[27]

Second, he insisted that life could be prolonged to the maximum only if the balance between the intake of nourishment and the output of physical activity was minutely regulated. Essentially, his recipe for long life was to keep both input and output as low as possible. His interest in the balance of nourishment and exertion led him to pay attention to the differing effects of different foodstuffs. Very nourishing foods should be taken in very small quantities; more could be allowed of foods that were less nourishing.[28] But Galen was seriously at fault because although he had advised reducing food intake in old age, he had not similarly adjusted his recommendations about exercise.[29] Cardano was convinced that vigorous exercise, which increased the appetite, shortened life.[30] Instead, he recommended passive exercise (i.e., being carried in carriages or boats), particularly advocating sea voyages. Perhaps as the fruit of experience during his own two channel crossings, he thought seasickness had a rejuvenating effect.[31] The notion is a good example of a recurrent trait in Cardano's medical thinking, indeed his ideas in general. He was not the first to advocate being carried or rocked as a form of passive exercise.[32] But in this as in other instances he made the idea his own by simultaneously pushing it to a disconcerting extreme and linking it to the world of his own experience.

In actual practice, he seems—no doubt prudently—to have recommended his revisionist dietetics to his elite patients only in modified versions. Even though *consilia* are edited products of a literary genre and can seldom be taken as a direct record of medical activity, two of Cardano's here illuminate the gap between prescriptive treatise and practice. The regimen for Cardinal Morone, which may have been written when the cardinal was in his fifties, simply suggests plenty of sleep and the avoidance of fatiguing physical exertion, although it adds the advice that if Morone has not slept, he should eat less and take less exercise; in those circumstances, too, "he should not get angry, he should not become sad, he should not be afraid [*Ubi non dormierit, minus comedat, et minus se exerceat, non irascatur, non tristetur, non timeat*]." It recommends a conventional list of temperate or hot foodstuffs (for example, veal "in moderate quantity," eggs) and advises avoiding some cold ones (muddy fish, shellfish). A *consilium* for an elderly nobleman goes somewhat further: it warns against the dangers of vigorous exercise, offering the movements of a carpenter, varied but not too strenuous, as an example of beneficial activity. Perhaps Cardano had in mind the turning of ornaments on a lathe, a pastime combining manual skill and artistry that was much favored among Renaissance and early modern nobility. The same *consilium* advises the patient to reduce his food intake "a little [*ut paulo minus cibi assumat*]," but the long and varied list of foods shows no signs of an orientation toward the cold and humid, except perhaps for the recommendation that snails are good.[33]

THE PROLONGATION OF LIFE

As one might expect, given his astrological and other occult interests, Cardano was aware of speculations about the possibility of extending the human life span and eliminating the disabilities of age by various occult means. In Europe, ideas of this kind seem to have emerged in the thirteenth century, especially in the context of Latin alchemy but also in some medical works, and had wide circulation. As Michela Pereira has noted, alchemical discussions of prolongevity associated with the names of Roger Bacon and (pseudo-)Lull involved the theory that the elixir would extend life by bringing about perfection of temperament.[34] The extent to which Cardano was aware of alchemical teaching about prolongevity is unclear (although, as noted, he was much interested in the idea of perfect temperament); his own recommendations for the elderly do not appear to have included the use of alchemical preparations. But he knew and cited Ficino's *De vita*, with its rich mix of dietary, magical, and astrological recipes for the revitalization of aging scholars. Cardano was fascinated by this work but somewhat uneasy about it; he thought that "the prodigious and almost magical kind of living that he followed in almost all his teaching could rightly have been condemned by me, were it not that I had heard that he lived to the age of 97 and his mother to the age of 117."[35] I have no information about Ficino's mother, but, as is well known, Ficino himself died in 1499 shortly before his sixty-sixth birthday.[36]

Cardano had read with interest the arguments of his contemporary and fellow physician Tommaso Rangone that the natural human life span was more than 120 years, and he himself thought human life might in very rare instances be extended to 150 years.[37] Nevertheless, he tried to put claims for great longevity to some kind of test. Although he repeated and gave some credit to the stories of 400-year-old men, ageless Indians, and people who prolonged their lives with quintessence that were staples of the prolongevity literature, his discussion of human life span rested on an attempt to gather multiple, recent, local examples. He stated as a matter of principle, "By our definition, a life is to be called long that is now established [as such] in Italy," not by ancient or distant peoples.[38] His anecdotal evidence about exceptionally long-lived individuals among contemporary or recently deceased Italians was flawed, since as we have seen in the case of Ficino, some of the information he got hold of was simply wrong. Although Cardano the astrologer sought out with care accurate knowledge of the birthdates (and times) of the many historical figures of recent past whose horoscopes he cast, his access to such information must have depended on many chance factors. He cast no horoscope for Ficino, perhaps precisely because he lacked secure information about his birthdate. But he also tried firsthand research on longevity, since he was convinced that one of his special gifts was the ability to judge age accurately.[39] Whenever he saw very old men, he would ask them how old they were and question them about their health; he recorded his conversations with a Paduan tailor, who said he was one hundred, a Milanese baker who said he was ninety-six, and a Pavian who claimed to be ninety-six, though Cardano estimated him to be only ninety because he was not as thin and his eyelids were not as sunken as those of the other two. All were fairly healthy, although the Paduan suffered from constipation and was forgetful—he kept coming back with the same questions day after day.[40] Cardano's conclusion was that in contemporary Italy human beings could live to almost a hundred, but only to about the age of eighty with both mental and physical faculties reasonably intact.

THE PHILOSOPHY OF DIET

The third approach to diet for old age on which Cardano drew, Alvise Cornaro's *Della vita sobria*, was, as its title suggests, diametrically opposed to the enticing promises of the earlier prolongevity literature.[41] Cornaro rigorously eschewed all alchemical, astrological, or magical means of extending life. Instead, he claimed that anyone at all—whether of good or bad temperament and whether rich or poor—could not only live to be a hundred or even older but also enjoy an old age that was healthy and active simply by adopting the correct "sober" diet. The recommended diet was sober indeed, since its main feature was that while food could be of any kind that suited the individual's temperament, the quantity allowed was very small; it has been estimated that the daily amounts of food and wine Cornaro suggested would add up to about one thousand calories.[42] Cornaro, who continued his active life of service to the Venetian republic into vigorous old age, claimed to be living proof of the success of his system. In one work after another he pointed to his own advanced age, reinforcing the message by allotting himself a few extra years.[43]

According to Cardano, *Della vita sobria*, which was first published in 1558, was "in everybody's hands."[44] Its appeal no doubt lay in a moralizing tone appropriate to midcentury taste and in the universality and simplicity of the regime prescribed. Moreover, although Cornaro's program appeared novel in its extremism and rigidity, the advice that the elderly should eat only small amounts of food echoed recommendations by the Hippocratic writers and Galen. The work made a strongly favorable impression on Cardano, who compared his own intellectual life with that of the more aristocratic author, remarking that both were part of the world of learning, Cornaro in a way "decorous for him as a Venetian patrician," Cardano himself in a way "decent for me as a professor."[45] Perhaps Cornaro's elevated social status helped to secure Cardano's favorable response to his book, which was highly unusual for a physician confronted with a vernacular work on a medical subject by a layman. He characterized Cornaro as "thrice wise" and asserted that he would not "disdain to make use of the example of his life and the *experimentum* of his work, even though Cornaro did not profess humane letters or medicine."[46]

But notwithstanding Cardano's admiration for Cornaro, in *Theonoston* he subjected his dietary recommendations to thorough and in some respects critical analysis. The characters in this dialogue, Philosophus, Eremita, and Civis, move from a discussion of whether it is possible to lead a tranquil life in the city in Book 1 to the subject of extending the life and preserving health of the body in Book 2, to immortality of the soul in Book 3, contemplation in Book 4, and the life and felicity of souls after death in Book 5. To the best of my knowledge, the dialogue as a whole has yet to be thoroughly studied and its full meaning remains opaque. It is clear, however, that the work incorporates strong elements of religiosity and spirituality and a great deal of reservation and ambiguity about the value of civic life (it was completed after the execution of Cardano's son).

In Book 2, Philosophus and Civis go to spend a week with Eremita, who is a member of a religious order, in his mountain retreat. On arrival, they ask him how he maintains his excellent health living in such discomfort at his advanced age. This opens a discussion on diet in which a main subject is the desirability of reducing food intake according to Cornaro's or some other scheme. Eremita, who was a medical practitioner before entering religion and has in any case just been reading Cardano's *De sanitate tuenda*,[47] is the expert, while Civis and Philosophus raise doubts and queries. Philosophus calls to mind various exceptionally long-lived people, who, though they ate moderately, did not do so in minuscule amounts (Ficino and his mother yet again), and points out that anyone who chose to consume his entire Cornaro food allowance in fruit and vegetables would be weakened for lack of food containing oil and blood.[48] Civis raises the horrid specter of "wasting of the stomach" and wonders if the sober life would not put an end to all conviviality, which he considers an essential aspect of every human society.[49] Eremita counters the last objection with some fairly depressing advice: the wise should meet for sober dinner parties together; alternatively, the sober guest could merely rinse his mouth out with wine and fill in with conversation the time in which everyone else was eating and drinking; finally, anyone who really could not do without dessert could have a wholesome treat, such as a small—a very small—amount of the "foam of milk," currently a fashionable dish among the nobility in Milan.[50]

Eremita reveals that he has reduced his own food intake to a minimum and strongly endorses this practice, which he regards as an invention of modern times on a par with printing and firearms.[51] Nevertheless, he has considerable reservations about the Cornaro diet. He notes that Cornaro had not made it clear whether he was talking about one meal a day or two (something that still puzzles Cornaro's most recent editor), that he had not given many details about kinds of food, and that his allowance for wine was more than for solid food. He adds that in any case, it would be dangerous to go on the Cornaro diet suddenly, and that he personally would recommend reducing intake gradually over a period of six months. Certainly, anyone attempting the diet should follow Cornaro's advice and eat an egg yolk every day; furthermore, it would be dangerous to combine this diet with any exercise more vigorous than walking.[52] When Eremita comes to describe his own diet, it becomes clear that, though exiguous, it is distinctly more moderate and flexible than Cornaro's. Between the ages of sixty and eighty, the food intake, while small, is greater than Cornaro allowed, the proportion of solids and fluids varies according to the season (with more liquid in summer), and the amount of food according to religious feasts and fasts and periods of exertion (harvesting grain, collecting wood).[53]

Two separate arguments emerge from this discussion. In one of them, Eremita and Civis represent opposing points of view, which Philosophus will presumably have to balance. The austere Eremita, at once medical expert, holy man, and aged person, approves a highly restricted diet, such as was recommended by both Cornaro and Cardano in his own person in Book 4 of *De sanitate tuenda*. The more sociable or self-indulgent (and perhaps younger) layman Civis objects. But at another level both Eremita and Civis jointly raise the problem that the "one size fits all" model diet proposed by Cornaro is not in fact equally suitable for different social categories. In Civis's view, such a diet would make impossible social gatherings essential to the civic life for which Cornaro designed it; in Eremita's it is unsuitable even for a religious hermit if his solitary life demands physical activity. Eremita (and Cardano) agreed that the diet of the elderly should indeed be restricted, but the restrictions should be different from those recommended by Cornaro.[54] Thus, ultimately, Cardano's approval of Cornaro was qualified. He approved the principle of dietary restriction for the elderly and praised the Venetian patrician for publicizing it; but where dietary details were concerned, he was not prepared to yield his professional expertise to a layman.

Both Eremita and Cardano in his own person in *De sanitate tuenda* go into much more detail than does Cornaro about mealtimes, menus, means of preparation, and the merits and demerits of particular food-stuffs. The last topic displays to the full Cardano's propensity to ambiguity and indeed contradiction. Although he situated *De sanitate tuenda* in the context of his theme of "medical contradictions" by opening the work with a reference to the contradictions of other writers on the subject,[55] his teaching on diet includes some flagrant contradictions of its own. Book 4 gives the conventional Galenic advice that the cold and dry elderly should eat humidifying and heating foods that were also well concocted and easy to digest, such as eggs, oil, milk, and certain meats, and should avoid fruit and vegetables;[56] but the proem claims that the best diet for longevity is a vegetarian one consisting of bread, nuts, and sugar water and excluding eggs and wine as well as meat.[57] The solemn warning against eating snails, fungi, and roots in the same preface reads oddly in light of the elaborate account in *Theonoston* of the dinner of snail soup and "tubers"—that is, probably, fungi—served by Eremita to his guests. Of this menu, Civis, urbane to the last, managed to remark, "It was never revolting, O well-born man [*Nunquam piguit, o generose*]." Eremita kindly obliged with the recipe, describing the appearance, habitat, and seasonal cycle of the best kind of snails and explaining in detail how to clean and cook them.[58]

There is probably no way of knowing whether these contradictions are the result of complete openness to all traditions, skeptical intentions, playfulness (*Theonoston* contains several remarks about joking),[59] or simple carelessness. Perhaps the inference is merely that any kind of wild food available is appropriate for the hermit life in a rugged outdoor setting.[60] But whatever the case, the effect is to undercut the value of all dietary advice, since the ultimate implication is that choice of foodstuffs does not really make much difference to either longevity or health. And indeed, when Cardano reflected on the relations among temperament, diet, health, and longevity in philosophical and moral terms, he was explicit that in reality nature and society were at least equal and perhaps more powerful determinants of the "natural" life span of individuals. Cardano's advice on diet, like Machiavelli's on political conduct, offers instructions and examples about behavior, while simultaneously assuming that the characteristics of individuals are in fact largely fixed. Civis in *Theonoston* surely spoke for the author of the work when he said that a person's life span was largely determined by natural physical endowment, the stars, inherited family traits, and the region inhabited (these are precisely the elements that Cardano listed at the beginning of his autobiography as affecting his own life). Thus, as Eremita put it a little later, knowledge about diet is like command of musical technique, which helps to fulfill the potential of someone with a naturally good singing voice but does nothing for the tone-deaf.[61]

Cardano indeed saw human life span and its stages (the "ages of man") as part of a cosmic order that also fixed the life spans of dynasties and states, all of which "not only have a terminus but a certain one, nor can it be set aside, but in states life is ended by circuits of times, just as the life of animals is." In this vein, he paralleled fourteen generations of biblical history with fourteen ages of man. His unusual scheme of fourteen divisions ignored traditional divisions into four or seven ages with their links to cosmological and religious ideas.[62] He included two stages after "senectus," with names indicative of the likely quality of human life prolonged to the physiologically possible limit: from 80 to 100 is "decrepitude" and from 100 to 120 "can be called memento mori."[63]

But despite the universal governance of the stars, multiple secondary causes and chance also operated to affect individuals, human societies, and the world of nature.[64] Cardano's recognition of such factors is in line with the teaching of both the Hippocratic *Airs Waters Places* and Ptolemy's *Tetrabiblos*, two texts to which he attached great importance and on which he wrote major commentaries. Both emphasized the influences of region and climate (each in turn astrally determined). Thus local variations in the physical environment explained why the Florentines "indulged themselves less with food"—as well as being more given to mathematics—than the Milanese.[65] His emphasis on the multiplicity of secondary causes may also owe something to his reading of Pico della Mirandola's critique of astrology, despite his rejection of Pico's main argument.[66] In the context of such ideas, diet could never be more than one among many secondary causes having some effect on the length of an individual's actual life.

Moreover, Cardano emphasized social factors affecting health, diet, and longevity in the medical *De sanitate tuenda* as well as in the philosophical *Theonoston*. He insisted that actual longevity required not only a cold and moist temperament but also freedom from anxieties arising from participation in public affairs. He maintained that most people who lived to be very old were either ascetic religious or poor and insignificant; and that their longevity was due both to temperament and to being unburdened by public affairs and consequent worries. At this point, his remarks seem as much a recipe for survival in times of war, absolutism, and confessional rigorism as a physiological theory. But he also gave consideration to the negative effects of poverty on longevity. People could not live long if they were starving, cold, or forced to do heavy physical labor; moreover, when they reached old age, they needed to have children who would not neglect them but supply them abundantly with necessities. In reality, however, very few people met all these criteria; and, in any case, multitudes died prematurely as a result of wars, famines, and epidemics.[67] One person who did meet most of Cardano's natural and social criteria for longevity—with the notable exceptions of absence of worry and anxiety and the presence of helpful children—was himself. He was a small, thin man from a long-lived family, who for much of his life was not at all well off.[68] Perhaps, too, these inquiries into the physiological basis of the "best" life (*optima vita*), in which he seems so clearly to have his own scholarly temperament in mind, should be associated with his interest in the nature, and possibility, of "perfect" temperament discussed in the previous chapter.

In his view, moreover, if relative poverty was at least potentially favorable to long life, true poverty was certainly unfavorable to health: the poor might have to work while ill, lack the resources to obtain the proper diet, and live in a place where the air and water were bad; thus "poverty is a great evil, which itself brings diseases, and death, and mourning [*Et ideo magnum malum est paupertas, quia ipsa adducit morbos, et mortem, et luctus*]."[69] This profoundly pessimistic and socially grounded view stands in sharp contrast both to medical (that is, Galenic) dietetics, with its goal of ameliorating the temperaments of individuals—in actuality, inevitably, prosperous individuals—and to the optimism of the alchemical, astrological, or magical prolongevity literature. Implicitly, it also casts doubt on Cornaro's idea that people of distinction could be preserved for long service to church, state, and the republic of letters.[70] Cardano's poor people and thin pale nuns with no public role constitute an image of old age very unlike Cornaro's model of the robust old male patrician guiding public life to the end.

These opinions about the social distribution of longevity and health together with the religious setting of the dietary debate in *Theonoston* provide clues to ethical or moral attitudes that underlay Cardano's assertions about the merits of a sparse diet. In the place of Cornaro's stress on the *vita activa civile*, Cardano seems to substitute connections with traditions of religious asceticism, a deeply disillusioned view of society and public life, and a reaction against courtly display. Similar feelings are summed up in his remarks about Platina's *De honesta voluptate*: Platina "wrote a book called *On Decent Pleasure*, which gives more information about cooking and the pleasure of drunks who frequent lavish banquets and are given to gluttony and the belly than about preserving health by art. He put all his study into the art of preparing a variety of luxurious and harmonious dishes and sweetmeats for the table, greatly to the detriment of human health; indeed, he followed pleasure, not utility. This is indeed a pernicious art. . . ."[71] Yves Pélicier has suggest a dual typology for the Renaissance concept of the meal as either Dionysiac or frugal.[72] When he wrote in the capacity of medical adviser to the elderly or as a moral philosopher, Cardano left no doubt as to his preference for the frugal. But these were not the only roles in which he addressed the subject of food and diet. Cardano the natural philosopher and Cardano the recorder of his own experience had different stories to tell.

THE NATURAL HISTORY OF FOOD

The substantial portions of *De sanitate tuenda*—almost all of Books 2 and 3—that consist of separate chapters on plants and animals used as food show a very different side of Cardano's interest in the subject. These chapters are, to be sure, squarely in the tradition of much medieval and Renaissance dietetic literature, a tradition that extends back through the *Tacuinum sanitatis* and similar handbooks to Galen.[73] In each chapter the reader is provided with a description of the food item in question, its complexional properties, and its nutritional benefits and dangers. But the same chapters also show Cardano participating in the grand endeavor of Renaissance natural history to confront every surviving ancient account of animals and plants with an expanding contemporary knowledge of fauna and flora. While many of the individual descriptions in all categories are of interest, they are far too numerous to summarize in any effective way. Instead, it seems preferable to consider the one category of foods to which Cardano devoted most attention, namely, fish.

In these books of *De sanitate tuenda* Cardano devoted more space to fish than to any other single major category of foodstuff: fifty chapters, as compared to twenty-three for vegetables (including herbs, gourds, roots, and fungi), twenty for fruits, fourteen for grains and legumes, and nine for meat.[74] Moreover, many of the fish chapters discuss more than one species. This special emphasis on fish can be traced to several causes. One of them—by now familiar to the reader—is Cardano's habit of incorporating his reading of recent scientific work in all fields. He had responded with his usual enthusiasm and rapidity to major new works on the natural history of fish that appeared during the 1550s. Other reasons for special attention to fish include the particular circumstances of his life in the 1570s, as well as, no doubt, the actual use of a large number of varieties of Mediterranean fish for food.

Cardano's response to the work on fish of contemporary naturalists can be measured by the difference between the discussion of fish in *De subtilitate* and in *De rerum varietate*. In keeping with the general tenor of the former work, published in 1550, its few pages on fish are mostly given over to ancient and other accounts of monstrous, strange, or very large sea beasts; by contrast, when *De rerum varietate* appeared in 1557, it contained a lengthy and informative chapter treating fish from the standpoint of natural history, as well as a shorter one on their (mostly marvelous or remarkable) properties.[75] Between these two dates, several of the most important sixteenth-century natural histories of fish appeared; moreover, Cardano's knowledge of the European community of naturalists was no doubt greatly enlarged by his travels in northern Europe in 1552. When he passed through Lyon, where he was already in touch with two publishers who had printed works of his own,[76] Rondelet was known to be at work on the text and illustrations shortly to appear there as his *Libri de piscibus marinis*.[77] At Paris, where Cardano met Fernel and other leading physicians and doubtless was told of recent books of interest, Belon's *L'histoire naturelle des estranges poissons marins* had been published just one year previously.[78] On his circuitous return journey from Scotland, Cardano went to Zurich to visit Gesner, a meeting that further stimulated his interest in natural history.[79]

By the time he came to complete *De rerum varietate* Cardano had thoroughly absorbed Rondelet's book, which was published in 1554. As Cardano said, the works of Rondelet and Belon were now as fundamental to the study of fish as those of Aristotle and Pliny.[80] The long chapter on fish in *De rerum varietate* is, indeed, heavily dependent on Rondelet, although, perhaps because Cardano had noticed Rondelet's slighting remark about the confused account of the mythical *remora* in *De subtilitate*, also strongly critical of certain of his views.[81] Eremita, in *Theonoston*, is made to express a preference for Belon over Rondelet, noting—justly enough—that the former knew more than the latter about the internal anatomy of fish.[82] Nevertheless, much of the chapter in *De rerum varietate* amounts to a summary of the opening sections of Rondelet's work, which, along with Belon and Pliny, is freely and for the most part favorably acknowledged throughout. The chapter is structured, in the Aristotelian manner adopted by Rondelet, around the differentiating characteristics, parts, and physiology of fish, with discussion of some species as examples. Also included are a number of references to experiences of Cardano's own in northern Europe—among them, his meals of salmon in Scotland and various remarkable fish that he saw at Dieppe and at the house of one of his hosts in Paris.[83] In a striking tribute to Cardano's newly acquired knowledge of the subject, in 1558 Gesner cited him as one of the scholars who had been particularly helpful when he was preparing the volume on fishes of his own great *Historia animalium*.[84]

The chapters on fish in *De sanitate tuenda* draw heavily on *De varietate rerum*, but with significant changes. Some of these are simply modifications to shift the focus to diet. The later work compresses general exposition of the *differentiae* and parts of fish into two pages, but greatly expands the discussion of individual species. It introduces information about fish as food, both in the shape of a general introductory chapter and for each species. Thus the description of salmon in *De sanitate tuenda* repeats the parallel passage in *De rerum varietate* word for word but adds a paragraph on its tender, fatty flesh and ways of cooking it.[85]

Other changes, however, reflect Cardano's response to his situation at the time of writing, when he was living out his last years in Rome on a papal pension. A notable feature of the fish chapters in *De sanitate tuenda* is the attention given to vernacular nomenclature. In zoology, as in botany and anatomy, nomenclature was a major and problematic aspect of Renaissance descriptive science. Authors sought both to identify species described by ancient writers and to establish a consistent relation among Latin, Greek—and in some cases Hebrew and Arabic—and vernacular terminology. As Gianfranco Folena has pointed out, the problem was particularly acute as far as Italian vernacular names for fish were concerned, both because of the large number of Mediterranean species and because of the many variant regional names for them in different parts of Italy.[86] In the fifteenth century, indeed, the difficulty of naming all the kinds of fish became something of a topos: Michele Savonarola remarked that "it would be exhausting and almost impossible to name all the fish that are eaten," and Luigi Pulci claimed that describing all the different kinds of fish would be as difficult as counting flies and mosquitoes.[87]

In *De rerum varietate* Cardano noted a few, mostly Venetian, vernacular names for various species of fish, but vernacular nomenclature was by no means a focus of his attention.[88] By contrast, in *De sanitate tuenda*, in addition to identifying a few by Venetian, Bolognese, or Milanese names, he identified at least twenty-one species by their Roman names, an emphasis that is doubtless the consequence of residence in Rome at the time of writing. However, the work on Roman fish of Paolo Giovio and the physician and anatomist Ippolito Salviani aroused the enthusiasm of Aldrovandi at Bologna in the 1550s and was very likely already known to Cardano before he left for Rome.[89] He almost certainly drew on the extensive tables of nomenclature in different languages compiled by Salviani for his large and beautifully illustrated volume on fish, which combines natural history, literary allusions, and a good deal of culinary information. These tables included several vernaculars but strongly emphasized Roman terminology.[90] Salviani's work, written under the patronage of a cardinal,[91] seems particularly suited to the clerical humanistic culture of Rome, given the elaborate preparations of fish customarily served at the tables of wealthy clergy on fast days. Of course, Cardano, too, in his last years was a hanger-on of that culture.

WHAT TO EAT ONESELF?

Finally, what of Cardano's own dietary practice? No one will be surprised to learn that it was not always as austere as some of the views he expressed in his prescriptive writings. His own reports of his dietary experiments present him as someone who was brought to realize the practical importance of permanently reforming his diet by two crises: an illness and the onset of old age. Until his fifties, according to his own account, he frequented luxurious dinner parties, chose foods on the basis of taste, overate, ate too fast, rushed out of the house with his meal undigested when he ate at home, and drank rather copiously (*potus uberior*).[92] His very well informed description, presumably gathered during his travels, of beer making in Germany (ingredients, recipe, varieties, strengths, flavors), and perry and cider making in Brittany implies a more than academic interest. Notwithstanding his belief that a hangover from beer was worse for the health than one from wine, he reminisced pleasurably about the exceptionally good ale he had drunk on the Scottish border.[93] As he remarked, "although beer seems unpleasant at first taste, it grows on one with use."[94]

A bout of illness in 1554 led to his first decision to change his eating and drinking habits. The regime he settled on was to eat breakfast later and omit lunch; in general, to eat less; to give up foods that were cold in complexion together with meat, eggs, fish, and cheese. The only specific menu mentioned is for breakfast, which was to consist of bread, honey, nuts and raisins, one piece of fresh fruit, and sometimes salted fish roe and green salad. His account of this episode makes no overt allusion to old age (although he mentioned being somewhat less busy than formerly), but the decision to give up cold-complexioned foods would constitute a Galenically appropriate response to its approach. We may note that Cornaro's *Della vita sobria* had not yet been published at the time of the illness, and that this narrative appears not in a medical treatise but in a work of edification, *On the Usefulness to Be Gained from Adversity* (in this instance, the adversity was the illness that caused the change in diet).[95]

Twelve years later he embarked on a period of much more intensive dietary self-regulation. The new diet, explicitly a regime for the elderly, limited food to small, precisely measured quantities, an emphasis that probably reflects a reading of *Della vita sobria*. The first version, introduced in 1566 when Cardano was sixty-five, was as follows: breakfast—four ounces of bread in meat or fish broth; midday snack—raisins and diluted wine; evening meal—two days a week a small amount of meat or fish with five or six ounces of bread (crusts cut off); other days a somewhat larger quantity of meat, eggs, or fish, and less bread. The meats allowed were doves and partridges, chicken livers, and organ meats. The following year he decided to put his diet "in balance" and became even more precise about quantities and cooking methods and restrictive as to ingredients. The midday snack has disappeared and supper consists of fish, organ meats, or chicken livers. Breakfast was to consist of the bread allowance soaked in a broth that had been used to cook "turtle, chopped snails, or some fish," sometimes with a little of the fish or snails. The last three foods were all considered cold and humid, and thus represent a turn toward Cardano's allegedly contra-Galenic theory that the elderly should strive to maintain a cold and humid complexion. Evidently, this diet also puts into practice the idea dramatized in *Theonoston* that snails, conventionally excoriated in diet books as gross and viscous, are in fact an excellent food.[96] These dietary recommendations are presented with the full weight of medical authority; they are included as an example in his *De tuenda sanitate* with the additional information that the author of the book and practitioner of the diet was professor of medicine *supra-ordinarius*.[97] One is, of course, reminded that Cornaro too had presented himself as a successful example of the results of his own regime.

But the effects of Cardano's dietary conversion experiences were soon modified by conflicting theoretical considerations, practical problems, and, one hopes, simple hedonism. In 1570 he moved slightly in the direction of Galenic conventionality by proposing to allow some stewed meat in the evening menu, and praising turtle meat in preference to snails, because of the "putrefaction" associated with the latter.[98] The main practical problem with the bread and snail broth mixture was that his maid did not cook it to his satisfaction and the only result of his nagging her about it was to make her lose her temper. He ended up in the kitchen, preparing the mixture himself from ordinary meat broth cooked for the household at large.[99] By the time he came to write the last account of his diet, in a chapter of the autobiography written in 1575, he was eating three meals a day with a varied menu that included eggs, salad, fruit, fish, meat, and "sweet new wine." Snails are explicitly dismissed as poisonous "unless purged" (as, indeed, is necessary). What is more, it is evident that the main basis for choosing many of the long list of foods in this chapter is taste and personal preference: the verbs are *delector, oblector, gaudeo, praefero*.[100]

Yet it is doubtful whether this last diet represents, at last, a move to practice unmediated by theory. It can still be accommodated within the endlessly flexible system of complexion theory. A diet based on preference could be justified on the ground that, as Cornaro had suggested, one would be able to learn from experience which particular foods were appropriate for one's own complexion.[101] Indeed, the central concept of dietary theory based on complexion—that it must be carefully matched to the individual's temperament—is profoundly appropriate to an autobiographical work. Furthermore, the content of Cardano's last diet is appropriate to an encyclopedic natural philosopher, a Hippocratic physician, and a person who believed himself to be endowed with special occult gifts: the emphasis on fish as a food of choice, and the long list of favorite

PART THREE

The Old and the New

Chapter 5

THE USES OF ANATOMY

IN HIS autobiography, Cardano listed anatomy among laudable disciplines that he knew only very slightly, since "many things deterred me" from it. Given that he here grouped anatomy with the ability to recognize plants, the practice of agriculture, and composing poems, and stated in the same chapter that he had no experience in surgery, it seems likely that he had anatomical practice—that is, dissection—in mind.[1] The comment probably does not misrepresent his practical experience. As far as can be determined, this was confined to attendance at public or private anatomical demonstrations and participation in some autopsies of his patients, in which it is unlikely that he did the actual dissecting. Nor did he write extensively on the subject. But these remarks gloss over an enthusiasm for the contemporary anatomical renaissance apparently first sparked in the 1540s by his reading of Vesalius and energetically renewed in the milieu of the University of Bologna in the 1560s.

Cardano's interest in anatomy is well known to the extent that his horoscope for and scattered allusions to Vesalius have many times drawn the attention of medical historians as well as of biographers of both men.[2] Much less attention has been devoted to the subject of the present chapter, namely, the way anatomy—and what aspects of anatomy—fitted into his philosophy of nature, prophetic/astrological worldview, and profession as a Hippocratic and Galenic physician. Cardano approached anatomy as a branch of natural knowledge to be mastered by a combination of study and experience (in this case, attending dissections). But despite some experience, most of his own knowledge came from books; certainly most of the uses he found for anatomy involved the interpretation of other books, both ancient and modern. But he also held that anatomical knowledge had practical usefulness for physicians, although the kind of usefulness he had in mind was chiefly rhetorical advantage in situations of professional competition. Yet he was strongly drawn to anatomy, perhaps primarily because he perceived autopsy as a technique of retroactively interpreting signs. As such it was comparable to medical prognosis, a "predictive" discipline that could look backward as well as forward—as indeed could the other predictive science to which Cardano was most strongly committed, that is, astrology.[3]

The chapter of *De vita propria* just quoted seems a good starting point for an inquiry into the uses Cardano made of anatomy, because it purports to distinguish between disciplines that he had in reality fully mastered and branches of knowledge in which he had the reputation of being competent. The self-analysis and meditation on the difference between representation and reality are insightful, but, like much else in *De vita*, conceal and contradict as well as reveal. In addition to understating the attention to the "laudable" subject of anatomy evident to any reader in several of his already published books, Cardano firmly denied ever having touched a list of "harmful disciplines" even though he had previously published a work on one of them, namely, physiognomy.[4]

Whatever the reasons for these reticences at the time he wrote *De vita*, the uses Cardano made of anatomy exemplify an important aspect of the sixteenth-century anatomical renaissance. In medical and other circles, response to the activities and publications of innovative anatomical practitioners and authors occurred rapidly and was relatively widespread. Despite some celebrated controversies, much of the response was favorable. But physicians and others who looked at, read, or read about anatomical books or witnessed anatomical demonstrations tended to take from anatomy just as much as fitted their own specific purposes, preconceptions, and preoccupations. Such was certainly the case with Cardano, who drew on Vesalian and post-Vesalian anatomy in a variety of ways, depending upon context, genre, and his changing personal situation. The present chapter will explore a few examples of the uses that he found for it.

Anatomy in fact appealed to a diverse public, both erudite and popular, for many reasons. It touched on several traditional disciplines (natural philosophy, medicine, and surgery) and had a long-established, if formerly minor, place in the university curriculum in medicine.[5] At the same time, along with botany and natural history, it was among the branches of knowledge most responsive to the general expansion of interest in collecting, inspecting, and describing particulars about the natural world.[6] Because it drew on a significant collection of Greek texts, in which major items had been recently recovered, it shared in the contemporary prestige of medical humanism or Hellenism. It was in several ways closely linked to contemporary artistic values and activities.[7] In addition, anatomy appealed to and strengthened existing philosophical and religious traditions of positive or negative moralizing about the human body.[8] Dissection provided a spectacle in which moralities could be enacted as well as curiosity about "the secrets of nature" satisfied. Indeed, the popular fascination that made some academic dissections into a public or semipublic spectacle has been plausibly related to the power of representation and theatricality in Renaissance culture.[9] Above all, as Galen had long ago proclaimed and as Vesalius echoed, human anatomy was testimony to the benevolence and design of the Creator.

Like other descriptive sciences of the period, anatomy combined observation, manipulation, verbal description, and visual representation of nature with meticulous attention to ancient texts. The striking enlargement of anatomy's practical, technical, and visual aspects is, of course, deservedly famous. As compared with its medieval predecessor, sixteenth-century anatomy was distinguished by more frequent dissections, improved techniques, more emphasis on personal observation, more attention to detail, and greatly enhanced standards of illustration. These changes involved contributions from many individuals and took place over many decades. Moreover, anatomy based on human dissection, perhaps even more than most other sciences, requires favorable social and institutional factors for its very existence as a legitimate activity. Thus the extension of anatomical practice depended in many ways on developments in the broader contemporary social and cultural context—in, for example, such diverse areas as artistic style and values, attitudes to the human body, patronage and connections among rulers, courtly and professional elites, and universities, and even patterns of crime and punishment. At the same time, the entire anatomical enterprise was largely shaped by study of the texts of ancient—that is, chiefly Galenic—anatomy, the availability of which was greatly increased through the efforts of humanist scholars, editors, and printers during the first third of the sixteenth century. Sixteenth-century anatomists challenged many specifics of Galen's anatomical teaching, but his works continued to define the nature of the subject, set the terms of debate, and provide an essential point of departure. In this respect, anatomy was just as bookish and classicizing as any other branch of learned culture. Furthermore, practicing anatomists rapidly produced a large body of new Latin literature on their discipline. Hence what distinguished Renaissance anatomy from its medieval antecedents was a notable enhancement of *both* practice *and* textual foundation, the latter both ancient and modern.

Within the university faculties of medicine, where most sixteenth-century anatomical teaching took place, the status and role of anatomy in the curriculum rose significantly over the course of the century. This was so even though the level of actual institutional commitment varied greatly in different parts of Europe and was not always permanent when made. In Italy, as is well known, various universities—most notably, of course, Padua and Bologna—increased emphasis on anatomical teaching, established professorial chairs in the subject, and, late in the century, constructed permanent anatomy theaters. But even in Italy the extent to which anatomy was actually taught varied from one university to another and even in major Italian centers from decade to decade. Often, the degree to which anatomy was pursued corresponded to the presence and interest of individual anatomists and the attitude of local authorities (on whom, among other things, the supply of cadavers depended). Much anatomy continued to be taught from books and from animals. The pursuit of anatomical research and investigation, as distinct from public or private teaching or the writing and reading of anatomy books, depended entirely upon the enthusiasm and private activities of a small community of anatomists.[10]

In part, the enhanced academic status of anatomy depended upon the perception of it as an aspect of the natural philosophical study of mankind. Vesalius himself punningly described his subject as "the *scientia* of the parts of the human body" and "a part [*membrum*] of [the corpus of] natural philosophy," thus associating it not only with philosophy, but also with the branch of medicine considered nearest to philosophy, namely, medical *theoria*.[11] Vesalius was here, implicitly, claiming the epistemological status of *scientia*, certain knowledge, for a descriptive discipline. But claims for the philosophical importance of human anatomy might also stress its significance for a religious and theological understanding of the place of man in creation; recent studies have revealed the extent to which Melanchthon's ideas of this kind influenced the formation of the Wittenberg medical curriculum.[12] At the same time, manual techniques, suppositions about practical utility, and, often, arrangements for the actual conduct of dissections continued to connect anatomy with surgery. At Bologna, the chair of anatomy was permanently separated from the chair of surgery only in 1570, while at Padua the two disciplines were taught together for much of the century.[13]

For both philosophical and pedagogical reasons, the subject of anatomical instruction was, as Vesalius put it, a "canonical," natural, and healthy human body. Essentially, this meant that a well-developed young man was taken as the ideal object of study (as the Vesalian illustrations demonstrate). In reality—as was well known to Vesalius and other anatomists who were simultaneously keenly interested in human diversity and variability—few of the actual cadavers of executed criminals, paupers, or friendless foreigners available for public dissection could have met the ideal.[14] But various other situations called for medical practitioners to inspect the internal organs of cadavers for physical abnormalities. In sixteenth-century Italy the practice of autopsy, which first developed in the late Middle Ages, appears to have been generally accepted and relatively widespread. Respectable families, including the families of physicians, sought autopsies for deceased members (especially, according to a recent study, wives and children) in order to safeguard the health of the lineage.[15] Individuals who died in the odor of sanctity, including Counter-Reformation Italy's two most famous saints, Carlo Borromeo and Filippo Neri, were examined for physical signs of their specially favored status.[16] Suspicion of poisoning or disagreement among physicians about the cause of death, especially where princely or eminent personages were concerned, provided yet other reasons for autopsy; such, for example, was the case with several of the eight sixteenth-century popes who were subjected to postmortem dissection.[17] However little was learned from most such inspections, both medical practitioners and those who engaged or permitted their services shared the belief that the postmortem appearance of the internal organs could reveal information about conditions that had affected a person in life or the cause of death. Moreover, as the sixteenth century wore on, reports of such inspections came to include increasing amounts of anatomical detail and close observation.[18]

From about midcentury, humanistically educated physicians incorporated their awareness of recent anatomy into works on a variety of other branches of medicine. The attacks of Hellenists on anatomical works critical of Galen continued for some time, and throughout the century anatomists themselves continued to build on and criticize each other's work and to engage in vigorous controversy. But in other, general, medical works new anatomy, especially as presented by Vesalius, seems soon to have ceased to be controversial at the price of being absorbed into the mass of bookish authorities. In some respects, the process parallels the synthesis of humanistic with scholastic Aristotelian philosophy that occurred during the same period—and is indeed part of a broader movement of synthesis characteristic of many aspects of Renaissance intellectual life. In the case of anatomy, a handful of examples must suffice to illustrate developments in the milieu of the Italian universities. For Giovanni Argenterio, who taught at Pisa, Naples, and Turin in the 1550s and 1560s, Vesalian anatomy served as a model and defense for his own radical critique of Galenic pathology.[19] But a generation later even a commentary written at Bologna on the part of Avicenna's *Canon* used in teaching medical *theoria*—presumably the most conservative book in the most conservative branch of the medical curriculum—included fifty pages on the anatomy of bones and muscles, presented a Vesalian account of muscular function, and proffered the advice that the *recentiores* should be followed on the division and structure of the bones.[20] By 1596, readers of a vernacular treatise on the duties of midwives encountered the authority of the "immortal" and "almost divine" Vesalius, along with that of the author's teacher at Bologna, Giulio Cesare Aranzio.[21]

Although intensified attention had been given to anatomy in advanced medical circles (including the University of Pavia) since the early years of the century, Cardano seems to have been too busy with his numerous other projects to take any interest in the subject before his reading of Vesalius's *Fabrica* between 1543 and 1545. His subsequent enthusiasm is striking testimony to the immediate impact of the *Fabrica* as a book and to the importance—even in Italy—of books and reading in disseminating the message of the new anatomy. At the time, Cardano was in the process of establishing himself as a professor of medical *theoria* at Pavia. As chapter 3 has shown, two of the earliest uses he made of his anatomical reading were entirely consonant with the role of a professor of *theoria* and the author of the in many respects scholastic *Contradictiones*. He allied himself with existing interest in anatomy teaching among the Pavia medical faculty by proposing the comparative textual study of the *Fabrica* and a Galenic anatomical work; and he asserted that the *Fabrica* and his own criticisms of Galen via the "method of contradictions" were parallel endeavors. But in the same year, 1545, he also brought anatomy into the context of medical practice with the claim that it was useful for internal medicine. In a chapter added to the second edition of *On the Bad Practice of Recent Physicians*, after denouncing physicians for failure to view human dissection, dismissing animal dissection as useless (an opinion he subsequently moderated), and briskly summarizing anatomical errors ascribed to Galen, Cardano asserted that *medici* ought regularly to dissect patients who had died of disease in the hospital in order to trace the specific effects of various kinds of disease; for this purpose, they should not dissect the entire cadaver but only the organs primarily affected—for example, in the case of phthoe, the lungs.[22]

The allusion to phthoe situates the suggestion in the context of Cardano's medical practice at Milan, rather than his teaching at Pavia. The hospital he had in mind was presumably the Ospedale Maggiore, a foundation he knew well because both he and his father before him had taught mathematics in the Piattine school, one of many charitable bequests administered by the Ospedale.[23] By the early sixteenth century, the Ospedale Maggiore and a network of subsidiary hospitals for the sick poor were by no means purely custodial institutions. Signs of medicalization included the employment of physicians and surgeons, a library of medical handbooks, and, for a few years at the end of the fifteenth century, some provisions for dissection. Furthermore, patients were segregated by type of illness as well as other criteria; for example, patients with phthoe were sent to the hospital of San Vicenzo for incurables.[24]

Various well-known Renaissance anatomists and artists are of course known to have worked on specimens from hospitals, most notably Eustachi at Rome and Leonardo da Vinci at Florence. It was indeed at one time suggested that Leonardo might have obtained human anatomical material from the Ospedale Maggiore during his first period in Milan, although this suggestion is now regarded as unfounded.[25] In any case, what is distinctive about Cardano's proposal is the idea of using a hospital not just as a general source of anatomical material, but specifically as a source of pathological specimens. The idea suggests a parallel with

Gianbattista Da Monte's actual use at Padua, also in the 1540s, of living hospital patients as material for his clinical lectures on disease.[26] It is also tempting to associate the proposal to dissect only affected parts rather than entire cadavers with ideas about sites of disease, but the remark may be no more than a pragmatic response to the difficulty of obtaining whole cadavers.

By 1547, Cardano succeeded in making indirect contact with Vesalius himself, since in that year the latter passed on to him a job offer from the king of Sweden; around the same time Cardano also cast the well-known horoscope which showed that Vesalius's stars were responsible for his manual dexterity, marvelous and profound *ingenium*, memory, studiousness, *scientia*—and numerous enemies.[27] Sometime before 1550, and as his remarks suggest probably after he was already familiar with the work of Vesalius, Cardano went to see Leonardo da Vinci's anatomical drawings. He lauded Leonardo as a painter who was also "a philosopher, an architect, and a craftsman of dissection," who many years ago had almost completed "an outstanding *imitatio* of the whole human body"; nevertheless, such a project really called for someone with even greater skill in dissection who was also "an investigator of the things of nature," such as Vesalius. In short, where the human body was concerned, *imitatio* of nature, however excellent, was not sufficient without accompanying investigation.[28]

These references to philosophy, *imitatio*, and investigation of nature as all three essential components of knowledge and representation of the human body are key elements in Cardano's discussion of the "most subtle" and "most noble" arts of painting and sculpture. In the same passage, moreover, he recorded his fascination with the technology of the plaster life or death mask as a way of achieving a precise representation of human features.[29] Yet apart from the brief mention of Vesalius just quoted, specific mention of anatomy as a natural philosophical or medical discipline is otherwise virtually absent from the encyclopedic works he produced in the 1550s. The books on mankind in *De subtilitate* and *De rerum varietate*, which wander through a vast array of human characteristics, moral, intellectual, and physical, have nothing to say about the discipline of anatomy as such.[30] But the central book of the twenty-one books of *De subtilitate* culminates with anatomy's subject, the perfect human body. Book 11 on "the necessity and form of man" concludes with an elaborately worked out list of the proportions of "the form of the perfect human body" (including, for example, the information that the opening of the nostril should be one quarter the length of the eye). The passage reflects the interest in Vitruvian proportion theory that Cardano shared with many of his contemporaries—among them

Vesalius.[31] Moreover, although anatomy is not explicitly referred to in the praise of medicine in Book 16 of *De subtilitate*, on sciences, it is implicitly present. The aspects of medicine here singled out for praise are prognostic powers connected with knowledge of weather and stars, notions that linked Cardano's conception of medicine to his central philosophical—that is, prophetic and astrological—concerns.[32] But, as will shortly become apparent, in other, later works he made it plain that he incorporated anatomy along with prognosis into a medical system of natural signs.

How much opportunity Cardano had, or took, for direct contact with anatomical practice in the 1540s and 1550s, either in an academic context at Pavia or in the form of autopsies in Milan, is unclear. It seems probable that his later insistence at Bologna on his power to interpret postmortem signs of disease reflected some prior experience; however, his own accounts of his practice at Milan, structured around the idea of cure, are uninformative about autopsies. But the move to Bologna in 1562 brought him for the first time to a major and flourishing center of academic anatomy. Three leading anatomists taught and dissected at Bologna during the years of his presence there. All three were a full generation younger than Cardano; his interest in their work constitutes remarkable testimony to his continuing eagerness for new knowledge at an advanced age. Giulio Cesare Aranzio held a lectureship in surgery and, later, anatomy, from 1556 to 1589; Costanzo Varolio began to teach in 1569. Volcher Coiter (1534–76) left his native Groningen in Holland with the evident intention of familiarizing himself with current work in anatomy throughout southern Europe. He acquired his doctorate in medicine from Bologna in 1562, after having previously studied with Rondelet at Montpellier and Falloppia at Padua; next, he went to Eustachi in Rome. He subsequently returned to Bologna, where he was friendly with Aldrovandi, and was appointed to a lectureship in surgery for the years 1564–65 and 1565–66. Sometime during his second appointment, however, he was arrested and briefly imprisoned by the Inquisition; subsequently, probably in the autumn of 1566, he left Italy for good.[33]

In the environment of Bologna, Cardano's interest in anatomy acquired several new dimensions. In the first place, he was involved as a witness and participant in anatomical events, joining in the noisy debates that were a feature of public dissections at Bologna and collaborating in autopsies with Aranzio and Coiter. Second, for the first and last time, he devoted a work of his own to the subject. In it and elsewhere, he considered the nature of anatomical science, how and to whom anatomy should be taught, and the merits of various anatomy books. Familiarity with more recent anatomical work modified his attitude to Vesalius; although still admiring, it became more detached and critical. Third, and probably in his view most important, he insisted and endeavored to demonstrate that anatomy was useful in medical practice because the skilled and gifted physician—notably Cardano himself—could use it to confirm diagnosis and prognosis. These three aspects merit further consideration below. His use of anatomy as a tool to explain Hippocratic texts is more properly reserved for another chapter.

ANATOMY, PUBLIC DEBATE, AND TEXTUAL KNOWLEDGE

While the annual formal public anatomy of winter 1562–63 or 1563–64[34] was being conducted "in the presence of the whole academy," an argument broke out over the course and structure of the bile duct. The subject was a matter of controversy because of challenges to the traditional belief, based on some qualified or ambiguous statements of Galen and on the early-fourteenth-century *Anatomia* of Mondino de' Liuzzi, that human beings had twin bile ducts, one emptying into the stomach, the other into the duodenum.[35] Consequently, when the lecturer, Antonio Fracanzano, first professor of practical medicine, maintained that a branch of the bile duct emptied into the stomach, he ran into opposition from the audience. Fracanzano supported his position by quoting from memory a passage in Greek. But Cardano quietly murmured that the quotation omitted a crucial negative. Fracanzano did not catch what Cardano said, but nearby students did. Immediately, they began to shout, "Send for the book." The book was most likely *On the Usefulness of the Parts of the Body*, the chief work in which Galen stated unambiguously that the bile duct emptied into the duodenum.[36] Naturally—since it is Cardano who tells the story in *De vita propria*—the book when fetched confirmed Cardano's correction, thus discomfiting Fracanzano and greatly impressing everyone else present, especially the students.[37]

The most immediately striking aspect of this post-Vesalian anatomy classroom is the superior authority of the Greek book to the dissected body either present or close at hand.[38] The professor of theory who can quote Galen correctly both scores a point off the professor of practical medicine during a dissection and is the possessor of actually more correct anatomical knowledge. But the anecdote is also suggestive of a certain ritualistic and repetitive element in the verbal exchanges that accompanied school anatomies. At Bologna, the Galenist Matteo Corti had emphatically made the same point about the bile duct in 1540, on the famous occasion when he lectured on the *Anatomia* of Mondino in tandem with Vesalius's dissection.[39] Long before then, both Alessandro Benedetti in his *Anatomice* (1502) and Berengario da Carpi, who taught at Bologna for many years, in his *Isagoge breves . . . in anatomiam* (1522) alluded to differences of opinion on the issue.[40] Both Massa and Vesalius had asserted that occasional instances in which a branch of the bile duct entered the stomach were anomalies.[41] To be sure, at the time of Cardano's triumph over Fracanzano, Falloppia had very recently (1561) published a full account of the structure, relationship, and function of the bile duct and related parts.[42] Nevertheless, it is hard to avoid the impression that in the situation of a public anatomy, the bile duct had become something of a topos—an opportunity for routine taking of positions and marshaling an expected small set of Galenic citations.

ANATOMY, MEDICINE, AND PEDAGOGY

Probably in about 1565, Cardano tried his own hand at a work on an anatomical subject. He chose to comment on the *Anatomia* of Mondino de' Liuzzi, perhaps because he hoped to give a course of lectures on that venerable work.[43] To do so would not have been particularly anomalous. The contributions to knowledge of post-Vesalian anatomists, like the Galenic revival of their predecessors, continued to be made through private investigations, the results of which were demonstrated to a larger audience in private and public teaching dissections. But their enterprise, like much else that was new in Renaissance universities, took place alongside and was partially incorporated into a formal medical curriculum still largely based on lectures on traditional texts. In this situation, discussion of rapidly changing contemporary sciences in commentaries on traditional textbooks became standard practice. Mondino's book continued to be prescribed as a base text for anatomy in various European universities for much of the century, although in some places it gave way to a work of Galen. There was also a significant recent local precedent for lectures on Mondino by a professor of medical theory, namely, the lectures by Matteo Corti that had accompanied Vesalius's anatomy at Bologna.[44]

For Cardano's proposed anatomical lectures, Corti was in a very specific sense both the model and a former rival to be surpassed. Corti had lectured on Mondino in the company of the most famous of modern anatomists, as Cardano surely knew, and his lectures had been transformed into a successful book. The sharp criticisms of Mondino from a Galenic standpoint that filled Corti's exposition ensured its publication in two successive editions in 1550 and 1551.[45] Nevertheless, Cardano's objectives were very different from Corti's. Although he expended some energy in demolishing Corti's commentary and defending Mondino as the victim of poor translations of Galen,[46] his main goal was to demonstrate the usefulness of anatomy for internal medicine; he announced that he was writing an exposition of anatomy that would be useful to physicians in curing diseases.[47]

Whether because of his departure from Bologna or for some other reason, Cardano's commentary remained unfinished and was presumably never delivered as a set of lectures. Although in addition to the *Fabrica* he cited a wide range of other modern anatomy books and authors— among them Gabriele Zerbi, Berengario da Carpi, Guinter of Andernach, Estienne, Realdo Colombo, Falloppia, and Vesalius's very recently published reply to Falloppia's critique of the *Fabrica*[48]—the anatomical content in the body of his commentary is insubstantial. Attention to the details of anatomical argument is much more evident in a group of questions in the *Contradictiones*, in which Cardano embarked on a comparative verbal analysis of the teaching of Galen, Vesalius, and Falloppia on the tunics of the veins and stomach and the structure and action of muscles, than in the commentary on Mondino.[49] But Cardano used the lengthy proem to this commentary as an opportunity to develop his reflections on the nature of anatomical knowledge, the purposes and methods of anatomical teaching, and the history of the discipline.

As noted previously, his interest in the epistemological status of disciplines based on empirical attention to particulars most certainly extended to anatomy. In general lectures on medicine some years earlier, he had already briefly addressed the question of whether anatomy was *scientia*, *ars*, or merely sense cognition. At that time, he came to the conclusion that anatomy fitted Aristotelian definitions of both art and science: it was an art because it involved learning from experience how to do something correctly; but when it involved rational demonstration and knowledge of causes, "it crosses over into a science."[50] As such, it was useful to and should be known by physicians. He offered as an example the difference between observing the eye and its parts and grasping by a process of reasoning about vision that "the eye is the instrument of the soul and that therefore the soul sees through the eye." In the latter instance anatomy—here understood as physiological and teleological argument about the functions of parts of the body similar to Galen's in *De usu partium*—is "a *scientia*, and an outstanding one."[51]

By contrast, he began his preface to the study of an anatomical text by stressing that anatomy was an art, and as such required a different type of introduction from the sciences, because "the arts ought to teach not only a sure way of teaching and finding out, but also a manner of doing."[52] Anyone who proposed to lecture or comment on an anatomical text, or teach anatomy, or practice dissection should first have mastered five things: anatomical information, appropriate procedures for conducting dissection, what animals could be substituted if human cadavers were unavailable, information about the text to be used, and how to represent anatomy. Unfortunately, in Cardano's view, in reality "this art has been very badly taught right up to the present day, not only because every art, and especially a very difficult one such as this, may daily receive an addition to knowledge, but because those who taught it lacked the art of dialectic, which I myself did not attain until I was fifty-seven. Therefore since with only one rule of dialectic Ptolemy constructed three most beautiful works, namely, the *Almagest*, the *Tetrabiblos*, and his divine work on music, anyone may consider how much we could profit from forty-four rules (for this is the number I found, for the art itself teaches itself, just as in the mechanical arts a smith makes a hammer and anvil for himself)."[53] The comment simultaneously presents anatomy as a cumulative endeavor and associates it with the precision, prediction, and cosmic significance that Cardano attributed to astronomy and astrology. Yet the subject is defective because those who teach it, presumably the youthful practicing anatomists of his acquaintance, lack the skills in reasoning that age and experience—and the inspiration that enabled him to write his work on dialectic in seven days—have brought Cardano. Consequently, he used the proem to sketch out his own ideal program in the subject.

Thus his outline of anatomical content to be mastered is decidedly oriented toward medical practice. The student should, of course, command the names, connections, and functions of all the parts and organs of the body. In addition, it "would be very beautiful and very useful for medicine" to show by anatomy the "mutual sensations and linkage" of the principal parts (brain, heart, liver) and the other parts in the bodily systems that these organs, respectively, were held to dominate, although Cardano lamented that "all anatomists, no matter how diligent, have omitted this, I think because of its difficulty."[54] Students should also learn how to both diagnose and cure diseases that depended on the structure of the body, by which he seems to have meant chiefly intestinal obstructions, bladder and kidney stones, and various kinds of tumors.[55] In the body of the commentary, he included an example of a patient whom he himself had diagnosed with a renal calculus, "out of the science of anatomy," and, he claimed, cured in only six hours.[56] At the same time, he insisted that the actual or potential usefulness of anatomy for internal medicine was fully consistent with the higher significance of the discipline: "If we dissect a human being for the sake of healing bodies, anatomy is part of the art of medicine; but if we do so in order to contemplate the diligence of nature and the wisdom of the Ruler and the majesty of God, and the care of ourselves and all things, it is natural philosophy and divine and even theology . . . therefore the work of dissection, which occupies a place of dignity in three of the greatest disciplines, should in no way be classified as mediocre."[57]

His directions for the proper conduct of dissection are largely conventional as far as site, audience, season, and dissection subjects are concerned, but in this context too he emphasized links between anatomy and the diagnosis and cure of disease. Dissections should take place in late December and early January in a specially constructed wooden anatomy theater. The shed should be open to the wind to carry away offensive odors and designed to accommodate as many spectators as possible. Proper instruments should be provided. Six cadavers, of which one should be that of a pregnant woman, should be dissected. If no pregnant woman were available, the body of a pregnant ape or cow could be substituted. Otherwise, he did not encourage the substitution of animal cadavers, in the case of a shortage of human ones. He thought it preferable to teach from sheets of diagrams or drawings (*foliata*). As a distinct enterprise, he called for much fuller studies of comparative anatomy than had hitherto been undertaken, alluding to the Aristotelian works on animals (a remark that reflects a growing interest shared by natural historians and anatomists in the second half of the sixteenth century).[58] Human dissection subjects "should not have been killed by some new and more terrible kind of death for the sake of a spectacle" (Cardano also considered hanging unacceptably cruel, preferring drowning as a more gentle death—a judgment with which not everyone will agree).[59] The *ostensor* should not discuss diseases and symptoms, because this must be done by the professor of medicine; the professor had also to teach any cure that depended on anatomy, but the dissector should show how to perform it (I am not sure whether the *ostensor* and dissector are meant to be two separate people—but evidently Cardano, like many of his contemporaries but unlike Vesalius, did not think it necessary for the professor to perform his own dissections).[60] Moreover, although anatomical anomalies should not be emphasized, attention could be drawn to abnormalities resulting from disease.

By way of an *accessus* to Mondino's text, Cardano situated it in the context of a history of the discipline and a comparative evaluation of other texts. The historical sketch included no mention of the early tradition of anatomical teaching on the human cadaver at the University of Bologna, the aspect of Mondino's activity subsequently best known to medical historians. Of the historical Mondino de' Liuzzi (d. 1326), who had been a professor of practical medicine at Bologna and the author of several learned commentaries besides the anatomy book, Cardano knew only that "he was a Florentine and I think a surgeon [*fuit Florentinus ut reor chirurgicus*]" who had lived about the time of Turisanus, "although none of this is certain." Instead, Cardano presented a classicizing account that began with Marinus (since Aristotle and Hippocrates were imperfect in this art), moved rapidly on to Galen, and lumped all subsequent Greeks and Arabs together as Galen's followers. The next event of major significance in the history of anatomy, according to Cardano, occurred thirteen hundred years after Galen, when Vesalius published the *Fabrica*.

Despite this reductive view of anatomy's history, Cardano's evaluation of Mondino's book was relatively sympathetic; Mondino was a man of good judgment and erudite to the extent that the conditions of his time and the anatomical texts and information then available allowed; his work was indeed full of errors but so was that of those who criticized him. Vesalius, who had studied anatomy with the greatest diligence, was also not immune from mistakes. Of other older anatomical works besides Mondino, only those of Galen were worth reading, but they were flawed because based on dissections of animals other than human beings and lacking illustrations. Moreover, the surviving books of *On Anatomical Administrations* were mostly about bones and muscles, and thus not very useful to physicians. Cardano's account of the anatomy of his own century is, as by now the reader will have come to expect, focused mainly on Vesalius. In contrast to the laudatory remarks about Vesalius scattered through Cardano's other works, the account here includes critical elements as well as praise. The *Fabrica* is characterized as "a beautiful description" in both text and pictures. But although Cardano discounted particular errors, which he regarded as inevitable in a book of such length and complexity, he claimed the work had some general faults, of which the chief was a tendency to carp excessively at Galen.[61] As will shortly become apparent, he also found the illustrations wanting in some respects.

Much more strikingly negative is a capsule biography of the *Fabrica*'s author. Cardano's interest in shaping and reshaping the story of his own life also extended to the lives of others. The narratives that accompany his horoscopes, for example, frequently summarize or characterize the subject's life. Shifts, contradictions, and revisions are as likely to be present in these estimates as in any other aspect of Cardano's thought. In the case of Vesalius, almost all Cardano's references to him are laudatory. In the *Contradictiones*, he gave Vesalius the highest of Renaissance accolades, describing him as "a man redolent of ancient ingenuity."[62] The horoscope, written about 1547, fills out the picture, adding favorable references to moral characteristics of studiousness and serious intent. The horoscope of Vesalius, in the sense of the actual astrological chart, was given to Cardano by the German astronomer and astrologer Georg Joachim Rheticus sometime in the mid-1540s. The accompanying narrative is, however, almost certainly Cardano's, and certainly expresses the opinions he wished to publish as his in 1547. These encomia, written when Vesalius was alive and in a position to do Cardano favors, are echoed in his autobiography written in 1575, long after Vesalius's death. There Cardano described the anatomist as "a most distinguished man and my friend" (of course, claimed friendship with Vesalius could also be useful even after the latter's death). In between comes the attack on Vesalius's character in Cardano's commentary on Mondino. These accounts cannot be read either for Vesalius's "real" character or for Cardano's "real" opinion. But they do throw some light on the different contexts in which Cardano came to terms with Vesalius's career and personality.[63]

The passage in the commentary on Mondino moves from listing defects in the *Fabrica* to criticism of the author. According to Cardano, two of these defects were omission of depictions of complete limbs and joints (that is, for example, showing the foot complete with bones, muscles, blood vessels, and nerves in a single illustration) and failure to teach how to treat tumors and ulcers. The second deficiency was explained by Vesalius's own incompetence in this area, which resulted in his botching the treatment of a cardinal's foot.

> I would not say this so that I might detract from the glory of Vesalius, whom I will call not divine (far from it), those people say that kind of thing who during his lifetime used to adulate him excessively with that sobriquet, but attacked and contradicted him on real issues: but I will call him a man of higher than human condition and admirable for his discoveries who lacked only the capacity ever to be satisfied in wealth and ambition, in which he resembled other outstanding men, and which turned out badly for him. For he had more than enough glory among mortals, not only more than he would have hoped but more than he would have desired, as the medical doctor of the emperor and of King Philip, the most powerful of all the kings that are recorded, having preserved Carlos, his only son, from imminent death, so that he really could be said to have snatched him from the jaws of death. But then annoyed by the irritations of envy, he undertook a wrongheaded voyage and died a little over the age of fifty, childless,[64] deprived of literary studies; he was cheated of his glory, he dispersed his wealth, and it is very likely that he was burdened by a great mass of sins; these things are the fruit of royal courts and immoderate greed, such uncertain goods.[65]

In this account, therefore, Vesalius is convicted of surgical incompetence and excessive ambition, in addition to being made to serve as almost a moral exemplum of the evils of cupidity. The most immediate stimulus to construct this narrative was probably the arrival of a report of Vesalius's death at Zante on the way back from his pilgrimage to Jerusalem. Conceivably, the report in question was either one of the letters on this subject written by Jean Matal from Cologne in April and May 1565, or some intermediate source deriving therefrom, since Matal attributed Vesalius's death to avarice (which had led him to allow inadequate funds and supplies for his journey).[66] The fresh impression made by this or another report, the self-appointed task of preparing a critique of the *Fabrica* from the standpoint of education for medical practice, reading of Falloppia's criticisms of Vesalius, and association with anatomists a generation younger than Vesalius might well combine to produce such an evaluation. The reference to Vesalius's journey to Jerusalem as wrongheaded (*praeposterus*) is at once ambiguous and provocative: was the journey wrongheaded because it was a pilgrimage or because it was poorly supplied? One would always like to know more about the nature of Cardano's relations with Erasmian ideas and his Protestant contacts—in this instance again including Coiter.

But Cardano's own self-presentation is also at stake here, since his accounts of himself are replete with ambiguity and tension over issues connected with money and the desire for money. On the one hand, he dwelt on his rise from youthful poverty to prosperity in middle life and expressed pride and satisfaction in the large sums paid or offered for his services.[67] On the other, he stressed his continuing relative poverty and indifference to material gain. The description of himself as bearing poverty with a cheerful face that he put into the mouth of his interlocutor in the unpublished prison dialogue *Carcer* (supposedly written in 1570 at the time of his own brief imprisonment) is quite characteristic in this respect.[68] The wills he made in Bologna and Rome show him in fact to have been modestly prosperous at the end of his life, although it is clear that he spent money on his intellectual interests as fast as it came in—for example, in collecting talismanic gems inscribed with occult symbols.[69]

Notwithstanding the defects he found in both Galen and, now, Vesalius, Cardano believed that *De usu partium, On Anatomical Administrations,* and the *Fabrica* were the most important books on anatomy.[70] But the order in which the contents were arranged in these works was not ideal for an anatomy useful to medical practitioners. For anatomy considered as an art, the order of the *Fabrica*, beginning with bones and muscles, was both perfect in itself and greatly preferable to what Cardano thought Galen's lack of order. But from the standpoint of the *scientia* of medicine, only the last three, physiological, books of the *Fabrica* were valuable to physicians, bones and muscles being the province of the surgeon. Hence Mondino's "order of dissection," beginning with the viscera, appealed to Cardano not only for the obvious pragmatic reason having to do with putrefaction, but also because it fitted in both with Galenic physiology and with his ideas about the kind of anatomy that was useful in medical practice.[71] However, in a comment highly revealing of the intimate association of anatomy with the judicial process, he remarked that one caveat about the use of Mondino as a textbook was that it was important to remember to begin the lectures four or five days before the condemned person was executed. In that way, preliminary generalizations that Cardano (perhaps unlike practicing anatomists) thought essential would not be skipped over in the rush to dissect before putrefaction set in.[72]

The representation of anatomy was in his view achieved by four means: *oratio, ichnographia, foliatum, sceletum,* none of which could stand alone. By *oratio* he meant anatomical narrative or description in words. The distinction between *ichnographiae*—a term also used in the sixteenth century for city plans—and *foliata* appears to be between anatomical drawings in books and diagrams, drawings, or paper constructions on independent sheets. The literary style of anatomical narrative was important: it ought to be continuous, well ordered, clear, and diffuse. By this standard, although neither author was perfect, he preferred Galen's "Asiatic eloquence" to Vesalius's style—"arid, brief, succinct, rough, with intent mind rather than smooth eloquence." What Vesalius needed was another Vesalius to lecture on and interpretatively expand his text. Cardano must surely be the only person ever to have found the more than six hundred folio pages of labyrinthine Latin prose in the first edition of the *Fabrica* excessively succinct. He put Vesalius's stylistic failings down to youth; Vesalius had written the *Fabrica* at an age when he, Cardano, "had not written a page that I did not commit to the flames, or wish to."[73]

Instructive *foliata* ought to be provided as subordinate accompaniment to complete and well-expressed anatomical narrative. Cardano optimistically planned to accompany his own commentary with an exceptionally complex set of eight hand-colored sheets, each showing a different region of the body and the connections of the organs within it, so that even the dullest intellect could see the three-dimensional relation of the parts.[74] Characteristically, the idea is a somewhat impractical elaboration of a known device. Hand-colored three-dimensional paper constructions are a striking feature of some sixteenth-century printed scientific books, especially in astronomy. Anatomical illustrations intended for students were sometimes issued as separate sheets designed to make it possible for the user to cut out and paste subsidiary pictures of individual organs in the right position. The most famous examples are those included by Vesalius himself in both the *Fabrica* and the *Epitome*, on pages that were originally available unbound as well. Vesalius also published separate sheets of anatomical diagrams—the *Tabulae anatomicae sex*—for student use. In addition, from the 1530s until the seventeenth century, various printers produced another kind of fugitive anatomical sheet, evidently intended to satisfy popular curiosity about the body: these instructive and entertaining toys (as Andrea Carlino has termed them) featured attractive illustrations that opened and closed combined with much simplified vernacular texts.[75]

Once the student had mastered the diagrams or constructions that Cardano proposed to provide, he could pass on to the plates in the *Fabrica*.[76] The preliminary study of Cardano's *foliata* was necessary because although the Vesalian plates were perfect as far as *ichnographia*—that is, presumably, the artistic representation of human anatomy—was concerned, Cardano found them lacking for instructional purposes. He complained that they did not depict all the parts of the human body, that the lettering was hard to read (as it is), and that they did not sufficiently show the movements, density, size, color, substance, location, and relations of the parts. Comparing them to other anatomical illustrations, he noted that Estienne's plates, although in all other respects inferior, were much better labeled (Estienne drew lines from each part to clear lettering placed outside the outline of the figure).[77] On the other hand, Leonardo's anatomical illustrations were beautifully drawn but scientifically worthless. Revising his previous judgment, he now completely dismissed their anatomical usefulness and denied Leonardo the status of a "*philosophus*" in anatomy that he had formerly attributed to him; Leonardo's drawings were "very beautiful and most worthy of such a famous artist, but indeed useless; he did not even know the number of the intestines. He was a pure painter, not a *medicus* or a philosopher."[78]

Even more ambitious was his suggestion for the improvement of teaching from the skeleton. "What indeed could be of the greatest use besides books, although an arduous and extremely difficult task . . . would be the construction of a skeleton, not the ordinary kind of the human bones, but of the whole body, so that nothing indeed was left to be desired. Therefore it would be necessary to make it out of hard material, lest so much labor of so many years and so much expense should perish in a short time, but it should also be malleable so that the smallest parts can also be shaped and bent and directed in any way. Therefore it should not be made from stone, or wood, or ivory, or wax, or clay, but from metal." After discarding lead, iron, gold, and silver (the last two because their value might tempt a prince who was "less attentive to glory and philosophy and the common good and the convenience of the human race" to melt the model down), Cardano settled on bronze as the most suitable material. The model was to be colored red, white, and other colors—presumably in imitation of nature—by alchemical means taught in "the book of secrets." The model was to have removable parts that could be taken away one by one, "just as in dissection," and then put together again (how to achieve this was also to be found in the book of secrets). Admittedly it would take an exceptionally learned *medicus* and a sculptor of great skill and subtlety working in collaboration to make this model, but the result would last for twenty years and "certainly be a work worthy of some outstanding prince." As it was, most princes spent their money "on useless rubbish . . . some of them on untimely wars, in which besides the slaughter of men and the burning of noble buildings nothing appears of convenience or profit, others in heaping up great piles, others on magnificent buildings, others on machines that show the motions of the heavens—they pour out immense treasures neither for useful purposes nor with knowledge of a certain end." Once more combining the themes of the philosophical significance and medical and surgical usefulness of anatomy, he continued with mounting enthusiasm: "What more generous, more outstanding, more beautiful, more useful than this construction that would make it possible to see how all the viscera, senses, and penetralia of nature are inside; and it could even be shown to students of philosophy and truth, seeing that there is no more illustrious and admirable spectacle under the moon than the human body, and also to physicians so that without any horror or danger of stench of vileness they could see daily not only how useful and healthful, but also necessary to the health of the sick, of whom the majority perish owing to the ignorance of the doctors, are those things that pertain to the composition, site, harmony, and size of the internal organs. Then indeed so great is the necessity for surgeons of this knowledge. . . ."[79] The passage concludes with a list of disasters caused by anatomically ignorant surgeons who leave patients paralyzed, lame, deformed, or scarred, or inadvertently cause them to bleed to death.

The enticing vision of a life-size,[80] anatomically accurate, model human being with a complete set of detachable internal parts, colored according to nature, is yet another example of the way in which Cardano's technicolor imagination seized on, enlarged, and transformed more sober ideas and techniques that came within his range of experience. As already noted, his interest in precise three-dimensional representation of parts of the human body went back at least to 1550, when he described the technique for making plaster death masks in *De subtilitate*. At Bologna, however, he came into close contact with a pioneer in the use of three-dimensional models to teach anatomy, namely, Volcher Coiter. Although wax models were made earlier by artists, the use of écorchés (muscle figures) and other types of three-dimensional models in wax, ivory, wood, or bronze by anatomists in teaching seems to have begun in the second half of the sixteenth century.[81] Coiter's interest in this method of teaching was more than casual. His pride in his model—which was probably his own work, for he was a competent anatomical artist—led him to have his portrait painted with it. He stands, appropriately, in front of a shelf of learned books, in the act of dissecting an arm.

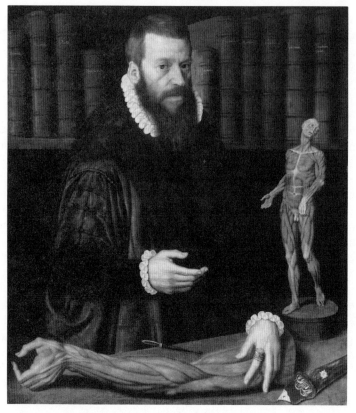

Portrait of Volcher Coiter with his anatomical model. When Coiter was at Bologna, his interest in anatomical modeling may have attracted Cardano's attention. Subsequently, from 1569 to 1575, Coiter held the position of town physician of Nuremberg, where this portrait was painted. Attributed to Nicholas Neufchatel, who painted the portraits of a number of Nuremberg patricians, it is dated 1575 and was donated to the Nuremberg Stadbibliothek in the same year. Photography courtesy Museen der Stadt Nurnberg.

On the table beside him is placed an écorché resembling one of the muscle men in the *Fabrica* (perhaps Plate 1 of Book 2). It looks to be about two or three feet high and is colored red and white; it is impossible to tell the material, though the color suggests that wax is likely. There is, of course, no way of knowing whether the actual construction of the model took place in Italy or after Coiter's return to the north. The portrait was painted at Nuremberg (where he held the position of city physician for several years) in 1575, almost a decade after his departure from Italy.[82] Whatever the case, his interest in the subject was doubtless already aroused during the period he was at Bologna. Coiter's model looks to have been a practically useful aid for teaching about the superficial muscles. But Cardano's imagination raced ahead of the limitations of small size, immobility, and restriction to one layer of the male body inherent in Coiter's actual achievement to an alchemically achieved perfect simulacrum of mankind.

MEDICAL SIGNS: DIAGNOSIS, PROGNOSIS, AUTOPSY

Medicine, like astrology, was a science of interpreting signs. Central to Cardano's belief in the usefulness of anatomy for internal medicine was his conviction that autopsy could yield clear signs in certain confirmation of previous diagnosis and prognosis of the living patient. Just as a retroactive horoscope of a historical personage—of which Cardano cast many—would reveal the underlying astral causes that had shaped his or her life, so a physician who studied postmortem appearances in the interior of the body of a former patient would find hitherto hidden evidence to support conclusions that he had previously arrived at via the patient's story and inspection of the body's exterior interpreted in the light of medical teaching. Perhaps Cardano's confidence in his ability to interpret postmortem signs was strengthened by a reading of Fernel's *Medicina*, first published in 1554, which was to become one of the most influential medical works of the century. Cardano's admiration for Fernel, whom he met in Paris in 1552 and with whom he shared a number of interests (see chapter 7) has already been noted. Fernel, too, was a forceful advocate of learning anatomy from direct study of the dissected cadaver; the information thus obtained was, he thought, as essential a prerequisite for medicine as geography was for history. Moreover, Fernel's writing on pathology spoke directly to one of Cardano's main interests as a practitioner: a chapter on diseases of the lung provided a series of correlations between clinical observations of respiratory disease and signs at autopsy together with notably full description of abnormal appearances in the dissected lung.[83]

At Bologna, Cardano was given or made the opportunity to put his ideas about autopsy into practice. In his several accounts of an episode or episodes that took place in 1565–66 both the roles of the actors and the purpose and nature of the autopsies shift and blur. His final version of the story ran as follows: "There are two things that I used to promise publicly at Bologna. . . . The second (this time reserving the right to accept any particular case or not) was that if anyone was about to die, I would show the site of the disease, and if after the person had died it was shown that I had been wrong, I would have to pay a penalty of a hundred times the fee I had received [for the diagnosis]. Therefore since at first many people were openly hoping that I could be shown to be wrong, they dissected bodies, for example, those of Senator Orso, Doctor Pellegrini, and Giorgio Ghisleri. . . ."[84] In this version, the focus is on the demonstration of Cardano's special powers, not on any general usefulness of autopsies. The context is that of a public challenge, paralleling his other undertaking to cure all comers. The initiative in actually undertaking the autopsies is not his but that of colleagues, whose chief motivation is a mixture of hostility to Cardano and acquisitiveness (they evidently share his fondness for a wager). As a result, they become witnesses to a series of triumphant demonstrations of his skill in diagnosis.

This distillation of the most personal and harshest elements in the story comes from *De vita propria*. But in another version, written very soon after the events, Cardano incorporated his experiences of autopsy into a wholesale revision of the doctrine of medical signs.[85] Here, too, professional competitiveness and his own superior powers are major themes. The thrust of the argument is, however, to establish interpretation of signs in the cadaver as a standard category of medical knowledge, not to claim it as a uniquely private gift. Hence he maintained that the use of autopsy to confirm previous diagnosis constituted a third kind of medical interpretation, alongside the traditional pair, diagnosis and prognosis. Moreover, this third category was not only persuasive in arguments among physicians but also more effective than either of the other two in establishing the authority of medicine before the laity. *Pathognomicon* (diagnosis) could seldom be based on symptoms sufficiently unambiguous to convince the laity: "[it] is not much valued because there is nothing about these things that can be shown by sense perception to ordinary people, just as if [a physician] were to say, 'this man is suffering from an obstruction or an ardent fever,' the common people and the unskilled reply 'Who knows? [The doctor] says this because one can't argue about it. God knows, perhaps it is so, perhaps not.'"[86] Consequently, if the patient dies, the physician is blamed for not having properly diagnosed the disease; and if he or she recovers, it is said to be by chance, and the physician may still be accused of misdiagnosis, often by a colleague. In the context of the doctor-patient relationship, prognosis too, for all its centrality to Hippocratic medicine and parallels with the other predictive art of astrology, had its limitations. Although prognosis "is indeed famous and in this the art of the physician is shown, yet it is of little use for the authority of the physician." The lack of proper respect for prognosis was, he thought, largely due to its limited actual utility to the sick but also came about because many people did not believe that "divination of this kind" existed in medicine.[87]

Thus the new third category of sign constituted by postmortem appearances in the dissected human cadaver, although unknown to Hippocrates and Galen, emerged as the "noblest" of all. Signs in this category Cardano termed "evident." In seeking out signs in the cadaver to confirm previous diagosis, "I was extremely fortunate and, first in my own time, and perhaps the first of all who went before us, I introduced it and dared to give it a prominent central role and test it; that is, I would say from what disease a patient was suffering, or in what part of the body, or in what member, so that if one of the other physicians objected to my treatment, when the patient died I would be able to show by dissection of the cadaver that I had been right and that the patient had died through someone else's fault. Since I often and often did as I have said, it turned out, very happily, that all those who could be cured were cured, and afterwards I would treat the sick with no one contradicting me."[88] The claim to priority does not, of course, relate to the performance of autopsies, but to public displays of diagnostic prowess. Whatever the truth of the claim, one model for Cardano's "tests" seems likely to have been Galen's public anatomical demonstrations, also conducted as theatrical displays with a view to illustrating the errors of opponents.[89] But whereas the demonstrations of Galen—and his Renaissance imitators—were of anatomical skill and knowledge, Cardano appears to have been trying to devise similar and equally impressive public performances for internal medicine.

With no mention of any wager or specific public challenge, the multiplication in 1565–66 of opportunities for such tests appears in this account as purely a matter of luck. The *necessarii* had offered him more bodies and had indeed even asked for bodies for him. Furthermore, he added with satisfaction, "these were not just bodies of vile persons handed over for the sake of the barber's fee, but they were all noble cadavers." The remark confirms the likelihood that private anatomical activity on occasion involved the purchase of the bodies of the destitute. Quite different was the case of noble bodies, the availability of which for inspection was, as Cardano explained to his readers, due to the aristocratic custom of opening the body in order to remove the viscera and brain for the sake of embalming.[90] Autopsy's signs are thus noblest not only because they are "evident" but also perhaps because they are frequently found in noble bodies. One example was Giorgio Ghisleri; when this Bolognese patrician was dying, he showed intestinal and gastric symptoms that led Cardano to pronounce that his stomach was injured and his liver burned, totally putrefied, and black. Ghisleri's body was dissected in the church of S. Francesco, which had also been the site of Vesalius's public anatomy in Bologna in 1540.[91] The organs were found in the state Cardano had predicted, to the admiration of three *medici* present, one of whom was Aranzio who presumably performed the actual dissection.[92] As this example shows, the arbitrary and obscure char-

acter of both diagnosis and the description of "evident" signs in autopsy
could facilitate the claim for a relation between the two.

Cardano concluded his lecture on signs by reasserting not only the
value of the "evident signs" to be found in the cadaver but the benefits
for all physicians of acquiring skill in interpreting them. "[I]f someone
is proficient in signs of this kind, his statements will be taken for oracles
in the art, even by his rivals; nor is there any comparison between this
category of 'evident signs' and the other categories."[93] His account is
highly suggestive of some of the factors contributing to "proficiency" of
the kind he had in mind and no doubt possessed. Among them, one
would certainly be inclined to give a prominent place to the physician's
persuasiveness and ability to impress (and no doubt Cardano was correct
in the conviction that his own powers were superior), to the role of collective and individual memory in the transition from diagnosis to autopsy, and to the willingness of the witnesses to confirm one another's
agreement that particular appearances in the abdominal or thoracic cavity could be correlated with, or interpreted in terms of, current disease
theory.

In addition to the record of public challenge and personal triumph in
De vita propria and the teaching on medical signs just summarized, Cardano left yet another account of one of the same group of autopsies,
that of Gianbattista Pellegrini. Cardano's lengthy description of the illness and death of this friend and colleague is one of his most detailed
medical narratives and as such will receive fuller analysis in another chapter. But the story includes an account of Pellegrini's autopsy that presents it, not in terms of a public demonstration of mastery of medical
signs, but as a private collaborative investigation in which Cardano was
intimately involved. Pellegrini died at the age of forty-eight after a lin-
gering illness that Cardano, contrary to two other attending physicians,
believed to be an affliction of the lungs.[94] Thereafter,

> It was therefore asked if I might dissect the cadaver, and I undertook it
> with the outstanding German anatomist Volcher who was a professor of the
> subject and we dissected [Pellegrini]. No hard tumor was found in the
> muscle of the right part, nor in the liver, nor in any of the inferior viscera,
> nor anything hard, only we saw the liver was of rather languid and pale
> color, that is tending toward white, but it was not attached to the di-
> aphragm by the usual transverse adhesions as in the rest of men, but it was
> almost wholly connected to it by other adhesions, so that that whole part
> was joined to it; similarly his stomach was also connected by ligaments of
> an unnatural kind to the diaphragm. Again the whole lung in the bottom
> part was joined in the same way by adhesions to the diaphragm, and to the
> membrane surrounding the ribs in front at the back and on the sides, which
> indeed Volcher himself said he had observed in many others, especially

those who died from phthisis. Besides the lung was very large so that it occupied almost the whole chest, and joined to the pericardium. But it was all full with hard swellings [tubercles] and blisters full of water.[95]

This autopsy report, striking in its immediacy, was written on September 7, 1566, the day after Pellegrini's death. In it Cardano bore public witness to his appreciation of Coiter, notwithstanding the latter's brush with the Inquisition, which had taken place before that date. Probably soon after Cardano wrote these words, Coiter left Italy forever. The passage is a record of a harmonious collaboration between Coiter and Cardano, apparently in private, which seems to have begun within a year of their arrival in Bologna. Probably in late 1563, Cardano wrote of observations he had made during "some" dissections, "with Volcher, a skilled German, doing the cutting [*secante Folcherio viro Germano perito*]."[96] Moreover, if the language of the description of Pellegrini's autopsy is to be taken literally, on this occasion Cardano the physician actively participated in dissection ("*Rogatum igitur ut dissecarem, accessi . . . dissecuimus*"). In turn, Coiter the anatomist was able to offer his own informed comments on clinico-anatomical correlation. Presumably as a result, the description is much more anatomically specific than in the case of Ghisleri, in which, it would appear, the judgment was all Cardano's and Aranzio's role was reduced to cutting and expressing *admiratio*. Pellegrini's autopsy was undertaken to demonstrate the correctness of Cardano's diagnosis, but it is not presented as part of a systematic program of such demonstrations. Rather, it has more the character of an investigation, for which the principal motivating factors appear to be his personal interest in Pellegrini's case, his long-standing involvement with phthisis and similar complaints, and his regard for Coiter. One might indeed speculate that Cardano's spell of intensified interest in and increased practice of autopsy precisely in 1565 had much to do with his admiration for Coiter and the latter's openness to collaboration.

Cardano's endeavors to show the usefulness of anatomy for internal medicine were, of course, ill-founded. It is a truism that Renaissance anatomy had little or no relevance to or impact on therapy, except in the case of arguments about phlebotomy. As far as diagnosis was concerned, only a few correlations between symptoms in life and postmortem findings were, or could be, securely recognized. Perhaps, indeed, his confidence in his ability to point to such relations initially sprang from knowledge (from personal experience or reading) of abnormalities in the lungs of some phthisical patients. But his adoption of Vesalius as a model for his own criticisms of Galen, his ready participation in anatomical debate, his schemes for improving anatomy teaching, his confidence in autopsy as a means of enhancing medical authority and individual reputations, his continued reading of new works as they were published—all testify to the seriousness of the attention he gave to contemporary anatomy and its significant impact on his ideas and activities, including his teaching. His remarks placing autopsy among medical signs and his full description of Pellegrini's autopsy come from a course of lectures delivered in his capacity as a professor of medical theory.

Some aspects of his treatment of anatomy are typically Cardanesque in their extravagance: the insistence on his own powers of diagnosis and recognition of postmortem signs and the floridly imagined model man. But much else is fairly characteristic of the ways in which new understanding or presentation of anatomy was partially absorbed, modified (or distorted), or put to serve specific needs within the general ambience of Renaissance medical culture. There are analogues in contemporary publishing projects: the proposal to make anatomy useful to physicians by way of Mondino plus three-dimensional diagrams and the Vesalian illustrations is not so different from Thomas Geminus's actual combination of Vesalius's plates and indexes with a text that ultimately derived from the anatomical portion of the early-fourteenth-century work on surgery by Henri de Mondeville.[97] In the classroom too, Cardano was by no means alone among learned professors of medical *theoria* in incorporating allusions to the new anatomy into his lectures on ancient books. In general, *theoria* was far from as isolated from current developments as is sometimes supposed. Few, however, were as eager as Cardano to press Vesalian anatomy into service in expounding Hippocratic texts. To Cardano as interpreter of Hippocrates it is now time to turn.

philosophy, as already noted in chapter 3, he used Hippocratic texts as a
source and endorsement of some of his key ideas. He directed his interest in history to the question of the authenticity and chronological sequence of the Hippocratic writings. In medicine, he portrayed himself as
a Hippocratic physician; moreover, Hippocratic texts provided key
sources and inspiration both for his attention to diet (discussed above in
chapter 4) and for endeavors to derive rules for use in diagnosis, prognosis, and therapy that would accommodate both general laws and the
particulars of experience. As a medical author, he planned to comment
on the entire Hippocratic corpus and actually produced a substantial
body of exposition that included major treatises seldom selected by other
commentators. As a commentator, he claimed both to understand Hippocrates' true meaning more accurately than Galen had done and to link
Hippocrates and Vesalian anatomy in mutual endorsement. But despite
the undoubtedly personal nature and unusual extent of Cardano's interest in Hippocratic medicine, his interpretation was in reality largely
shaped by existing medical, that is, Galenic, tradition. Cardano is seldom
more like Galen than when he claims—against Galen—to be the best interpreter of Hippocrates. Accordingly, the goal of the present chapter is
to explore some of these uses and meanings that Cardano found in Hippocratic medicine and investigate his endeavor to claim it for his own.

For many reasons, that claim turned out to be as chimerical as his endeavor to find clinical applications for Renaissance anatomy in internal
medicine. Indeed, as was just noted and will become further apparent,
his anatomical and Hippocratic enterprises were closely connected. But
just as much as his anatomical interests, Cardano's Hippocratism represented an enthusiastic response to contemporary developments. Some
Hippocratic works had been components of the Latin medical curriculum since the early Middle Ages; their author enjoyed general veneration
as a founder of medicine and the author of famous, if obscure, medical
books.[7] Humanists began to turn their attention to Hippocratic treatises
in the late fifteenth century.[8] But Fabio Calvo's Latin translation of the
corpus, which appeared in 1525, and the Aldine edition of the Greek in
the following year revealed in print the scope of the collection as a
whole, as well as making such major works as the complete *Epidemics*
and the Hippocratic writings on surgery generally available for the first
time.[9] New Hippocratic editions, translations, and commentaries continued to appear throughout Cardano's lifetime, most notably the Greek
edition (1538) and Latin translation (1546) of the corpus produced by
Janus Cornarius.[10] Moreover, interest in the Hippocratic books as witnesses to an early stage in the development of Greek language and Greek
science extended beyond medical circles: the young Joseph Scaliger
sharpened his critical skills on *On Wounds to the Head*.[11]

Although knowledge and appreciation of the Hippocratic texts became wider and deeper among university-trained physicians as the century progressed, nevertheless for most of them Galen, not Hippocrates, remained the principal authority in medicine. Moreover, Galenic medical ideas and Galen's commentaries on Hippocratic books shaped the way in which the Hippocratic texts were understood. Indeed, since Galen had proclaimed himself a follower of Hippocrates, the teaching of the two authorities was seldom distinguished.[12] Reevaluation of the relative merits of Hippocrates and Galen was an extremely slow process, which was only just beginning in the second half of the sixteenth century. In northern Europe, Paracelsus's praise of Hippocrates as opposed to Galen would subsequently be influential, but Paracelsus's view of Hippocrates was very little known before 1575.[13]

Cardano's Hippocratic enterprise thus forms part of a broader Renaissance Hippocratism, a subject about which much still remains to be learned. But, as usual, his approach was both personal and idiosyncratic. Hippocrates was for him at once a key figure in his planned renovation, mastery, and integration of natural knowledge and a vehicle for the justification of his own medical practice. He tried to do for the Hippocratic corpus what he believed he had done for Ptolemy's *Tetrabiblos*: for the true ancient medicine as for the true ancient astrology, he would clear away misinterpretations and explain and reestablish the authentic rules of the discipline. The result was a body of Hippocratic commentary that— in length and in the importance he himself attached to it—constituted one of his principal scientific enterprises, in or out of medicine. Only its most significant themes can be examined within the scope of this chapter. But first, an account of the genesis and fortunes of Cardano's Hippocrates project.

THE PROJECT

The origin of Cardano's special interest in Hippocrates seems to be yet another example of the rapidity with which he seized on significant new books. With his usual indifference to self-contradiction, he described the collection of accounts of diseases at Sacco that he began in 1526 first as "the size of the Hippocratic *Epidemics*" and subsequently as "rather slight and unworthy to be compared to the narration of Hippocrates."[14] Yet the two statements agree in implying that the Hippocratic *Epidemics* served him as a model. If in fact he originally made the comparison in 1526, rather than only in hindsight, it may have been based upon a reading of Calvo's translation, in which the complete *Epidemics* first became available in print, within a year of its publication.[15] The Aldine edition is not in question, since Cardano had not mastered Greek in 1526.

However, he could perhaps have gained an idea of the nature of the *Epidemics* from his reading in Galen or Arabic authors even before he encountered the complete work.[16]

The *Epidemics* was one of the most important "new" Hippocratic works to become available. It remains deservedly famous for the individual case histories that constitute some of the most notable examples of Greek observational science. The case histories were, however, only one of several features that appealed to sixteenth-century readers, since the *Epidemics* also contained much material about the relations among disease, climate, and region, and appeared relevant to the art of prognosis. In contrast with his spontaneous and independent interest in the *Epidemics*, Cardano's appointment to a professorship in medical theory at Pavia brought with it the responsibility of lecturing on the *Aphorisms*, one of the Hippocratic texts traditionally central to medical teaching about diseases, symptoms, and their outcome, and the subject of a chain of commentaries stretching back to antiquity.[17] Before he left for Scotland in 1552, he had written his own commentary on part of the *Aphorisms*, probably basing it on the translation by the most celebrated of medical humanists, Niccolò Leoniceno.[18]

Shortly after his return from Scotland, Cardano began to work up his material on the *Epidemics* and the *Aphorisms* into a digest and exposition of all Hippocratic teaching. By so doing, he claimed, he had "completely covered four arts in one volume each"—previously arithmetic, astrology, and music, and now medicine.[19] Whether or not the one-volume digest of Hippocrates (of which no trace survives) was ever in fact finished, by 1561 it no longer satisfied its author. By then, he was projecting a complete exposition of the entire Hippocratic corpus, in which "the text will take up about three hundred *chartae* and there will be twelve hundred *chartae* of commentary, so that the work will have to be published in two volumes."[20] By *chartae* he probably meant folio sheets printed on both sides, in which case his figures translate into six hundred and twenty-four hundred pages.[21]

Cardano confidently expected his grand work on Hippocrates to appeal to a wide, socially elevated, and humanistically educated audience both in and outside the medical community. He believed that his most important scholarly contributions were in the four arts named in the last paragraph, although he recognized that his encyclopedic and philosophical works had broader appeal.[22] No doubt correctly, he attributed the small audience for his work in mathematics, astrology, and music both to the inherent difficulty of these technical disciplines and to social factors: the low status of most mathematical practitioners, the criticisms that had been leveled at astrology (he probably had Pico della Mirandola in mind), and the unintellectual character of most musical performers.

By contrast, "these commentaries on the entire teaching of Hippocrates, in addition to embracing the whole of the art, give pleasure with *historia* and are also useful, and are written for erudite, noble, and rich people. The art [of medicine] itself is held in veneration, and the fame of the author is outstanding."[23]

The two handsome folio volumes, so precisely and fondly envisaged (perhaps as vivid in his mind's eye as the red, green, and gold cover of *De rerum varietate* shown him in a dream),[24] never appeared. Nor did Cardano interpret all the works ascribed to Hippocrates, although he continued to work on them almost up to his death.[25] But he did produce more than twelve hundred printed folio-sized pages of Hippocratic commentary. The extent of this body of work becomes even more striking when contrasted with his meager output of commentary on other medical authors.[26] Besides his interpretation of Hippocrates, Cardano's Hippocratic commentaries exemplify his ideas about proper methods and goals in medical commentary as a genre. Cardano was as fully committed as any of his contemporaries to the idea that one of the main obligations of a scholarly physician and professor of medicine was to provide sound expositions of authoritative texts. But implicitly—and often explicitly—he was highly critical of most of the ways the task had been carried out. As will become apparent from what follows, at different times, and for different reasons, the objects of his criticism ranged from Galen himself through scholastic authors and leading sixteenth-century medical philologists. Some of these criticisms may spring from his own experiences, first as a medical student attending lectures and later as a practitioner endeavoring to wrest a medical meaning from volumes of academic exposition. Yet in their final form his own commentaries, too, are in most respects conventional academic productions for their time and place.

In the versions finally published, all but one of Cardano's Hippocratic commentaries are based on academic lectures given at Bologna, where it is evident that he systematically devoted most of his teaching to Hippocrates.[27] He began in 1562–63 with the *Aphorisms*.[28] In 1563–64, he taught Books 1 and 2 of the *Epidemics*;[29] in 1565–66, *Prognostic*;[30] in 1567–68, *Airs Waters Places*;[31] in 1568–69, *Aliment*;[32] and in 1569–70, *Regimen in Acute Diseases*.[33] Perhaps realizing that his glowing advance description of the complete commented Hippocrates in a massive two-volume set had failed to attract the attention of patron or publisher, he published these expositions as independent volumes. Four of the lengthy commentaries just mentioned, plus a shorter exposition of *On the Seven Month Child*, appeared in the decade between 1564 and 1574.[34] Only his commentaries on *Regimen in Acute Diseases* and the first two books of the *Epidemics* remained to be published posthumously.

CLASSIFYING THE CORPUS

Writing in an age in which traditional schemes of the arts and sciences were beginning to be disrupted by new disciplines and new philosophies of nature, Cardano gave considerable thought to the place of the Hippocratic corpus in the system of natural knowledge. He experimented with at least four different classifications of its treatises. In three Hippocratic commentaries and a work on practical medicine, all written within the space of a decade, he arranged the corpus twice as a collection of medical texts, each differently ordered; once as an encyclopedia of moral and natural philosophy and medicine; and once in supposedly historical or chronological sequence. Each of these shifting classifications served a plausible purpose in its specific context, a sign perhaps of the increasing fluidity or even pragmatism of disciplinary concepts after midcentury. Conceivably, a little work by Sylvius on the classification of medical books, first published in 1539, which listed some fifty Hippocratic titles, might have provided general inspiration for these endeavors. But Sylvius's classification is very unlike any of Cardano's; it intermingles works of Hippocrates and Galen and uses an entirely different system of division.[35]

The simpler of Cardano's two medical schemes, prefaced to his commentaries on the *Epidemics*, divided the Hippocratic corpus into introductory, theoretical, and practical works. In the division into theory and practice, though not in the allocation of individual treatises, this scheme matched the standard categories of the university curriculum. Since it also classifies the *Epidemics* as a theoretical work on prognostic, it seems likely that its intended function was to justify the suitability of some books of the *Epidemics* as texts in the curriculum in medical theory and the basis for lectures by Cardano, professor of medical theory at Bologna.[36]

The second, and more refined, medical scheme took as its starting point the statement attributed to "Suidas" that Hippocrates wrote sixty works in addition to the *Oath*, *Prognostic*, and *Aphorisms*.[37] Cardano divided the total of sixty-three (which he held included sixteen lost works) into nine sets of seven, assigning a different medical subject to each set: medical ethics; principles of the subject of medicine, namely, the human body; parts of the body; diseases, diagnosis, and general prognostication (the *Epidemics* and *Airs Waters Places* are both in this set); specific prognostication; diet; therapy; surgery; and a miscellaneous category. In this scheme, the only exception allowed to the purely medical classification of the corpus is the statement that some parts of the *Aphorisms* belong more to divination. Furthermore, the scheme takes for granted the controversial position that the subject of medicine is the human body (rather than health), and subsumes anatomy and physiology completely under medicine.[38] Prefaced to his commentary on *Airs Waters Places*, the scheme had of course the advantage of justifying the presence of the extensive geographic and ethnographic content of that work in a medical curriculum.

By contrast, in a preface to a section of his commentary on the *Aphorisms*, a core work of the standard university curriculum, Cardano presented Hippocrates as the author of an encyclopedia of moral philosophy, natural philosophy, and medicine for physicians. This time, the works on medical ethics belong to moral philosophy. Hippocratic natural philosophy concerns "the beginning of all things," that is, the teaching on material immortality, the three elements, and celestial heat in *De diaeta* (*Regimen*) and *Fleshes*, which, Cardano once again took the opportunity to note, he had adopted as his own;[39] "the principles of mortal things," namely, the four humors and the primary qualities, first taught by Hippocrates in *On Human Nature*, "from which the whole Peripatetic philosophy flowed down";[40] the simple and composite parts of animals (that is, roughly, tissues and organs); reproduction; and the nature and customs of peoples, expounded in *Airs Waters Places*.[41] The remaining books, defined as purely medical, are divided into four groups (each further subdivided): the nature of medicine; "removing superstition from medicine," a category containing only *On the Sacred Disease*; regimen in health, diseases (internal, dental, gynecological, epidemic, acute), and surgery; prognostic and maxims. In this scheme, anatomy and physiology are part of natural philosophy and *Airs Waters Places* has turned into a treatise on anthropology. The *Aphorisms* itself, however, is categorized as purely medical. The arrangement seems masterful. On the one hand, it manages to perform the traditional task of reminding students engaged with a core text in medical theory of the intersection between their branch of medicine and the dignity of natural philosophy, while neatly obviating philosophical discussion of the *Aphorisms* itself—something Cardano wanted to avoid, since he thought of the work as a practical medical handbook (see further below); on the other, it pointedly reinforces his claim that his own idiosyncratic natural philosophy was based on correct principles drawn from (other) authoritative Hippocratic texts.

The fourth classificatory scheme, which occurs in a practical handbook of diagnosis and therapy, reveals both Cardano's strong personal interest in history (which he described as one of his chief pleasures)[42] and the assumption, typical of humanist medicine, that philological or historical investigation of ancient medical texts and practical usefulness in medical education were one and the same. Renaissance approaches to the history of the Hippocratic corpus rested on premises almost diametrically opposed to those of twentieth-century scholarship: Hippocrates, about whom a good deal of reliable biographical information was available, was securely the author of a large body of texts, usually held to include his correspondence.[43] Nevertheless, awareness grew that statements by Galen showed that not every book ascribed to Hippocrates was actually by him. Girolamo Mercuriale's *Censura Hippocratis* (1584), which assembled references to individual Hippocratic treatises by various ancient authors, has been called, perhaps deservedly, the beginning of "serious modern interest in the question of authenticity among the works attributed to Hippocrates."[44] But twenty years earlier, Cardano was already giving thought to the problem of establishing criteria for the identification of genuine works of Hippocrates. He—and indeed Mercuriale— may have been encouraged to do so by the attention drawn to the topic in a commentary attributed to Galen on the Hippocratic *De humoribus* published in 1562.[45]

According to Cardano, there were three valid criteria for the attribution of a written work: an author's own testimony; the witness of contemporaries, or of someone of good judgment who was very familiar with the oeuvre—in this case Galen; and style. In judging style it was, however, necessary to be aware that the same author might write differently in different genres or at different times of life. Armed with these criteria, he divided the Hippocratic corpus into twelve classes, ranging from works that were "highly authentic [*germanissimi*]" and of the first importance for medical education to those that were "useless but enjoyable [*inutiles, sunt tamen lectu iucundi*]." *Airs Waters Places* headed the list, standing alone in the top class. Then came a class consisting of the *Aphorisms, Regimen in Acute Diseases, Prognostic*, and Books 1 and 3 of the *Epidemics*. The supposed correspondence of Hippocrates occupied the last place, at the bottom of the twelfth class.[46]

THE CHOICE OF TEXTS

The selection of Hippocratic works on which Cardano lectured at Bologna and on which he left written commentaries thus largely coincided with his own list of the most important and authentic Hippocratic works. With the exception of the *Aphorisms*, which as already noted was prescribed in the statutory curriculum, probably all of the treatises on which he taught represented his own choice.[47] In some cases, however, his choice was conditioned by or coincided with a long tradition of the schools. From the twelfth century to the 1530s or later, *Prognostic, Regimen in Acute Diseases*, and the *Aphorisms* had been closely linked in Latin medical teaching, since the three were major components in the collection of basic texts that came to be known as the *articella*.[48] By the mid–sixteenth century, the *articella* was no longer being reprinted, all three texts and Galen's commentaries on them circulated in humanist rather than medieval translations, and much more attention was being devoted to the *Aphorisms* than to the other two treatises. Nevertheless, all three were traditional teaching tools, although Cardano's approach to them certainly was not. He was, of course, by no means alone in using commentary on traditional medical textbooks as a vehicle for his own views. For example, at Padua in the 1540s Gianbattista Da Monte had endeavored to press portions of the *Canon* of Avicenna into the service of integrated medical teaching that would overcome some of the disadvantages of the traditional curricular division into theory and practice.[49]

By contrast, the *Epidemics, Airs Waters Places, Aliment,* and *On the Seven Month Child* were highly unusual choices, each of which, in one way or another, responded to Cardano's particular interests. The attraction of the embryological treatise, on which there seems to be only one other sixteenth-century Latin commentary, was probably its potential for astrological interpretation. Such, at any rate, is suggested by his explanation that the formation of a viable fetus required more than six months because the sun, "the author of the life of all things, as Ptolemy also teaches [*vitae omnium author . . . ut etiam Ptolemaeus docet*]," had to get beyond the opposite zodiacal sign from the sign at conception.[50]

His interest in *Aliment* was a late development. As he admitted, he forgot even to include this compilation of exceptionally obscure philosophical and physiological maxims in his discussion of the authenticity of Hippocratic works. His exposition was written after, and perhaps partially in response to, the appearance "in everybody's hands" of a commentary by his former rival at Bologna, Antonio Fracanzano.[51] But once his attention was focused, Cardano claimed to find in *Aliment* the fundamental principles underlying his own views on nutrition, physiology, and longevity (described in chapter 4).[52]

By contrast, the *Epidemics* was a lifelong interest. Cardano's efforts to interpret and apply these books, pioneering in 1526, were still unusual in the 1560s and 1570s when he wrote his expositions of Books 1 and 2, even though two other leading medical figures, namely, Fuchs and Da Monte, had by that time preceded him in commenting on parts of the work.[53] Although Cardano wrote commentaries only on Books 1, 2, and part of 3, he read and perhaps intended to comment on all seven books of the *Epidemics.* He wrote a preface to the work as a whole in which, in addition to attempting to differentiate the chronology and authors of the seven books (chiefly on the basis of information from Galen), he also discussed differences in their content; and in various places he cited Books 5, 6, and 7.[54] Clearly, the accounts of particular cases and outbreaks of disease appealed to his interest—historical and medical—in the record and narration of particulars.[55] He evidently perceived in this Hippocratic work a model for his own method, in all disciplines that he held to be somehow conjectural, of collecting examples from which predictive rules might be extracted or confirmed. At the same time, trained in a Galenic medical system, he unquestioningly accepted Galen's picture of Hippocrates as the author of universally valid basic medical precepts. Thus Hippocrates had written the *Epidemics* because he wanted "to constitute the foundations of the art from *experimentum*," but, simultaneously: "Since the whole work is all prognostication, it concerns expectation of the future and divination, which is also the divine part. And indeed . . . he who foresees the future really seems to be divine." Yet the *Epidemics* did not teach rules for prognostication in any simple or direct way; rather, it "narrates only the essence of the thing and does not teach what should be done."[56] The extraction of rules required effort and a methodical approach, but could be accomplished in two ways. First, the physician could go through the Hippocratic case histories looking for common elements: thus he could, for example, collect and categorize examples of abnormal varieties of urine and see with what diseases or symptoms they were associated. "The second utility is something I used to practice in my youth, trying for myself, and it was that I would read whatever had happened to a sick man without the outcome and judge whether he would die or not, and when; and if a man follows this in a few cases, how much glory he will hope for in medical practice, and if in many it is better, and if in all and fully then he will know he is already perfect."[57]

Alone among the Hippocratic works on which he commented, *Airs Waters Places* offered Cardano the possibility of fully integrating medicine, astrology, and philosophy of nature. Its teaching about the effects of weather, climate, and region on health and its enumeration—similar to that also found in Ptolemy's *Tetrabiblos*—of the characteristics of peoples inhabiting particular regions set forth ideas that became fundamental to ancient, medieval, and Renaissance understanding of the relation of human beings to their environment. Both books asserted with examples that the physical environment—celestial, climatic, and geographic— shaped the characteristics of peoples. In one form or another, this type of environmentalism was, of course, a standard part of cosmological theory in western Europe from the twelfth to the seventeenth century. The concept received a notable Renaissance reworking at the hands of Jean Bodin, who applied it to the European societies of his day.[58] But few or none of Cardano's contemporaries rivaled the attention he devoted to the Ptolemaic and Hippocratic texts; indeed, he seems to have been the only author who commented on both of them.

Airs Waters Places was, in Cardano's words, "extremely useful to physicians, philosophers, geographers, and astrologers."[59] But perhaps because of this multidisciplinary character it was not part of the standard medical curriculum and was not tackled by Latin commentators. He had therefore every reason to expect that his projected commentary would be the pioneer interpretation of an important work. He was somewhat disconcerted when, in 1557, the French physician Adrien L'Alemant published his commentary on *Airs Waters Places*, whole pages of which came—with acknowledgment—from Cardano's own commentary on the *Tetrabiblos*.[60] Cardano dealt with the situation with his usual aplomb. He instructed his students and readers, "I want every one of you to have a copy of the *vulgata commentaria* [of Alemanus] for easy consulting, in case our exposition seems to someone to be rather serious or difficult for beginners."[61]

Much more than any of Cardano's other medical works, the exposition of *Airs Waters Places* gave scope to his historical and anthropological interests and, indeed, his random curiosity. For example, among the topics that caught his interest were the identification of places and peoples named by Hippocrates (such as "the Sarmatae, whom we now call Muscovites and Poles"),[62] free cities in antiquity and the present, military and political conduct of the ancient Romans, the French habit of accompanying small snacks with a lot of wine, the poverty that forced some Italian parents to neglect their children, and the marvels of Africa according to Leo Africanus.[63] In one passage, he indulged in a burst of orientalist enthusiasm for the alchemical, erotic, and magical expertise of the East—Cianglu and Ciangli, Pianfu and Pazanfu—where "they cultivate three arts, chymia, lymia, and hymia. Chymia is what we call alchemy for transmuting metals and gems, which they know much better than we do, even though they cannot make gold or silver; however they change some gems so that you cannot tell them from real ones, but metals with great difficulty. Lymia is the amatory art, of which there is scarcely a trace among us, yet it is extant and I think it is in use among the Turks. Scymia is conjuring, at which they excel, nor do they only do conjuring tricks to deceive the eye, but they are so proficient in it that it is almost magic, controlling winds and rain and averting hail."[64] These aspects of the exposition, like the fairly frequent citations of the Aristotelian *Problemata*, link it to Cardano's encyclopedic writings and doubtless explain his expectation that it would appeal to a broad audience.[65]

The central focus is, however, philosophical, medical, and astrological. As one might expect, Cardano enriched the Hippocratic text with technical geographical and astronomical explanation, including tables and diagrams. He also introduced a number of criticisms of Aristotle's meteorology. He noted that the brief comments about stars and weather in the text seemed to come from Hesiod,[66] and supplemented them with an account of precisely how the stars affected health (maintaining that they exercised not only manifest influence on the weather through their light and motion but also occult influences via elementary qualities).[67] He insisted on the practical medical importance of awareness of the influence of different climates and customs with highly specific and local examples. A good physician ought to travel and would enjoy doing so: "there is so much of pleasure in it."[68] He should know local diseases (catarrh and melancholy at Bologna, pestilential fevers and diarrhea at Milan) and local remedies. He must be aware of the impact of a change of environment in order to recognize that an Italian in Spain would need different medical treatment from an Italian in Italy. He must know the customs of peoples—for example, that he could not prescribe pork to a Jew, even though it was very good for the stomach. He should be aware of deleterious local health practices, such as the Bolognese custom of using *fontes* (small surgical incisions, made and deliberately kept open solely to allow for the drainage of bad humors).[69] And, in the personal confirmation to which Cardano always ultimately returned, he noted that the Hippocratic author's description of the rigid, pertinacious, and contumacious inhabitants of bare, meager places lacking in water and with few changes in the weather was "very apt for the little town where our family comes from, Cardano . . . twenty-four miles from Milan."[70]

But although he unhesitatingly endorsed and amplified the Hippocratic author's environmental determinism for practical, medical purposes, he was also acutely aware that it involved difficult theoretical issues. The assertions about environmental influence on physiology and psychology in *Airs Waters Places* provided a series of opportunities to discuss the philosophical problem to which he so often returned, namely, the relation between fate, the power of the stars, or natural law on the one hand and chance, contingency, or human will on the other. Thus Jackie Pigeaud has called attention to Cardano's discussion of the implications for the relation of soul and body of the text's attribution of moral characteristics (e.g., cowardice and bravery) to the influence of region and climate.[71] In discussing nature and culture, he also raised the question of the origin of evil and the extent to which education and laws could change human nature for the better.[72] His conclusion concerning the latter was that "Christian law alone makes people really good, if it is applied to simple or to truly wise people; but sophists are made tricky, deceitful, and crafty."[73]

In the exposition of *Airs Waters Places*, Cardano returned to the question of how to extract usable medical rules from Hippocratic precepts, an issue that in some sense underlies his entire approach to Hippocratic medicine. This time, his discussion was both fuller and more explicit and decidedly less optimistic than in the preface to the *Epidemics*. The maxims in *Airs Waters Places* about environmental factors affecting physiology, physical characteristics, health, and mores[74] constituted much clearer and more direct precepts or rules than did the case histories in the *Epidemics*. But in any given case of illness, multiple factors supposedly operated simultaneously—climate, region, weather, the astrological situation, the patient's temperament, age, sex, ethnic identity, diet, and many more. Cardano the mathematician and mathematical astrologer was struck by the impracticality of working out how *all* the rules, in all their possible permutations and combinations, applied to *every* particular sick patient. By his calculation, a proper consideration of every possible astrological, environmental, and physiological influence responsible for a case of disease would involve taking 2,936 factors into consideration, a number that he subsequently upped to 3,194. Thus the multiplicity of these precepts made them effectively useless as a way of determining outcome or even estimating probabilities. The only practical medical solution for the dilemma that he was able to suggest was to assume that Hippocrates meant the physician to limit the environmental factors actually taken into account to changes in diet and exercise: to inquire, for example, into the effect on an Englishman of being forced to eat lightly and take a lot of exercise or on a Milanese of being compelled to subsist on vegetables in a time of dearth.[75] The central issue was thus to find a way of extracting usable rules that could be employed to guide therapy and predict outcome (or describe it retroactively). Looked at in this light, the problems of correctly interpreting the rules of Hippocratic medicine and the meaning of horoscopes do indeed appear very similar.

To make the matter even more difficult, the rules taught by Hippocrates in any case applied only to what was within the power of human knowledge to grasp: things that were evident and happened according to rule as well as a few obscurer things. Part of what did not occur according to rule (*"quae non ordinibus constat"*) fell into the category of conjectural knowledge for human beings. But only "better beings than ourselves have knowledge that extends not only to all peoples but also to individuals, and single events, and chance happenings, but these are understood with infinite reasons . . . and that knowledge of these infinite things is possessed by incorporeal beings, from which [they know] fate and causes of natural things and particulars and times and the way things happen and events, about which we do not have even conjectural knowledge."[76] The passage reveals how profoundly Cardano's Hippocratic medicine, like his Ptolemaic astrology and his autobiographical writings, is concerned with issues of certainty, chance, and probability—and, indeed, with the world of the daimons or angels.

HIPPOCRATIC MEDICINE / CARDANO'S MEDICINE

As noted earlier, Cardano habitually represented himself as the exponent of a medicine that was practical in several senses. It focused on disease and treatment, it was ratified by Cardano's personal experience with many patients, it purported to provide efficacious remedies and valid prognostications, and it avoided irrelevant or extraneous subject matter. In his Hippocratic writings, but especially in the commentaries on the standard teaching texts *Aphorisms* and *Prognostic*, all these claims are made on behalf of Hippocratic medicine as interpreted by himself. The main thrust of much of the exposition is to defend the medical validity of specific recommendations for treatment found in—or believed by Cardano to be substantiated by—the Hippocratic text, and to explain away any philological problems, inconsistency with other Hippocratic statements, or opposing views. In addition, Cardano endeavored to convince his readers that the text of the *Aphorisms* constituted a complete and systematically ordered manual of medical practice. He alleged that the *Aphorisms* had been assembled as a digest of all the teaching contained in other Hippocratic medical treatises.[77] He habitually pointed out topical connections between groups of aphorisms and asserted that "those who deny that these *Aphorisms* form a continuous work deserve no forgiveness."[78] And with the remark "No book of Aristotle or Galen is written with so much order,"[79] he claimed that the *Aphorisms* was actually superior in organization to the works of the two main academic authorities in natural philosophy and medicine. With the aid of Cardano's exposition, this supposedly systematic treatise could serve as both a handbook of practice for students and a justification and explanation of his own procedures as a practitioner.

He further proclaimed that his exposition of the *Aphorisms* would exclude speculative discussion of first principles that was irrelevant to medicine.[80] As already noted, the university curriculum in medical *theoria*, to which the *Aphorisms* belonged, retained strong ties to natural philosophy. Thus another major Hippocratic commentator, Antonio Musa Brasavola of Ferrara (1500–1555), found it entirely appropriate to begin his lectures on the *Aphorisms* by stressing his philosophical qualifications and approach; Brasavola explained that he had formerly taught natural philosophy, and now "we will begin to interpret the same natural philosophy under another name, for certainly the most distinguished men have judged medical theory to be part of natural philosophy."[81] In Cardano's view, irrelevant dialectical and metaphysical discussions had been introduced into the exposition of the *Aphorisms* by Galen and his followers: "I don't know what may be the good, or help in learning medicine, of those questions about first principles that are neither absolute nor sufficiently firmly established. The cavilings of Swineshead would be more useful, since they are more about real things than those arguments dealing with things about which there is as yet no agreement as to what they are."[82]

Only the application of this particular criticism to Galen and the appreciative twist to the remark about Swineshead put Cardano's own stamp on a sentiment that in other respects was far from original. Applied to fourteenth- and fifteenth-century scholastic physicians, denunciations of excessive devotion to speculative philosophy and disputation were a common theme in sixteenth-century medical rhetoric. Cardano further asserted that the cause of error in diagnosis and treatment by "Galen, Paul of Aegina, Avicenna, and all the professors of medicine today" was an excess of purely intellectual contemplation allied with insufficient experience in treating patients. But he was equally dissatisfied with less pretentious practitioners: "those who actually do treat patients neither engage in speculative thought, philosophy, and dialectic nor, being overwhelmed with such a multitude of sick people, do they notice similar or dissimilar things common to many of them." Hence the best professor of medicine, and the one most like Hippocrates, was one who began to teach after long experience of practice as Cardano himself had done.[83]

In holding up Hippocrates as, above all, a guide to medical practice, Cardano tended to assimilate Hippocrates' experience to his own. The idea appears overtly on the title page of the 1568 edition of the commentary on *Prognostic*, where it is asserted, "These men, Hippocrates and Cardano, besides the best doctrine, both had remarkably long and happy practice in the works of the art, since each of them wrote these things when he was over sixty years of age." The phrasing here may be the publisher's, but Cardano himself repeatedly expressed the same thought. Hippocrates, like himself, had written down in old age the things he had observed in his youth, recording those particulars of his own experience from which good rules of practice could be constructed.[84]

Similarly, Cardano referred to the ease of learning, from his commentary, "the art of medicine as it is transmitted by Hippocrates and by us."[85] His repeated claims of superior, Hippocratic, method and skill for himself were paralleled by denunciations of the erroneous ideas and ineptitude of his medical colleagues; at one point he remarked that of those who did not die by violence, two-fifths perished because of the errors of physicians.[86] In a preemptive strike against counterattacks on the grounds that his treatments were not, in fact, always successful and that his prognostications were highly inconsistent, he again compared himself to Hippocrates. He noted that Hippocrates had had no rich patients and much ill fortune, whereas Taddeo Alderotti had amassed great wealth;

"should we on that account put Hippocrates after Taddeo [*ob hoc Hippocratem postponemus Thadeo*]?" In his own case, the patients whom he had failed to cure did not want to be cured; and he had realized that accurate prognostication was impossible because a patient's recovery depended on so many factors beyond his, Cardano's, control, such as the actions of the attendants, the pharmacist, other physicians, and his own assistants.[87] Thus Cardano did not—evidently he could not—claim that employment of "Hippocratic" medicine would automatically guarantee actual therapeutic or prognostic success in all cases. Rather, the *Aphorisms* and *Prognostic* were of practical value because of their focus upon diagnostic and therapeutic essentials and their provision of correct principles of action.

In reality, even within the context of the knowledge of Hippocrates available in the mid–sixteenth century, Cardano's claim to teach and practice Hippocratic medicine was true in only a very limited sense. Although he evidently knew many treatises of the corpus thoroughly, his understanding of them—and presumably therefore his use of them as guides to medical practice—was deeply colored by the medical needs, contributions, and debates of his own day and by his reading of later medical authors, ancient and modern. For all his criticism of Galen as an interpreter of Hippocrates (see further below), his estimation of the authenticity of Hippocratic texts rested on Galen's information and judgment. Both the attentiveness and the limitations of his reading of Hippocrates are encapsulated in his discussion of Hippocratic bloodletting. With insight extremely unusual for the mid–sixteenth century, Cardano recognized that bloodletting is seldom advocated in the Hippocratic corpus.[88] But he was evidently unable to envisage good (and therefore truly "Hippocratic") medical practice without this essential therapeutic tool of Galenic medicine. Accordingly, he reacted to his own observation by explaining and harmonizing it away: "Since Hippocrates in his age shrank more from bloodletting than from purging . . . he did not let blood either in fevers or in large fractures, but rather prescribed hellebore and rigorous fasting. . . . However, in old age he adhered more to bloodletting, because he saw that the patients could not stand that severe lack of nourishment. Therefore he used to let blood when the patient was in danger of *phlegmone*. And from this the harmony of Hippocrates with Galen and Erasistratus appears."[89]

INTERPRETIVE METHODS

A good commentator, held Cardano, should neither simply explain the text, omitting any other account of the subject matter, nor use commentary as a pretext for expounding the subject matter without any reference to the actual content of the text, "the way Julius [Caesar] Scaliger did when he commented on Theophrastus." The proper procedure was first to explain the mind of the commented author, then to give a general account of the subject, and finally to bring the two together "so that we understand the thing itself through Hippocrates and accommodate the thing itself to Hippocrates."[90] The result would presumably be a Hippocratic medicine that was simultaneously true both to the ancient texts and to current medical realities.

In fact, Cardano's Hippocratic medicine gave more weight to medical ideas than to textual scholarship. Although his knowledge of medical Greek was considerable, it did not equal that of leading sixteenth-century scholars in the field. Compared with some other contemporary Hippocratic commentaries, his are markedly less philological in approach. For example, Fuchs's commentary on the *Aphorisms* accompanies his own edition of the Greek text together with his own translation; the commentary is chiefly a guide to reading the Greek. Brasavola's commentary on the same work, although appended to a Latin translation, devotes much attention to the textual tradition and interpretation of the Greek and includes the Greek of a supposed eighth book accompanied by his own translation.[91]

Cardano's Hippocratic commentaries accompany Renaissance Latin translations of the texts, into which he occasionally introduced some emendations of his own.[92] He seems to have worked on the basis of consultation of the Greek text of the Hippocratic corpus in both the Aldine and other editions as well as in various Latin translations. Thus he compared the Greek text of *Epidemics* 1 in Cornarius's edition with the lemmata in Galen's commentary on *Epidemics* 1, as edited by Hermann Croeser.[93] With his usual confidence—not to say overconfidence—in his own powers, he assumed that this procedure enabled him to adjudicate between Cornarius and Galen as transmitters of the Hippocratic text, as well as among the translators.[94] On occasion, however, he could be a perceptive critic. Thus although he had at one time simply accepted (probably from the Aldine edition) the assertion that Galen had not thought *Aliment* was written by Hippocrates, when he came to comment on that treatise himself, he examined the question carefully. In the proem he vigorously defended Galen's belief in the work's authenticity by identifying a number of his citations of or quotations from it.[95] Of course, in Cardano's view, this also amounted to a defense of the proposition that the treatise was genuinely by Hippocrates.

In many instances, his primary preoccupation with medical issues rather than with text criticism and philology led him to turn philological discussion to medical ends and to resolve difficulties by medical, not philological, criteria. Particularly in the commentaries on the *Aphorisms* and *Prognostic*, he usually discussed the meaning of Greek terms or problems relating to the Greek text only when he believed that a question of medical significance was at issue. He was, however, committed to the notion that clarification of Hippocratic disease terminology would lead to greater precision in diagnosis. He devoted lengthy passages to such topics as the differentiation of diseases referred to by various Greek terms latinized as *cancer* or *carcinoma*, the explanation of how the term *lepra* had come to be used to refer to several separate diseases, and ways of distinguishing among various kinds of pustules, that is, contagious diseases producing skin eruptions. Thus he explained that "*lepra* of the Greeks" was *lepra simplex*, which he identified as a kind of *scabies* or severe *impetigo*. It could turn into the more dangerous *lepra media*, characterized by whiteness of the skin. However, Avicenna and the other Arab authors had applied the term to a different disease, lepra of the Arabs or elephantiasis, characterized by great change in the form of the body, foul stench, and a raucous voice. Lepra simplex was common in contemporary Italy, and lepra media occurred there, although so rarely that he himself had not recognized it at first when called to a case. Lepra of the Arabs, or elephantiasis, was rare in Italy ("although I saw it in the hospital in Milan") but common in France and even more so in Ireland on account of the large amounts of fish and milk consumed together in the local diet. That left the puzzling question of how to classify "lepra of the Jews"—that is, leprosy in the Bible—which after some discussion of the symptoms described in Leviticus he defined as a separate variety, mingling two of the other kinds. Following earlier humanist physicians, he also included *morbus gallicus* under the heading of a variety of lepra.[96]

As he struggled to clarify and refine the disease terminology found in the Hippocratic texts, Cardano habitually sought to relate his definitions not merely to subsequent medical tradition and other authoritative sources but also, as in the example just cited, to descriptions of specific, individual cases. He used accounts drawn from the *Epidemics* and from his own experience in about equal measure to illuminate other texts (one is reminded of Machiavelli's habit in *Il Principe* of using a mixture of ancient and modern examples). Thus he commented on a pair of aphorisms about the significance of different kinds of sediment in the urine with the aid of three examples of individual cases: the black particles in his own urine that had ceased to appear after his son was executed and which had therefore perhaps been ominous; the hairs emitted "in all his excrements and in his blood" by a Spanish nobleman who had been among his patients and whom he had successfully treated with medication; and the "scabies of the bladder" of the son of Theophorbus, described in *Epidemics* 5.[97] Cardano's interest in identifying and classifying individual manifestations of specific, named diseases or conditions and his attention to the issue of the appropriateness of ancient disease descriptions to modern manifestations link his expositions of Hippocratic texts to central concerns of mid-sixteenth-century medical debate.

In general, he almost never questioned the veracity or plausibility of the Hippocratic descriptions but merely sought to interpret the disease terminology or anatomy involved. Thus he endorsed a story from *Epidemics* 5, that of a youth who accidentally swallowed a snake while sleeping open-mouthed, by the addition of directions for luring the snake to leave in such cases and an anatomical discussion based on Galen and Vesalius of the muscles that open and close the mouth.[98] Occasionally, however, he criticized Hippocrates on the basis of his own experience:

> I knew a man from Brescia (he was a servant of mine) by the name of Ortensio who had been chained for eighteen years in a galley among the [North] Africans, who indeed got married. But when he closed his eyes and did not move any part of his body, he could not be said to differ in anything from a dead man. Pallor, emaciation, stretched skin, pinched nostrils, leaden and purplish color with a certain swelling near the eyes made him resemble a dead man. But it is obvious that someone who was like this was not healthy. Yet Hippocrates calls a man healthy who may perform the functions of the healthy.[99]

On occasion, however, he was prepared to treat the text in a highly arbitrary fashion in order to extract a meaning that seemed to him medically plausible. An example is provided by the aphorism that states, "If the part of the womb near the hip-joint suppurates, one must use *emmoton*."[100] Latin translators and commentators before the sixteenth century had made various guesses at the sense of the latter part of this aphorism. For example, Ugo Benzi (d. 1439), faced with a Latin translation that ran, "Si matrix in vertebro posita fecerit saniem necesse est commotum fieri," cautiously restricted himself to saying it meant medical treatment was necessary; Giacomo da Forli (d. 1414) opined that commotion would arise in the womb.[101] Fuchs stated that *emmoton* literally meant a (medical) tent, that is, a linen plug that could be spread or soaked with medication and placed in a wound or other cavity, but that it was preferable to interpret it as meaning medication appropriate to be used on such a tent; Brasavola, following Galen, simply asserted that the word meant tent; both added derisive comments about Ugo and Giacomo.[102] Fuchs's gibes on this score inspired Cardano to a burst of patriotic rhetoric. "Does a German call Italians barbarians?" Italians had contributed many more of the new translations of Greek medical works than had Fuchs, and it was the Italian Matteo Corti, not Fuchs, who had pioneered the restoration of Galenic method. As for the fifteenth-century Italian commentators, they were erudite and inventive men whose only fault was that they had lived in an unpropitious age.[103]

Cardano himself impartially rejected all previous interpretations—by Galen, by the Latin authors who wrote in the medieval tradition, and by Renaissance translators and commentators—in favor of his own explanation that *emmoton* meant a deep sinuous ulcer, that is, a fistula. He introduced this explanation with the claim that correct understanding of the aphorism's meaning would be reached not through the application of linguistic criteria but by the extraction of a sense consonant with medical experience. His idiosyncratic rendering was thus far from arbitrary; rather, it is a striking example of his determination to refer Hippocratic statements to conditions encountered in his own practice, no matter at what cost to the text.[104]

THE CRITIQUE OF GALEN

Criticism of Galen as an interpreter of Hippocrates was one of the underlying goals of Cardano's entire Hippocratic enterprise. His critique of Galen sprang from his realization that existing commentaries on the *Aphorisms* were the work of "people listlessly expounding Galen so that not even the shadow of the sense of Hippocrates seems to be followed."[105] Cardano assured his readers that, as a result of his own efforts to disentangle the "true" Hippocrates from the pervasive influence of Galenic interpretation, "you will hear Hippocrates for the first time speaking with a new and different tongue, no less new than you think the things we have discovered in geometry and arithmetic to be." His claims were in fact quite similar to those Galen himself had made for his own "faithful" interpretation of Hippocrates as opposed to that of his rivals.[106]

These remarks reflect more than simply the general perception that Galen had understood Hippocratic texts in the light of his own medical ideas. Cardano had specifically in mind the wide current influence of Galen's Hippocratic commentaries. As is well known, in midlife Galen had embarked on a systematic program of commenting upon Hippocratic books.[107] In the Latin West his expositions had accompanied *Aphorisms*, *Prognostic*, and *Regimen in Acute Diseases* since the Middle Ages.[108] The recovery, editing, and translation into Latin of most of his remaining commentaries in the 1530s and 1540s was an important part of the endeavor of Renaissance Galenism—and Hippocratism.[109] So highly prized were these commentaries by Galen that Renaissance forgery obligingly supplied several missing ones.[110] The authors of new commentaries on Hippocratic books took it for granted that their task included attention to Galen's commentaries, where available. Thus, for example, Fuchs's translation and commentary of the *Aphorisms* included annotations to Galen, while Brasavola titled his work *Commentary and Annotations on the Aphorisms of Hippocrates and Galen*, and printed both texts.

Cardano's Hippocrates project was thus simultaneously a highly Galenic enterprise. Galen was as much his model for systematic commentary on the Hippocratic corpus as for medical autobiography and autobibliography. In this, as in so many other instances, the ancients set the program for Renaissance science. But as autobiographer and autobibliographer, Galen was a model whom Cardano admired, as well as emulating and perhaps seeking to rival. By contrast, his attitude toward Galen as a Hippocratic commentator was fundamentally negative. In undertaking the *Aphorisms*, which for centuries had traditionally been considered in conjunction with Galen's commentary, he pledged to expound only the Hippocratic text without reference to Galen's exposition, which he described as simultaneously inadequate and prolix (a promise not always kept when opportunity to criticize Galen arose).[111] In his exposition of *Epidemics* 1, he vigorously and repeatedly attacked Galen's recently recovered commentary on the grounds that it oversimplifed obscure passages, obfuscated clear ones, or just misunderstood the text.[112] And he boldly assured potential readers of his commentary on *Epidemics* 2 that with his exposition at hand, "you will not feel the immense loss of Galen's commentaries [*ita nos egisse, ut Galeni commentariorum amissorum immensam iacturam non sentiatis*]."[113] In practice, he frequently turned to other works of Galen for help in expounding *Epidemics* 2 (for example, by referring to Galen's discussion of simulated illness to explain an obscure Hippocratic allusion to fear).[114] Moreover, in works published in his lifetime on Hippocratic books for which Galen's commentary was not available, he did not claim to be providing an equally valuable substitute; rather, he either expressed the hope that a lost commentary by Galen would be found or noted its absence in neutral terms.[115]

Cardano objected to Galen's whole approach to the task of commentary, ascribing to him—and indignantly repudiating—the idea that a commentator's responsibility was not to demonstrate the truth of the statements in the text at hand but only to explain their meaning.[116] In any case, he denied that Galen had any special or superior insight into the meaning of the Hippocratic books; instead, he had imposed his own views on Hippocrates. "Galen could only conjecture what Hippocrates meant: he was a man and could be deceived about many things. But . . . whenever he lays down what Hippocrates would have wished, we know what Galen would have wished."[117] Cardano could only conclude that in reality Galen "greatly envied the glory of Hippocrates, even though he seems to extol him."[118]

He also repeatedly criticized particulars of Galen's interpretation. The thrust of these criticisms was primarily that Galen's readings disseminated erroneous medical information and recommendations. For example, Galen was delinquent because he had not endorsed the Hippocratic injunction to restrict diet in severe illness strongly enough, thus allowing "murdering modern physicians" to overturn this excellent counsel. Galen fell into "insoluble knots of contradiction" over whether or not humid foods contributed to longevity. Because he assumed Hippocrates was referring to vital forces when really he meant innate heat, Galen produced an explanation that was "totally absurd"; as a result, Galen's precepts about the amount and frequency of food in illness "accord neither with his own principles, nor with Hippocrates, nor with experience."[119] In his last Hippocratic commentary, the brief exposition of twenty-two cases from the *Epidemics*, he went so far as to make sweeping claims that Galen lacked clinical experience: "Galen saw few *experimenta* of internal diseases and made fewer observations about them"; "Galen indeed does not attain to any of the difficult things"; and "on account of his [Galen's] excessive erudition and study in those things [grammar], he exercised himself less in serious and more useful things."[120]

An area in which Cardano claimed to identify particularly important discrepancies between Hippocratic teaching and Galenic interpretation was the doctrine of critical days, that is, the concept that an illness would reach a crisis and turn toward death or recovery a certain—calculable—number of days after onset. The Hippocratic writings, particularly some of the case histories in the *Epidemics* and *Prognostic*, were an important source for the theory, which doubtless also had roots in ancient ideas about ominous days; it underwent much subsequent elaboration, notably at the hands of Galen, as well as becoming linked to astrology. The doctrine of critical days was, for example, the principal subject of an astrological handbook for physicians published in 1546 by Cardano's astrological rival, Luca Gaurico; in it Gaurico collected and critically reviewed a variety of previous expositions of the subject.[121] Cardano believed that full and precise understanding of critical days demanded technical command of astronomy and the calendar that Galen and his followers simply did not possess. In another context, he had characterized Brasavola's confusion over the rising and setting of the stars as laughable;[122] of a problem relating to critical days he asserted, "I say therefore that no one can solve this difficulty unless he understands the Hippocratic art of Ptolemy."[123] Accordingly, in his commentary on *Prognostic*, he provided a comprehensive summary of the doctrine of critical days proclaimed to be "according to truth and the opinion of Hippocrates, which Galen wrapped falsely with so much nonsense and inconsistency that those who might seek it would never be able to get to the bottom of the matter."[124] Actually, Cardano heaped upon his readers a mass of astronomical detail not even hinted at in the Hippocratic text.[125]

The freedom with which Cardano criticized Galen as a Hippocratic commentator and the frequency with which these criticisms turned into attacks on particular aspects of Galenic medical theory and therapy do not, of course, mean that he was a wholehearted anti-Galenist. It must be emphasized once again that he was as much a product of a generally Galenic framework of medical learning as any of his colleagues. Approving citations of works and opinions of Galen abound in the Hippocratic commentaries as well as elsewhere in his writings. He himself characterized his own position as an endeavor to undermine uncritical reliance on Galen's authority, not to repudiate all Galenic doctrine.[126] He believed that students of medicine should prefer Hippocrates to Galen, but that some Galenic treatises remained indispensable. The important thing was to learn to discriminate among Galen's works: "When you have thoroughly understood all the books of Hippocrates, then I order you, not just advise you, to read Galen's *On the Affected Places, On the Usefulness of the Parts, Method of Healing,* and . . . [portions of] . . . *On Simple Medicines* and *On Composite Medicines.* If you abstain from the rest of his books, not only will you gain the time that you would have spent, but you will be less perplexed about the things that are handed down clearly by Hippocrates."[127] In a similar list that he included in a general handbook of medicine, rather than a commentary on Hippocrates, Cardano urged his readers to study Vesalius's *Fabrica* first, then selected major works of Galen, then Hippocrates.[128]

In certain respects, Cardano's critique of Galen as a Hippocratic commentator suggests parallels with the somewhat similar undertaking of Giovanni Argenterio (1513–72). He, too, was responsible for a concentrated attack on Galenic doctrine in one specific area, in his case that of the causes, varieties, and symptoms of disease. In a set of treatises on disease, first published in 1550 while he was a professor at Pisa, Argenterio closely followed the subject matter and organization of Galen's works on the subject, while vigorously dissenting from their content. His critique played a part in the complex sixteenth-century debate about disease, although its impact was limited by the evident lack of any more satisfactory system of pathology with which to replace Galen. Both Argenterio and Cardano were independently stimulated by the success of the revision of Galenic anatomy to extend the critique of Galen to areas that they perceived as immediately connected to medical practice. Argenterio, too, explicitly invoked the Vesalian model that was never far from Cardano's mind.[129] Yet the context of their endeavors—as indeed of Vesalius's own—was the generally improved knowledge of Galenic texts and teaching supplied by the efforts of medical humanists. Retaining vast influence, Galen was nonetheless by the 1560s an ambiguous figure subject to both praise and blame.

HIPPOCRATIC MEDICINE / VESALIAN MEDICINE

Cardano's Hippocratic medicine thus encompassed the goals of making Hippocratic books yield usable rules of medicine, illuminate and be illuminated by "the thing itself," and serve as medical manuals. To attain these goals, the brief and frequently obscure texts needed not only to be purged of irrelevant or erroneous commentary but also supplied with truly authoritative expansion and clarification. To a considerable extent, he presented his own medical knowledge and experience as authoritative for those purposes. But he also drew repeatedly on findings of modern anatomy to amplify and confirm the maxims attributed to Hippocrates. In this way, he made Vesalian anatomy and Hippocratic medicine into symbiotic—and indeed synchronous—systems, mutually verifying one another. The assimilation of the ancient and modern authorities was doubtless facilitated by the terseness and, often, ambiguity of Hippocratic language and ideas, which, as Vivian Nutton has pointed out, "could easily accommodate new discoveries and new trends."[130]

The association of Hippocrates and Vesalius allowed Cardano to connect the Hippocratic texts (and his own readings of them) with Galen's single most successful modern critic, and with the area of medical knowledge for which the most striking and unambiguous recent—and therefore post-Galenic—advances were attested. Furthermore, the use of modern anatomical exposition to fill out Hippocratic brevity was a device that enhanced the comprehensiveness and, in Cardano's view, the practicality that he claimed for these treatises. He acknowledged that Hippocrates had not practiced human dissection (". . . *anatomia corporum humanorum ignota Galeno, atque Hippocratis aetate sic amissa* . . .).[131] Yet he took for granted perfect harmony among Vesalian anatomy, Hippocratic medical doctrine, and the best actual medical practice. As noted in the previous chapter, he was also convinced that current knowledge of anatomy had useful medical applications. Numerous passages therefore attest to his belief that the truths of Vesalian, and post-Vesalian, anatomy could illuminate the truths of the Hippocratic books. For example, the aphorism "When a patient has a spontaneous discharge of blood and urine, it indicates the breaking of a small vein in the kidneys" is explicated by way of a summary of Vesalius's description of the kidneys and Falloppia's corrections of Vesalius's account of those organs, illustrated with a schematic diagram. Another aphorism, "Those with an impediment in their speech are very likely to be attacked by protracted diarrhea," called forth both a long disquisition on speech defects (which has parallels in and may be partly dependent upon Brasavola's commentary) and a summary of Vesalius on the hyoid bone and larynx, complete with diagram. The statement in *Prognostic* that "Acute pain of the ear with continuous high fever is dangerous, for the patient is likely to become delirious and die" produced an account of the formation of abscesses with reference to the anatomy of the ear, a description of the three small bones of the ear, and mention of the anatomical discoveries of Eustachi.[132] In the commentaries on the *Epidemics*—in which very few modern authorities are cited apart from editors and translators of the text and Vesalius—a long disquisition on hernia is made to rest on Vesalius's description of the testicles.[133]

Cardano's treatment of the account of the Amazons in *Airs Waters Places* offers a particularly striking example of his confidence in the utility of modern anatomy to explicate Hippocratic texts. According to the Hippocratic author, Amazon mothers used a special bronze instrument to excise their infant daughters' right breasts, subsequently cauterizing the wound to prevent the breast from growing. As a result of this procedure, strength was transferred to the right arm and shoulder, so that the girls grew up able to bend the bow.[134] In Cardano's exposition, both main elements in the story—gender role reversal and sexual mutilation—received extended analysis. After the historical note that Tartar women do not now follow this practice, he turned to the philosophical and practical problems raised by the idea of women warriors. He did not have much use for soldiers of any kind and, as one might expect, still less for female ones. Military training would prevent women from developing the qualities they needed for child rearing and domestic administration, since no soldier was ever gentle or prudent. The arrangement was particularly puzzling in the case of the nomadic Scythians, who had no houses that they might need to fight to defend.[135] Yet he noted that in a crisis, women might indeed be needed to join in fighting to defend the *patria*, as they had occasionally done even in modern times, and added a summary and citations of Plato's advocacy of military training and duties for the female guardians, together with the observation that female animals fought just as much as male ones. No doubt his reading included some of the contributions to the widespread ongoing debate over the position, virtues, and abilities of women—perhaps, for example, Heinrich Cornelius Agrippa's *declamatio* on female superiority, or one of the Italian treatises influenced by that work. Cardano evidently also shared the Renaissance fascination with fighting heroines—provided that, in most instances, they were suitably far removed in time, distance, or literary fiction.[136]

But he also read the story as an account of a surgical operation, which he analyzed in the light of Vesalius's description of the anatomy, blood supply, innervation, and development of the breasts. He assured his own readers that although Vesalius "teaches that there is much glandular flesh in adults but little in small girls, yet around the region of the nipple there is a fairly large gland, and surrounding it many other small ones." But Vesalius's account showed that the procedure described by the Hippocratic author, although not necessarily life threatening, was far from being a minor event comparable to circumcision; the removal of "so many glands, veins, nerves, arteries, occupying an ample space" would be major surgery.[137] What, then, could the Hippocratic author have meant in this context by infancy—a newborn, who would feel less terror and pain, or a seven-year-old, who would have strength to endure such an operation? Moreover, in an adult woman the surgical removal of a breast would be likely to weaken rather than strengthen the arm and shoulder; the Amazons must really have acquired their strength through compensatory exercise during girlhood, not from this operation.[138]

The reconstruction of Amazon surgery with the aid of Vesalian anatomy was, of course, as hypothetical technically as it was historically. Its starting point was the unquestioning acceptance that every detail in the Hippocratic account was true. The Amazons had also been described by Herodotus, modern travelers mentioned women warriors in the New World, and the case was proven.[139] The anatomical description slips insecurely between the area around infant nipples and the adult female breast. The realistic-seeming surgical analysis is a back-formation from the reading of an anatomical text, layered over with Cardano's imaginative sympathy for the young victims, awareness of the effect of exercise on muscles, and even his archaeological interest (why a bronze surgical instrument? was it because they had no iron?).[140] In this way, here too, Hippocrates and Vesalius could be made to confirm one another.

Cardano's hopes for the reception of his work on Hippocrates were not, as far as one can tell, fulfilled. Of the Hippocratic writings, only the commentaries on *Prognostic* and *Aliment* went into a second edition before being included in his collected *Opera*.[141] By contrast, the popular encyclopedia *De subtilitate* went into edition after edition. The content of the Hippocratic commentaries was, with the exception of *Airs Waters Places*, probably too closely tied to the context of medical education to attract wide attention outside the medical profession. In medical circles, knowledge of and interest in the Hippocratic corpus was a growing trend in the middle decades of the century. But in the 1560s and 1570s, when the commentaries were published, endeavors to separate Hippocrates from Galen had barely begun. Cardano's attacks on Galen as interpreter of Hippocrates, especially when allied with his personal claims to be a Hippocratic physician who understood Hippocrates better than Galen had done, were likely to evoke the hostile response exemplified by Camuzio's attack on the commentary on the *Aphorisms*. Camuzio, who wrote at the official request of the rector of the University of Pavia, was alarmed by the dissemination of Cardano's version of Hippocratism among students and "even some graduates who are not ashamed to cite Cardano like the oracle of Apollo against Galen's opinions."[142] As this remark suggests, the subsequent spread of new ideas about the relation of Hippocrates and Galen may have owed something to Cardano; but as a European phenomenon it owed much more to Paracelsian radicalism.

Moreover, even though Cardano deserves to be remembered as one of the pioneers in the endeavor to disentangle Hippocrates from Galen, and even though he commented on a wider range of Hippocratic texts than almost any of his contemporaries and achieved a number of good insights, his Hippocrates did not really speak "with a new and different tongue." As several times noted above, his interpretation of Hippocrates remained in many respects thoroughly Galenic. Nevertheless, his Hippocratic commentaries merit more attention than they have usually received in accounts of his life and work. They splendidly illustrate his own apothegm (directed at Galen) that commentary is apt to tell more about the views of the commentator than about the commented author.[143] In his Hippocrates project as in other parts of his intellectual enterprise, he sought to master a reformed system of natural knowledge, incorporated his own experience, and pursued his interest in prognostic arts. Hippocrates and Ptolemy were the two ancient scientists to whom he devoted most attention. One may suppose that they appealed to him for very similar reasons. Both appeared to offer hitherto misunderstood systems of knowledge that not only had ancient authority but, with proper techniques, were also practically useful and capable of verification. Furthermore, the Hippocratic works served to provide him with the most ancient and authoritative endorsement for his claims for his own medical practice and his ambivalent relationship with the Aristotelian and Galenic tradition of the schools. Hence he had no hesitation in using the authority of Hippocrates to endorse his own ideas, any more than he did in supplementing Hippocratic teaching with the findings of modern anatomists.

PART FOUR

Medical Wonders

Chapter 7

THE HIDDEN AND THE MARVELOUS

CARDANO'S gift of a nature especially suited to mastery of subtlety manifested itself in a variety of ways, of which technical command of mathematics, astrology, music, and medicine was only one. He was guided—at least some of the time—by a personal genius or daimon. His body was a theater of portents and strange manifestations: mysterious marks in his fingernails and specks in his urine warned of trouble to come. Omens in his external surroundings followed him throughout his life. He dreamed prophetic dreams.[1] He fitted these intimate personal experiences easily into his view of a universe ruled by God through the stars. But about other supposed marvelous or miraculous phenomena or events, he was at times profoundly skeptical, attributing them on occasion to natural causes, false report, human credulity, or fraud. His attitudes to and beliefs about occult causes and marvelous events, the natural and the supernatural, the celestial and the divine have attracted attention, but not yielded consensus, from his own day to the present. Some contemporaries characterized him as excessively credulous, others as prudently skeptical, and yet others as dangerously so.[2] The interpretation of his views, especially as regards their implications for religion, continues to be a subject of scholarly inquiry.[3]

In medicine, these aspects of his thought as a rule emerged overtly only when they were of specific relevance to particular medical topics. Although Cardano stressed the universality of his knowledge, he also preserved disciplinary boundaries. He wrote philosophy as a philosopher, mathematics as a mathematician, and medicine as a physician. This compartmentalization is particularly obvious as regards astrology and medicine. The relationship of these two disciplines was traditionally close, Cardano was a famous astrologer, and the governing role of the stars was fundamental to his entire philosophy of nature. Moreover, as the previous chapter has shown, he viewed medical prognosis and astrological prediction as sister disciplines, fundamentally similar at the deepest level. Yet, for the most part, his medical writings introduce details of technical astrology chiefly in the discussion of a range of specific standard medico-astrological topics—for example, as already noted, critical days in illness and months of fetal life. It is only when one turns to his analysis of his own health history in the light of his horoscope in an astrological work (see chapter 10) that the depth and scope of his attention to the heavenly bodies' role in health and disease become apparent.

For various Renaissance physicians, Cardano among them, occult causation and marvelous effects were authentic medical topics because of their obvious relevance to diseases and cures. Yet Cardano's views about such matters seem even more fundamentally ambiguous in medicine than in philosophy, perhaps because the practical and professional implications were more immediate. This chapter (which sets technical astrology aside) will explore his position on occult causes and marvelous effects in medicine as well as his medical presentation of his own concept of subtlety, which included a physiological component as well, perhaps, as the power to cure.

Although Cardano's particular combination of ideas on occult causation and marvels—as on so many other subjects—was personal, idiosyncratic, and in some respects highly unusual for his time and place, it also reflected both pervasive elements in the ambient culture and his reading in learned sources. The large presence of the occult in late medieval and Renaissance culture and society as a whole is by now too well known to require further elaboration here.[4] The philosophical basis of intellectual interest in and controversy about occult causes and marvelous effects was of course common to medicine and natural philosophy. The regular course of nature was considered to be defined by Aristotelian physics and the Galenic theory of humors, elementary qualities, and temperament (*krasis, complexio*). Things that appeared inexplicable in a universe ordered by these rules, whether such familiar experiences as the action of a magnet or exotic *mirabilia*, were the result of hidden causes. The concept could refer simply to the unknown causes of phenomena inexplicable in terms of Aristotelian physics, but recognized as natural and even (as in the case of the magnet) as regularly occurring. But other phenomena that aroused sufficient wonder to be regarded as preternatural marvels might, but did not necessarily, involve the manipulation of nature by angels or demons. True, supernatural miracles that actually changed the course of nature were the province of God alone.

The boundaries of the natural, the preternatural, and the miraculous were extensively discussed in the late Middle Ages. But from the late fifteenth century, interest in occult causes in nature and preternatural marvels was reinforced by the influence of the magical side of Renaissance Neoplatonism. This promulgated the concept of a spiritually elevating magic that would enable its practitioner to manipulate the sympathies and signatures linking macrocosm and microcosm and tap into the astral forces that governed the world. In the sixteenth-century climate of increasing religious and social anxiety, however, concern about the activities of evil demons was also pervasive. All these ideas permeated some medical as well as philosophical writings; indeed, Marsilio Ficino's instructions for invoking astral deities in Book 3 of his *Three Books on Life* were intended to aid the petitioner's health and well-being. Philosophical discussions of occult causation often invoked medical examples, just as medical authors invoked nonmedical ones, for instance, the action of a magnet; thus Pomponazzi's *On Incantations* takes as its starting point examples of use of incantations for purposes of healing.[5]

Nevertheless, in the context of medicine, and especially that of medical practice, the idea of occult causation took on a number of particular connotations besides the general association with diseases and cures. As a general rule of "rational" Galenic medicine, medicinal substances were supposed to work through the mixture of elementary qualities and to cure by contraries (so that, in the simplest possible example, a temperamentally cold herb would be a remedy for a disease resulting from excessive temperamental heat). Galen had, however, taught that not all remedies worked in this way, since some acted through a property inherent in their whole substance. In scholastic medicine this idea developed into a specialized theory of occult causation, the doctrine of action by specific form. As Arnald of Villanova (d. 1311), for one, explained, certain medicaments worked through a power inherent in their whole substance or species, a power termed occult because its cause could not be ascertained by human reason and its effects became known only by their occurrence.[6] More generally, for practitioners, the idea of hidden causes and marvelous cures could be used to express both the possibilities and the limitations of medical skill. Even more important, perhaps, for both practitioner and patient, the concept of *mirabilia* was intimately bound up with the desire for cure, whether by natural, preternatural, or supernatural, manifest or hidden, rational or other means.

These ideas played a part in fifteenth- and sixteenth-century endeavors to accommodate a changing disease environment, a new attention to particulars, and new explanations within a medical system that remained, for the most part, fundamentally Galenic. Practitioners simultaneously continued to draw on Latin scholastic medical tradition, believed that the improved knowledge of ancient Greek medical texts achieved in their own age gave them important new resources, and confronted apparently "new" epidemic diseases. In this complex situation, much medical interest in diseases, cures, or forms of disease transmission possibly falling outside the bounds of Galenic explanation relates to increasing concern with specific description, and to the confrontation of a wider range of ancient texts with unprecedented forms of current experience.[7] But some of the interest in unprecedented forms of pathology and hidden causes of disease reflects the fascination in the broader culture with magic and demonology as well as with the ever-expanding store of information about the novel, strange, or monstrous things in the world.[8] In medical texts, words such as *mira*, *mirabilia*, *miranda*, and *admiranda* and references to occult causes have various implications ranging across "unusual," "rare," and "extraordinary," to "wonderful," "marvelous," "magical," or even "miraculous." Different practitioners deployed the words and concepts differently and used them for diverse intellectual and professional purposes.

In terms of medical practice, moreover, "remarkable" or "worthy of wonder" is likely to have been a more or less open category as regards both disease and cure. Such openness seems a highly probable corollary of the indeterminate nature of the rational explanatory system that referred disease, therapy, and result largely to the theory of complexions or temperaments, that is, to the balance of the elementary qualities in the patient and in the medicaments. As a system of explanation the "rational" medicine of humors, qualities, and temperament seems usually to have been sufficiently flexible to accommodate almost any symptoms and almost any outcome. Furthermore, the relation between treatment and outcome—even allowing for a nonabsolute concept of cure—must frequently have been uncertain. Such circumstances evidently left a medical practitioner great latitude in judging whether a particular episode of internal illness or recovery in one of his patients belonged in the category of *mirabilia*, or was at any rate the result of causes other than temperamental imbalance, or was explicable by rational medicine. He was presumably guided only by his own experience and his interpretation of his reading.

Cardano's statements about subtlety, hidden causes, and marvelous effects in medicine and his decision to entitle a collection of his own cures *De admirandis curationibus et praedictionibus morborum* therefore need to be considered in the light of other examples of Renaissance medical thinking on similar topics. Here, considerations of space limit the comparison chiefly to two well-known works, namely, Antonio Benivieni's *De abditis non nullis ac mirandis morborum et sanationum causis* and Jean Fernel's *De abditis rerum causis*. Both Benivieni (1443–1502) and Fernel (1497–1558) were themselves celebrated practitioners and focused the larger part of their medical writings on practice. However, despite the similarity in their titles, the two treatises—both of which were known to Cardano—are very different in character. Benivieni's little book is a collection of cases personally encountered in the course of his practice. Fernel was the author of an influential general work on medicine but devoted this treatise to a theoretical account of occult causation in physiology and pathology.

Benivieni and the Limits of Medicine

According to Antonio Benivieni, "anyone who practices medicine for a long time sees many different kinds of things that are worthy of wonder." The reflection led him to collect material for a work that has given him a partially deserved but somewhat misleading reputation as a pioneer of surgical and postmortem pathology.[9] As he explained, Benivieni planned to issue three collections each containing an account of one hundred remarkable instances from his long experience in practice; at the time of his death, he had assembled most of the material for the first two.[10] With few exceptions, the contents are brief anecdotes about the illnesses of named individuals. Many of the accounts relate to surgical cases. Although there are some topical clusters, no overall order of arrangement is discernible.[11] Cures by nonmaterial means (prayer, incantations) are included alongside accounts of physical manipulation and treatment by internal and external medication. Descriptions of physical symptoms—often with a fair degree of specificity—are regularly present; there are a number of references to autopsy and a constant insistence on the author's personal observation. The word that recurs most frequently throughout may well be *vidimus*—"we [that is, I] saw." These last are, of course, the factors that account for Benivieni's reputation as a pioneer of pathology. At the same time, the apparently heterogeneous nature of the collection and the anecdotal quality of the separate accounts convey an impression of directness and artlessness unmediated by theoretical or rhetorical considerations.

But however Benivieni's intentions may be understood, it is most unlikely that his work is either philosophically naive or innocent of rhetorical artifice. He was a learned man who had studied rhetoric under Landino and philosophy and medicine at the University of Siena.[12] Together with his brother the poet Girolamo Benivieni, he moved among the erudite Florentine elite of the late Quattrocento, in a circle that included Ficino and Poliziano.[13] Apart from *On Hidden and Remarkable Causes*, the record of Antonio Benivieni's practice survives in the form of brief and conventional works on plague, therapy, and regimen, replete with recipes and citations of medical authorities.[14] It is clear that he was an extremely successful practitioner in one important sense: he earned the esteem and affection of exceptionally intelligent and influential clients.

By 1487 he had accumulated a substantial library, the contents of which reveal his interest in rhetoric, literature, and philosophy, as well as medicine.[15] Besides standard Arabo-Latin texts and commentaries and works on medical practice by thirteenth- to fifteenth-century Latin authors, his medical books included Celsus's *On Medicine*, of which he made pioneering use in *On Hidden and Remarkable Causes*.[16] Among his philosophical books were Ficino's translation of Plato and an extensive collection of Aristotelian philosophy, including such up-to-date items as the books on natural philosophy in Greek and the books on animals in the fifteenth-century humanist Latin translation by Theodore of Gaza.[17] He also owned many books likely to be useful for the study of hidden causes in nature. He was well supplied with the natural philosophical works of Albertus Magnus, whose views on the soul, the interior senses, and the heavenly Intelligences, derived from Avicenna as well as Aristotle, were often cited in discussions of occult causes. He had the major collections of natural *problemata*, or questions: those attributed to Aristotle, those of Alexander of Aphrodisias, and the commentary on the Aristotelian *problemata* by the physician and astrologer Pietro d'Abano.[18] He also owned Cicero's *On the Nature of the Gods* and Pliny's *Natural History*; his books on astrology included Ptolemy's *Quadripartitum* (that is, the Latin version of the *Tetrabiblos*).[19] One lacuna in this otherwise notably complete assemblage of works from which theories or examples applicable to "remarkable" phenomena could be extracted is the absence of Avicenna's *On the Soul* (known in medieval Europe as the *Sextus de naturalibus*), which was a key source of ideas about the powers to affect bodies of souls, imagination, and celestial Intelligences.[20]

Benivieni's *On Hidden and Remarkable Causes* has sometimes been associated with another work "on the causes of remarkable effects," also composed by a physician in Florence at about the same time.[21] The author, Andrea Cattani of Imola, taught philosophy at the University of Florence, where he lectured on Avicenna's *On the Soul*, and was supervisor of the city's major hospital, Santa Maria Nuova.[22] Taking as his starting point the Avicennan ideas just alluded to, Cattani developed theories to explain such supposed phenomena as prophecy and cures by incantations.[23] Thus, according to Cattani, prophetic dreams were the result of communication of the human soul, in sleep partially liberated from the body, with angels and Intelligences. Moreover, there are certain human souls so elevated and noble that through their natural capacity they can affect other bodies beside their own and thus either work miracles of healing or bring down calamities on sinful cities for the purposes of moral reform. A number of Cattani's assertions are highly unorthodox from a Christian standpoint. For example, he insisted that the oracles of ancient pagan deities might have been truths imparted by celestial Intelligences descending to inhabit appropriately prepared images.[24] He also attributed cases of apparent demonic possession to the action of celestial Intelligences, with only the slightest allusion to the possibility that some such beings might be malevolent.

As his plague treatise makes clear, Benivieni shared the standard medical belief in the influence of the stars on human disease.[25] But whether or not he knew of Cattani's work, it seems highly unlikely that he would have accepted its more extreme positions. Like his two brothers, Antonio Benivieni became a devout adherent of the religious reforms of Savonarola.[26] He was consequently committed to a rigorist form of Catholic belief and to the genuinely supernatural character and divine origin of the miracles and prophecies attributed to the intercession of Savonarola and some of his disciples. It therefore seems most improbable that he would have regarded the idea that oracles from pagan statues conveyed heavenly truths with anything other than unmitigated horror.

Benivieni's career and associations throw considerable light on the contents of *On Hidden and Remarkable Causes*. At least three distinct though interrelated programs, medical, philosophical, and religious, seem identifiable. Obviously, medical pedagogy is one major objective. At the most fundamental level, Benivieni's collection of examples informs readers—presumably understood to include practitioners or students of medicine without his own wide and long experience—of the existence and character of various more or less unusual conditions. Into this category may, for example, be thought to fall his descriptions of cases of various birth defects, of gangrene and its fatal course, and of what appears to be an instance of petit mal epilepsy.[27] Another fundamental lesson conveyed is that of the limits of medicine. A cluster of stories about practitioners who let blood carelessly or to excess, prescribed hellebore, or misidentified a type of fever illustrate the theme of the fatal results of incompetence.[28] But in other instances Benivieni the good practitioner does his best and the patient dies anyway.[29] Prescriptive statements about the limits of medicine are routine in medieval medical writing (they often derive from the Hippocratic list of organs to which injuries were always fatal),[30] as is the idea that bad practice can kill. But Benivieni's record of deaths among his own patients and personal acknowledgment of the limitations of his own ability to cure are highly unusual. It is perhaps the emphasis on death as a likely outcome rather than the presence of autopsy (not in itself particularly unusual at the turn of the fifteenth and sixteenth centuries) that marks off *On Hidden and Remarkable Causes* from most other medieval and Renaissance medical writing on disease.

At a different level of medical instruction, a number of cases seem designed simultaneously to relate a generalization to a specific instance and to show how terms encountered in the medical literature—especially in the still relatively unfamiliar work of Celsus—should be applied in practice. Some examples of this type also manifest an interest in distinguishing the common from the rare: "To be attacked by the disease of the small intestine that the Greeks call ileon is common, but it is unheard-

of to be attacked so severely that life is lost."[31] Two case histories follow—of an obese woman and of a peasant—in which this complaint was
in fact fatal. In both, subsequent autopsy allegedly revealed a break in
the intestine. Whatever its observational basis, the account is shaped by
both medical and social preconceptions, for the reader learns that the
peasant's autopsy disclosed that he had just eaten fresh grapes. Medieval
and Renaissance dietary theory held all kinds of fruits to be potentially
unwholesome, but they were regarded as especially unsuitable food for
peasants.[32] The connections of some of these stories, not all of which
Benivieni claimed as his own experience, with other types of social narrative also emerges in several anecdotes about cures that unexpectedly
occurred to rustics, servants, or women through accident, crass excess,
or comic misunderstanding.[33]

The final and most obvious medical purpose is the justification of
Benivieni's own practice. The reader is repeatedly informed that
Benivieni either understood a case better than did other physicians or effected a cure after other physicians failed. In some cases, his success is
attributed to superior understanding of causes; in others, either
Benivieni's superior understanding fails to prevent the patient's death, or
he finds effective remedies even though he fails to understand the cause
of the disease.[34] Thus, unlike his partial model Celsus, Benivieni made no
general claims for any necessary link between understanding and the
ability to cure.[35] Rather than asserting either that knowledge of causes
ensures ability to cure or that ability to cure depends on knowledge of
causes, Benivieni warned explicitly that "a wise man should not give any
judgment about uncertain and occult illnesses."[36]

This last remark links the medical with the philosophical and religious
aspects of the work. In his preface, Benivieni explicitly disclaimed any intention to "resolve the *arcana*" of medicine. Rather, he proposed only
to run through "the remarkable things that have been seen in our own
time" so that students could "recognize the hidden causes of nature."
That is to say, medical practice calls only for recognition, not for profound levels of explanation. Typical of his attitude is the comment "Nature does many things that seem remarkable to medical practitioners and
often calls a dying man from the jaws of death."[37] In *On Hidden and
Remarkable Causes*, references to astral causation or to the activities of
celestial Intelligences, central, for example, to Cattani's natural philosophical discussion of *mirabilia*, are conspicuous by their absence. As a
record of and guide to medical practice, *On Hidden and Remarkable
Causes* deals only in causes that are strictly terrestrial and corporeal or
wholly supernatural or diabolical.

Causes in the former category are hidden only insofar as they are internal to the human body, where they may or may not be uncovered by

a skilled physician. They are hidden causes in Celsus's sense of the term, part of what Celsus called "rational medicine" and "principles of our bodies."[38] Indeed, the birth defects, tumors, and traumatic injuries that make up a significant element in Benivieni's collection of "remarkable" diseases could equally well be interpreted as falling within the explanatory system of Galenic "rational" medicine as set forth in standard medieval medical textbooks. Although complexional imbalance served to explain most internal disease, separate categories termed *mala compositio* and *solutio continuitatis* encompassed, respectively, defects and trauma.[39]

The other causes comprise supernatural miracles performed by God in answer to the prayers of the pious and the activities of evil demons. Benivieni believed that there were two new and calamitous epidemics in his own age: the *morbus gallicus* and an outbreak of demonic possession.[40] For the latter affliction, in his view, only spiritual remedies would help. As far as other diseases were concerned, he several times returned to the idea that the only legitimate forms of treatment were the physical attentions of an expert physician or surgeon and the spiritual ones of a pious priest. The remedies of unskilled medical practitioners or empirics were ineffective or dangerous to the body. Incantations were medically effective, but dangerous to the soul.[41] Whereas Cattani had declared that the effectiveness of incantations in healing disease was due to the natural power of the imagination of certain specially gifted individuals, acting at astrally appropriate moments, over the bodies of others,[42] Benivieni's assumption was that incantations involved commerce with demons. Hence he surrounded the admission that he himself had successfully used a verbal formula to cure a toothache with a whole series of reservations. The patient was a woman (and hence as such especially susceptible to corporeal impressions received from her own imagination); she was not a regular patient but someone encountered casually in the street; Benivieni was a youth at the time; the magic formula he whispered over her was feigned; and he instructed her to recite the Lord's Prayer. As the title of the chapter informs us, moreover, it was in fact her faith—expressed in the prayer—that cured her.[43]

It thus becomes apparent that the handful of miracles described in *On Hidden and Remarkable Causes* are not, as has sometimes been assumed, peripheral or subordinate to the much more numerous "natural" cases. Instead, they are an integral, and perhaps a central, element in the work. As has frequently been noted, these are miracles that endorse the religious and political program associated with Savonarola. They are the result not of patients' prayers to traditional saints, participation in established cults, or visits to shrines but of "the will of God alone through the faith and prayer of that most holy man" Savonarola's disciple Fra Domenico of Pescia.[44] When a young Florentine in intractable pain was saved from suicide by religious conversion, he began to utter political prophecies, among them the exile of Piero de' Medici, whose departure in 1494 was followed by Savonarola's dominance over the city. Moreover, it is in the miracle stories that this strongly personal collection takes on its most insistently personal note of witness. Benivieni "not only saw but with my own hands grasped" a patient's miraculously healed knee; Giovannina Benci, who told him the whole story of the miraculous cure of her persistent diarrhea, was his near relative; and, in the most personal account of all, Benivieni told how he himself was healed by the prayers of his devout and loving brother.[45] Thus the notion of "hidden and remarkable causes of diseases and cures," both natural and spiritual, is presented in terms acceptable to a rigorist Christian belief. The pragmatic nature of the medical descriptions is in part a consequence of this attitude.

FERNEL AND THE REFORMULATION OF MEDICAL PRINCIPLES

The modest success of Benivieni's little book was far exceeded by the fame and lasting influence of Jean Fernel.[46] As recorded in chapter 2, Cardano was one of Fernel's earliest admirers, ranking the Frenchman the equal of Vesalius. Subsequently, he remembered a friendly encounter with Fernel in Paris as one of the high points of his northern European tour in 1552.[47] Fernel's characteristic theories about causes of disease, *spiritus*, and innate heat, which were to make him a symbol of neotericism to two generations of conventional Galenists, first appeared in treatises on physiology and on hidden causes published in the 1540s (*De naturali parte medicinae*, 1542; *De abditis rerum causis*, 1548). In these works he modified standard Galenic physiological concepts such as *spiritus*, or *pneuma*, and innate heat in ways designed to emphasize links between the human body and celestial and astral powers and the operation of occult causes in nature.

In 1554, Fernel published his pioneering general textbook, *Medicina* (an enlarged edition published after his death was retitled *Universa medicina*).[48] Incorporating his earlier physiological treatise, the work covered physiology, pathology, and therapy clearly and systematically in one convenient volume; it opened with anatomical description and insisted on the indispensability of dissection; and it contained a number of insights and observations about pathology.[49] These features ensured its widespread use, continuing long after controversy over Fernel's distinctive theories had faded or ceased to be of any particular importance. Although Fernel was still being held up as a symbol of neotericism at the University of Padua in 1587,[50] by the end of the century he seems to have been regarded in northern Europe simply as a sound medical author who represented a modern Galenic alternative to Paracelsus.

In Fernel, Cardano encountered a physician who matched many of his own ideals. Fernel had proclaimed the need for a reform of medicine; he too claimed that knowledge of anatomy was important for internal medicine and stressed attention to particulars in diagnosis and therapy.[51] Where Cardano attempted to record episodes of disease in Sacco, Fernel is said to have systematically studied the action of various purgatives in different doses for different patients and conditions.[52] Some aspects of Fernel's ideas about *spiritus*, which laid much emphasis on the role of the heavens, surely resonated with Cardano's astrological concerns; moreover, the emphasis on the exceptional refinement of *spiritus* recalled one side of Cardano's concept of subtlety. In addition, Fernel shared not just Cardano's astral worldview but his command of mathematics and technical astrology, having written several treatises on mathematics, cosmology, and astrology before concentrating on medicine. He is also said to have taught astronomy or astrology privately and constructed astronomical instruments. Although he is alleged to have turned away from astrology later in his life, he adhered to fundamental beliefs about celestial causation throughout his career.[53]

Exhaustive modern analyses of Fernel's attempted reform of principles of physiology and pathology have rightly stressed the connections of some of his ideas both with the religious and magical aspects of Renaissance Platonism and with the climate of interest in new, or supposedly new, diseases and in disease transmission.[54] His theories about *spiritus* have also been shown to bear some resemblance to medieval Christian philosophical and theological adaptations of ancient medical and cosmic pneumatology.[55] Essentially, Fernel maintained that in addition to the animal, vital, and natural spirits of standard Galenic medical teaching, celestial *spiritus* of divine origin flowed down from the heavens into the very substance of terrestrial things and were the bearers of form. Within the body these special divine *spiritus* were the carriers of innate heat and the source of all vital function. In some cases, however, the *spiritus* could induce "disease of the total substance," that is, a disease in which the entire substance and form was corrupted in a way that had nothing to do with temperamental imbalance. The idea of disease of the total substance was also to some extent an extrapolation from Galen's doctrine that certain remedies acted by their whole substance (or, in the scholastic version, their specific form) rather than by the balance of elementary qualities. Wholly speculative though the theory of "disease of the total substance" was, it had links with sixteenth-century epidemiological realities, since it served to express the special and total character of "new" diseases, notably the *morbus gallicus*. Fernel used the concept mainly to explain pestilential and epidemic diseases, but he also classified phthisis as a disease of the total substance.[56] These ideas were incorporated into his general work on medicine, but the underlying theory was expounded most fully (with philosophical background) in his dialogue *De abditis rerum causis.*

A substantial portion of that work is given over to an endeavor to demonstrate the harmony with Christian teaching of Platonic and Neo-platonic ideas about the role of the heavens in governing terrestrial things, the world soul, and the presence of ruling celestial spirits in all matter, including stones.[57] But these spirits are by no means impersonal. A long chapter listing the various kinds of governing spirits through which the world is administered amounts to a concise small treatise on angelology and demonology. It runs through the angelic hierarchies, the fallen angels, Platonic and Neoplatonic accounts of daimons, Socrates' daimon, and Roman beliefs in lares and penates. Finally, after warning against the tricks of demons and the dangers of having anything to do with them, Fernel envisaged "spirits flying and wandering through the whole world, incorporeal and immortal and sharing in intelligence; we cannot reach them by sense, but we feel our soul capable of intelligence and when it leaves the body it will join the spirit flocks."[58]

He also made clear in another lengthy chapter that for him the theory of disease of the total substance involved the belief that many diseases, which might appear natural, could in reality be inflicted either by God or by evil spirits, acting under God's permission and conjured by maleficent human beings. In particular, spells could make men impotent or bring on demonic possession. The principal case history recounted in *De abditis rerum causis* is that of a young man whose convulsions failed to yield to any ordinary medical treatment and were subsequently re-vealed to be the result of possession. The demon then explained that it was his strategy to make the doctors try so many different remedies that they would kill the patient. For such diseases, prayers and exorcisms were of course the proper remedy, but Fernel admitted that for ordinary illnesses charms and amulets invoking spirits could also seem temporarily effective, although they were "neither certain nor safe, but deceiving, captious, and dangerous [*nec certa, nec tuta, sed fallax, captiosa, et pericu-losa est sanatio* (p. 642)]"; charms and so on that did not invoke either God or spirits were, by contrast, completely useless.[59] Fernel's treatise on hidden causes thus deserves a modest place in the sixteenth-century literature of demonology and witchcraft, as well as in that of medical innovation.

Fernel's *Medicina* also presents his theories about *spiritus,* innate heat, and disease of the total substance, but in the context of a general med-ical textbook. Philosophical discussion is curtailed; demonology does not make an appearance; and the pathological and therapeutic sections are devoted to the diagnosis and treatment of disease, including diseases classified as "of the whole substance," by wholly rational and naturalistic means. In them, moreover, Fernel stressed the importance of medical attention to a very different kind of relation between the hidden and the manifest, namely, the use of the site and character of external symptoms (hardness, swelling, unusual excretions, and so on) as a guide to the site and character of internal disease: "Every investigation leads from that which is perceived by the senses to abstruse and hidden [*occultatas*] causes, because what is last by origin and order of causes occurs first to investigation. And this is true even of any manifest disease with a known symptom. For it would be either damaged function or unusual excrement or pain that either by its site or type led us to suspect what part was affected."[60] His attempt to link symptoms of phthisis in life with appearances in the deceased patient's dissected lung, mentioned in a previous chapter, shows his own careful attention to this type of relation.

The apparent contrast between *De abditis rerum causis* and the *Medicina* is so great that the former was once thought to be an early work that Fernel left behind him when he turned to a more pragmatic, observational, and "modern" medical science.[61] But in 1538 Fernel had already begun to write the treatise on physiology subsequently incorporated as the first part of *Medicina*, and he was still at work on *De abditis* in 1540.[62] The relation between *De abditis* and *Medicina* more closely resembles that between a statement of theoretical principles and their working out in practice. Fernel's undertaking, like Cardano's, seems simultaneously aimed at elucidating governing astral principles and taking account of particulars. There is probably no reason to suppose that Fernel or his contemporaries would have found anything incompatible about the two parts of this enterprise. As Fernel's devoted pupil Guillaume Plancy put it, *De abditis rerum causis* functioned to explain "the more difficult places" in Fernel's physiology, pathology, and therapeutics.[63]

CARDANO ON OCCULT CAUSATION IN MEDICINE

Cardano gave extended consideration to occult causation in medicine in several contexts. One of these was when he wrote the long chapter entitled "Superstitious Cure of Diseases" for *De rerum varietate*, which, he explained, comprised "marvelous causes of diseases . . . and marvelous cures [*causas morborum mirabiles amplectitur, et curas rursus mirabiles* (p. 165)]."[64] It reviews a series of medical marvels culled indiscriminately from ancient and modern medical authors, ancient history, medieval chronicles, recent travelers' tales, and local gossip. Some of the marvels are the kind of thing Benivieni collected, with the difference that Benivieni collected predominantly examples from his own practice: strange diseases, such as the condition of the unfortunate girl who excreted more than her own weight in urine every day (a story told Cardano's father by Giovanni Marliani, allegedly about one of Marliani's patients); anatomical peculiarities, such as those of the man at Bologna reported by Coelius Rhodiginus as having six fingers on each hand and six toes on each foot; physiological rarities, such as the two deaf-mute brothers still living at Milan and the absence of puberty in some adolescents. Many more, however, concern cures. A few of the marvelous cures involve medicines that are simply unknown or rare, for example, herbs used by the Indians of Peru. One is Cardano's own discovery that he could mitigate his toothache by lightly grasping the tooth with the thumb and first finger of his left (but not his right) hand. Most, however, can be classified as in some sense magical—they involve amulets, ligatures, verbal charms, or various forms of sympathetic magic (for example, a cure for leprosy that called for bathing the leper in water that had been used to wash a cadaver).

Like the work of which it forms a part, the chapter is not organized around an argument but has the heterogeneous character of one of Cardano's collections of particulars. Nevertheless, it is evident that the overall goal is much more to explain wonders by natural causes than to question whether wonders happen. In a few cases, Cardano expressed incredulity: if ointment applied to one knee of the doge of Venice cured his other knee, this was more likely due to physical contact between his legs than to occult causes; Marliani's patient probably recovered owing to a change in the weather rather than to any treatment that could have been given at a time when "good letters still lay hidden and with them the Greek [medical] authors [*bonae literae adhuc laterent, et cum his Graeci authores* (p. 168)]"; many people who thought they had warded off rabies from a dog bite with a charm were probably in no danger of getting it in the first place. But in the great majority of instances, Cardano accepted the phenomena without comment and attributed them (including such a traditional magical effect as the power of peony root) to natural causes, namely, astral influences, occult natural properties in gems, plants, or people, and occasionally the power of *imaginatio*. But the fecundity that enabled the flute-maker's wife who lived near Milan's east gate to have twenty-five children was equally a natural marvel, earning the comment "Many and marvelous are the hidden things of our nature [*Magna et miranda sunt naturae nostrae arcana* (p. 169)]." Not only did all these therapeutic or physiological marvels have nothing whatsoever to do with witchcraft or commerce with evil demons, some of them could produce moral as well as physical improvement. The three ways of reforming an erring son were parental vigilance, prayer, and medical treatment; the last usually involved purgatives, but a blood transfusion from a better conducted young man, if such a thing were possible, would change the delinquent's behavior.[65] Avoiding the Scylla of evil demons, Cardano thus drifted close to the Charybdis of Galen's physiological determinism.

But Cardano reserved his fullest treatment of the topic of occult causation in medicine for a medical work. "Whether Incantations Can Be of Any Use in Cures," included in the enlarged second edition of his medical *Contradictiones* (1548), is by far the longest item in the volume.[66] There, he addressed the topic somewhat more systematically than he had done previously, no doubt in part because of the constraints of the *quaestio* format, but also because he was explicitly engaged with Pomponazzi's *De incantationibus*. Cardano was indeed among the readers of that work while it was still in manuscript. In *De incantationibus* Pomponazzi had argued at length that there was no room for either demons or miracles in Aristotelian philosophy; marvels or exceptions to the regular course of nature were therefore due to natural causes, notably the stars, powers of the human soul, or occult qualities in things.[67]

Cardano began by assembling a catena of *mirabilia* from the most authoritative philosophical and medical sources, starting with Aristotle (the Aristotelian *mirabilia* come mostly from *Historia animalium* and include such items as the billy goat of Lemnos that gave milk and was declared a portent by an oracle [3.20, 522a14–19]—amounting to two *miracula*, one of nature and one of the oracle, as Cardano pointed out). From Dioscorides, he listed various instructions for using plants suspended or in ligatures to ward off poisons. He added examples from his own personal knowledge of apparently successful cures of toothache and wounds by charms. And he included an example each of demonic possession and miraculous cure from Benivieni's collection, remarking that "if they are true, they are very pertinent to our business [*quae si vera sunt, magnum nobis negotium praebent* (p. 470)]."

Yet, as he went on to point out, not only were magical cures incompatible with Aristotelian philosophy, prohibited by law, and condemned on religious grounds, there were also powerful medical arguments against their legitimacy and efficaciousness. Both Galen and Hippocrates, in *On the Sacred Disease*, had denounced medical incantations; to accept cures of this kind involved accepting that *circulatores* were good medical practitioners, which was plainly ridiculous; and if these things were true, there would be no need for any other kind of medicine, for all medical treatment would be performed with divine or demonic aid and would always work perfectly.

In considering the problem, Cardano set down as a basic premise that the innumerable phenomena in the world and the limitations of human knowledge made it necessary to inquire whether any apparent marvel could be a natural effect. Then, after rapidly setting aside as inadequate or partial explanations attributed to "the astrologers" and to Avicenna, he devoted many pages to the exposition and analysis of Pomponazzi's views. As Ingegno has pointed out, although Cardano rejected Pomponazzi's positions en masse as "not only false and impious but largely alien to Peripatetic philosophy and self-contradictory," he actually accepted a good many of them in slightly refined and modified versions.[68] Among those he explicitly endorsed were the existence of special occult properties in species of plants, animals, stones, and so on, the power of the human soul to change things (although, in Cardano's more physiologically oriented version, the changes it brought about in the body through *imaginatio* required the medium of *spiritus*), the universal rule of heaven, or celestial intelligence, and the stars, and the readiness of people to attribute to the supernatural any phenomenon of which the causes were not understood.

But he also introduced some significant changes of emphasis. He almost entirely eliminated discussion of the existence or nonexistence of demons, the main point of Pomponazzi's treatise. He repeatedly urged, in a manner highly unusual in the sixteenth century—and far from consistently sustained in his own works—that the first thing to ask about a supposed marvel was not what had caused it but whether it had happened.[69] And he added propositions that brought two specific categories of *mirabilia* within the scope of the discipline and profession of medicine. (A third category, amulets, he simply accepted as a type of medicament endorsed by Galen; other types of *mirabilia* discussed without reference to medicine here include divination, although elsewhere, as noted in the previous chapter, he emphasized parallels linking divination, medicine, and astrology.) One of these propositions maintained that occult properties in the human body depend to some extent on diet (p. 481), an assertion that reveals the interconnection between two of his favorite themes, the powers of specially endowed people and the effects of diet. At various times he attributed special gifts and properties of certain people to exceptionally good temperamental balance (see chapter 3) or to an endowment from the heavens (there is no reason to suppose that he would have regarded the two explanations as mutually exclusive). Either or both might be the source of such marvelous properties as his own prophetic dreams, and so on, as well as of remarkable ingenuity and the power to grasp subtlety. But since some marvelous physical properties that ran in families seemed to be the result of their diet—he gave the example of the healing touch of the French royal family, due, he thought, to their use of aromatics—it should theoretically be possible, Cardano hypothesized, to induce other desirable marvelous properties by manipulating the diet. For example, one might expect a boy nourished on verbena (traditionally a magical herb) to be gracious (p. 482).

Two other propositions concern cures supposedly resulting from spells or incantations: one classified all cures that work by substituting hope for fear as cure by contraries and thus part of rational medicine; the other stated that cures using charms were effective for only a small cluster of conditions. These were all ailments in which the *imaginatio* of the patient was particularly involved. The most notable examples of such cures were charms to relieve impotence and toothache, staunch bleeding, and extract barbs embedded in the flesh. Given the almost universal belief in Renaissance society in the power of spells to cause impotence, a problem from which he himself suffered for years at a time (see further chapter 10), Cardano's apparent reluctance to attribute impotence to preternatural causes is especially striking. He noted that men were sometimes impotent because they believed themselves to be enchanted; in such cases, supposedly magical remedies worked simply because they substituted hope for the patient's despair. Toothache charms seemed to work either because the power of the patient's *imaginatio* affected his or her *spiritus* or when the tooth became deadened (*"obstupescente dente"* [p. 481]); trust in the charm or a practitioner might relax the flesh so that it was easier to extract an arrowhead. Practitioners who used charms on ulcerated wounds might not seem to apply any physical treatment, but in fact they changed the dressings and removed detritus, and this constituted treatment (p. 484).

These explanations had specific professional implications. In the sixteenth-century Italian medical marketplace, all practitioners are likely to have encountered among their patients of every social level reliance on *circulatores* who provided amulets, magical charms, and so on; as Cardano noted, "there are many people now exercising this art in our part of the world quite successfully [*Nunc autem multi nostris in regionibus hanc artem satis feliciter exercent* (p. 470)]." Practitioners of "rational" Galenic medicine were not in a position either to claim consistently superior powers to cure or to dismiss magical medicine as invariably ineffective. To argue that cures apparently brought about by charms (and perhaps also by prayers) were due to hidden natural causes was to accept, not deny, the cures themselves. The effect of such an argument was therefore to legitimize all kinds of inexplicable cures, and *magia naturalis* itself, as part of medicine. At the same time, Cardano avoided yielding any professional ground to *circulatores* by emphasizing that their effectiveness was restricted to a small number of relatively insignificant conditions and that experienced physicians had all kinds of special skills and knowledge that seemed marvelous to patients.[70]

Yet Cardano's insistence in the *quaestio* on incantations in medicine that most occult cures were natural and nondemonic did not mean that he was convinced that cures by demons never occurred. Shortly after publishing that *quaestio*, he reported elsewhere the case of the Milanese noblewoman afflicted with burning urine and constant urge to urinate. The efforts of seven physicians (of whom Cardano was one) with as many diagnoses, several surgeons, and a prolonged series of treatments ranging from hot fomentations to surgery only made matters worse. The treatments were unpleasant enough to make it highly unlikely, in Cardano's view, that the patient was malingering. A professor of Greek who knew no medicine but had a reputation as a magician, whispering magic charms to the woman's son, induced the boy to look into a crystal and say that he saw three demons afflicting his mother, and then another demon driving them away. The woman recovered, "because she was healed either by the demon or by imagination and faith [*vel daemone sanata est mulier: vel imaginatione, fideque*]." But since the professor of Greek refused a fee and risked acquiring a damaging reputation as a magician whether or not the cure succeeded, "it is more likely that she was healed by a demon, and that there are demons and they wander about [*verisimilius est a daemone sanatam esse: daemonasque ipsos esse et vagari*]."[71]

On the subject of medical incantations, he concluded by sharply distinguishing the use of verbal formulas, such as those used by the professor of Greek, from magical cures that did not employ words. It was, he claimed, exclusively the use of verbal formulas that rendered such cures illegitimate. If the cures worked naturally, the words had absolutely no effect so that anyone using them was a fraud. But if, "in agreement with the law you say that the words do have force, then their power is from demons and the cult of demons is practiced, which cannot possibly be allowed. But if they are done without words, they are part of medicine if they pertain to health, and if to something else, for example, the remora [the ship-holding fish] or the magnet, they are part of natural philosophy. So there is no need to postulate another science [of magic]. Therefore magic is nothing unless you place it as part of either medicine or natural philosophy, and understood in this way magic is no more illicit than carpentry."[72]

Pomponazzi's naturalism, his recourse to the stars, and his insistence on the falsity of many of the beliefs that attributed effects to the power of demons clearly appealed to Cardano. For all his criticisms of details in Pomponazzi's arguments, these positions underlie Cardano's explanation of occult causes and marvelous effects in medicine in *Contradictiones* 2.2.7. Moreover, Cardano, too, claimed to be offering an Aristotelian explanation and, indeed, faulted Pomponazzi for philosophical eclecticism. On the last point he was right, though he was scarcely in a position to criticize anyone else on that score.[73]

But he did not endorse Pomponazzi's thoroughgoing philosophical repudiation of the existence of demons. Cardano was explicit that *magia naturalis* worked through understanding of sympathies and properties of things to change the human body or perceptions and did not involve demons.[74] Nevertheless, his astrally governed cosmos owed much to a Christianized Neoplatonism that gave a large role to spiritual beings. He identified the archangels with planetary gods: the virtues of Mercury, which ruled over the intellect and senses, were the virtues of Raphael, "that is, of the god of medicine."[75] Family and personal experience— always for him a test of reality—confirmed the existence of lesser spirits, most importantly his own guiding genius. The problem was thus that, although "it is difficult to defend with reasons that demons and souls of the dead are about everywhere; yet this agrees with experience [*experimentum*]."[76]

The way in which Cardano thought of his genius emerges from another of the medical *Contradictiones*, in which he sharply attacked Agostino Nifo's treatise on demons.[77] In an exercise in orthodox demonology of the kind that threatened both the intellectual foundations and the social viability of the entire tradition of learned natural magic, Nifo had asserted that demons existed and that they were invariably evil, not by nature but by will and obstinacy. His supporting evidence included the assurance he had received from the inquisitor of heretical pravity of the province of Padua that demons frequently enabled witches to become invisible.[78] In his critique of Nifo, as in various other contexts, Cardano attributed alleged demonic feats to fraud, credulity, or financial motives. He denounced Nifo for believing that demons could transport women from place to place (a belief "unworthy of a barber, let alone a philosopher [*ista sunt indigna tonsore nedum philosopho*]") and allowing himself to be conned by a Neapolitan alchemist; he likewise denounced alchemists for lying because they are unable to perform what they promise, and people who write magic books for profit and ascribe them to Solomon, Pietro d'Abano, Avicenna, Albertus Magnus, and other worthy characters who never thought of such a thing.[79]

But among evil demons Nifo had specifically included the daimon (in Cardano's terms, genius) of Socrates. In rebuttal, Cardano maintained that genii, like prophetic or meaningful dreams, were genuine evidence of God's knowledge of and care for individuals. People who had possessed a personal genius included Cardano's own father, who had never used his for gain, to harm enemies, or to get to know about the immortality of the soul. Among others were Avicenna, Averroes, and Algazel (yet another testimony to medieval Arab sciences). The genii of the latter two had been seen in disputation: Averroes' was small and blackish and Algazel's larger and more rubicund.[80] (This remarkable observation occurred on August 20, 1491, when the elder Cardano received a visit from seven daimons in Greek costume, who proceeded to conduct a scholastic disputation on the eternity of the world in which one of them showed himself to be an Averroist.)[81] Elsewhere, but not here, Girolamo reported another experience of his father's more readily reducible to terms of orthodox demonology. It occurred when Fazio Cardano was sitting up at night keeping vigil while a boy he had been tutoring lay sick in another room. A small, cold, invisible left hand, about the size of a ten-year-old child's, passed over his face and tried to put its fingers in his mouth. Fazio prudently kept his mouth tight shut, but the fingers were so cold that his teeth ached anyway. The sick boy died the next night.[82]

In his response to Nifo, however, Cardano provided a benign intellectual definition of genii. While vague as to their exact nature—they were either eternal spirits, or minds of men endowed with an airy vehicle, or something in us distinct from the soul—he made it clear that their primary characteristics were knowledge and memory of singulars. One's genius knew everything, including all the things one had once known and had forgotten.[83] The entire discussion links Cardano's beliefs and experiences involving genii and dreams very closely with his ideas about the soul and the power of human beings to know.

Yet he found the medical conclusions that Fernel derived from an astrally governed Neoplatonic universe alive with spiritual beings as unacceptable as Pomponazzi's complete dismissal of demons and Nifo's assumption of their universal malevolence. Despite his general admiration for Fernel, Cardano devoted the last of his surviving *Contradictiones* to a vigorous repudiation of Fernel's theory of disease of the total substance.[84] Fernel's arguments were "very beautiful [*pulcherrima*]," but nevertheless all the conditions he explained as a result of corruption of the total substance were actually the result of imbalance of the primary qualities.[85] Unlike Fernel, Cardano was not closely involved in the contemporary debate over epidemic disease and disease transmission, as his brief and conventional (despite the use of the terms *spiritus* and *contagium*) account of plague transmission shows.[86] He disliked Fernel's theories, not because of what they had to say about contagion or epidemics, but because they implied a role for demons in certain diseases and cures. Instead, Cardano insisted that "there is imbalance of temperament even in fascination and love and diseases of this kind." Once again he introduced the example of men who believed themselves bewitched into impotence and were subsequently relieved by simple magical remedies.

This time the explanation is even more elaborately naturalistic and physiological; rather than just asserting that the substitution of hope for fear constituted a cure by contraries, as he had done before, he now specified that the patient's own *imaginatio* caused inappropriate cooling of the affected part and overheating of the blood.[87] And here too he cited Hippocrates' *On the Sacred Disease* to the effect that many diseases have unknown causes, and yet they are not from God. As Cardano remarked on another occasion, "Platonists are remarkably addicted to belief in demons."[88]

Thus the fluctuations of opinion denounced by the skeptical philosopher Francisco Sanches and other sixteenth-century critics of Cardano's natural philosophical discussions of demons are also present in his accounts of occult causes and marvelous effects in medicine.[89] In specifically medical contexts, he registered his dissatisfaction with all three of the principal intellectual positions available: the total rejection of all possibility of demonic activity in disease or cure, the assumption that demonic intervention was widespread and universally malevolent, and the idea that demonic forces caused certain specific diseases or disabilities. He was no doubt, as has been suggested, trying to find a middle way between Aristotelianism and Neoplatonism, while maintaining religious orthodoxy (or the appearance of it).[90] His ambivalence on this difficult issue probably also relates to the importance he attached to *experimentum*, particulars, and the use of his own experience as a test case.

Yet although his position on occult causes in medicine, as on so many other issues, was eclectic and sometimes confused (or at any rate confusing), in general he presented his medicine as rationalistic. His medical theory and everything he reports of his practice combined Galenic rationalism with nondemonic *magia naturalis* in an astrally governed universe. His description of genii seems designed to remove any connotation of spirits invoked to do the will of a magus. His references to his own genius suggest instead an unbidden source of knowledge and memory linked with the heavens, which, like his dreams, helped to enhance his natural, but special and unusual, gifts of *inventio*, *ingenium*, and mastery of *subtilitas*.

THE POWERS OF THE PHYSICIAN-MAGUS

In theoretical discussions about medicine—the chapter on "superstitious cures" in *De rerum varietate* and the critiques of Pomponazzi and Fernel in the medical *Contradictiones*—Cardano fairly consistently attributed the power of healing charms and spells to natural causes. In describing cures that he performed himself using the tools of rational medicine, he employed the language of marvel. He entitled his collection of his own successful cases *On Wonderful [admirandis] Cures and Predictions of Disease* and used the term *miraculum* for some of them.[91] Discussion of this little work as medical and autobiographical narrative is reserved for a later chapter, but the sense in which it is a collection of wonders is relevant here.

Cardano's collection, like most of Benivieni's, is made up of cases encountered in his own practice. A common idea motivates both works, namely, that of the value of recording the "marvellous" or "wonderful" in medicine. Both Benivieni and Cardano made collecting and writing accounts of *mirabilia* that they claimed to have personally encountered in medical practice into an important part of their professional activity. But in the great majority of instances, Cardano's cases are not marvelous in either of the senses used by Benivieni: they are neither rare pathological conditions nor examples of supernatural intervention. Most of the patients suffer from conditions to which a standard name (*lepra, morbus gallicus, podagra*, tertian fever, etc.) can be attached. The challenge of these illnesses is not rarity or strangeness, but severity, long duration, and difficulty of cure. Much attention is given to detailed description of the means of therapy, which are invariably "rational": instructions for regimen, herbal medications, bleeding. Cardano's ingenuity emerges in his choice of particular remedies and improvements of the details of treatment.[92] The marvels that the reader is invited to consider therefore consist exclusively of Cardano's successes in achieving cures by selecting appropriate rational treatment.

But a certain ambiguity surrounds the source of these successes. His entire self-presentation as a Hippocratic physician required that they be the result of wisdom and skill, acquired by study, knowledge of good rules of medicine, and reflection on experience. Moreover, the collection contains abundant material to substantiate such a claim. For instance, he carefully explained that although a patient was astonished (*"admiratus"*) at his (Cardano's) ability to describe all the patient's symptoms accurately after one quick glance, the diagnosis was actually reached through the interpretation of observation, no doubt in the light of experience.[93] Yet the free use of the term "miracle" about some of the cures ("By a similar miracle, I cured Julia Rotora")[94] and the language in which some of them are described seems also strongly to imply that Cardano's power to heal was among the *mirabilia*, as he termed them, of his subtle nature.[95]

In recounting the case of an innkeeper whom he claimed to have cured of some form of paralysis, he used the following language:

> What happened to Gaspare Roulla . . . therefore seemed very close to a miracle to everyone and many people ran to see it. For it did not seem that he could be healed by any human power before he was healed by us. But it

will give pleasure to narrate the history. He had already been lying contracted in bed for an entire year, but for the last five months of that year completely immobile; he could not move his foot, his head, his arm, or anything else. Beside giving him great pain, his limbs were hard as a stone. And it was the middle of winter. Therefore it was agreed by me that this would be fully healed within forty days, not to the wonder but to the stupefaction of those who saw him. For some were saying he was star-struck, others smitten by divine wrath, others paralyzed, others possessed by the devil, so that prayers and execrations were not lacking.[96]

The range of possible causes invoked by the bystanders is, it will be noted, precisely that found in the erudite discussions of occult causes of disease considered so far: occult but natural astral influences; the action of God; the action of the devil; or factors internal to the human body.

Cardano decided that bleeding was necessary, "not only on account of the magnitude of the disease, but also because by consideration of his lifestyle and the disease itself I conjectured that the whole mass of blood was corrupted. Nor did the judgment made about this thing fail me in any part. Indeed all the blood that went out was putrid."[97] The innkeeper was accordingly bled three times and finally completely cured except for a twisted neck. Despite Cardano's explanation of the rational grounds for his choice of treatment, the language in which this cure is presented reads very like that of a miracle story. The paralytic disease, the emphatic description of symptoms, the assertion of the impossibility of cure by any human means, the expectations of the crowd, the allusions to the power of God and the devil, to prayers and curses all create an atmosphere more reminiscent of shrine healings or accounts of possession and exorcism than of the clinic. Even the numbers—forty days' treatment and three bleedings—might be thought to have religious or magical overtones.

No doubt, such language contains an element, possibly a large element, of the rhetoric of professional defensiveness and self-aggrandizement. No doubt, too, it may be influenced by Galen's florid descriptions of his own successes in *On Prognosis*, the acknowledged model for Cardano's *Wonderful Cures* (on these aspects, see further chapter 9). But the language also reflects Cardano's general usage of the word and concept "miracle." He did not, as has sometimes been alleged, deny the possibility that miracles could occur by divine power; rather, he used the term so broadly that he blurred the distinctions among supernatural phenomena to which religious significance was attributed, remarkable occurrences resulting from occult natural causes, and regular aspects of nature that aroused awe or admiration.[98] Moreover, he asserted that many events described as miracles in the religious sense were produced by occult causes in nature, by a disturbance of the senses of the people involved, or by human contrivance for reasons of avarice, power seeking, or self-justification. Thus people reported their rescues from sudden illness or injury as miracles because the fear of death turned the victims' thoughts to religion. In reality such sudden escapes could be due to the healing power of Nature, a change in the position of the stars, or, in many cases, the protection of a daimon, or genius. Meaningful dreams or visions, such as he claimed to have experienced himself, might, however, occur—either "through the will of higher powers or as a result of causes obscure to us but noble in nature."[99] As a result of this attitude, Cardano applied the word "miracle" (*miraculum*) not only to miraculous healings reported as religious events by Saint Augustine but also to the eruption of teeth in old age and the fact that every human face is different.[100] His application of the term "miracle" to cures he performed himself is an extension of this usage, with all its ambiguity. All of nature was a wonder, all wonders were in some sense natural—but, where cures were concerned, it was not given to everyone to perform wonders.

Hence Cardano's use of the terms *mirum* and *miraculum* for the cures he performed does not imply a claim that they were achieved by anything other than natural means. He rested his claims to success in medical practice on a combination of natural gifts—*inventio, ingenium,* subtlety of perception, capacity for mastery of subtlety—and skill acquired through study and experience. These were the characteristics that enabled him to find the various theoretical and practical improvements that he believed he had contributed to medicine. Although he professed to be unable to judge whether his power of medical prognostication was the result of "divine inspiration, a Harpocratic [that is, naturally prophetic] constitution, or a certain perfection of judgment and mind [(*seu divinus afflatus, seu Harpocratica constitutio, seu quaedam iudicii et mentis perfectio*]," he added immediately that he never made predictions without careful inquiry into the circumstances.[101] Thus he could lay claim to a *miraculorum ratio*, a reasoned (that is, natural) way of bringing about miracles of healing, just as he claimed the power to find a reasoned (that is, natural) interpretation of his meaningful, but natural, dreams.[102] Moreover, although his claim to "miraculous" power to heal looks very different from Benivieni's pragmatic awareness of the limits of medicine, it, too, may encode a rather realistic estimate of the random and arbitrary nature, in the Renaissance medical world, of apparent therapeutic successes. Nevertheless, Cardano's insistence on the way in which some of his cures seemed miraculous—to himself or others—suggests the aspect of subtlety that involved a unique sensitivity to occult forces in nature and the guidance of his genius. His ambivalence about the relation between acquired skill and special gifts that were arbitrary and perhaps impermanent emerges from the summing up of his "wonderful cures":

And these things are about the more notable patients who were cured by us from desperate diseases, although the passage of time and forgetfulness has abolished my memory of innumerable others. For I did not have a reasoned way of bringing about miracles [*miraculorum ratio*] of this kind until a few years ago. This one thing should be enough: I was always exceptionally happy in the works of the art, to the extent that just as some refer it to chance, so others do to the devil. But just as no one was happier with perpetual success in curing, so no one was safer from errors and adverse chances than I.[103]

Chapter 8

THE MEDICINE OF DREAMS

CARDANO believed himself an exceptionally gifted dreamer of prophetic dreams. One of his favorite examples was a nightmare that he had in Milan in 1536 which, he thought, saved him from certain death. In this dream a huge menacing serpent lay on the ground eying him hungrily. He awoke terrified but having no idea what the dream might portend. A few days later, he was summoned to attend Count Camillo Borromeo's small son. The little boy—at that time the count's only surviving male child—did not seem to be seriously ill and had obvious signs of worms, so Cardano prescribed a vermifuge with which at Sacco he had successfully treated many children of lesser lineage. The servant was on the point of leaving for the pharmacy with the prescription, when Cardano remembered his nightmare. In his recollection, the serpent in his dream bore a remarkable resemblance to the one on the Borromeo family's coat of arms.[1] Now recognizing that the dream had been a warning of danger for him in the Borromeo household should the child die under his care, Cardano hastily called back the servant and changed his prescription. For the strong vermifuge he substituted a milder medicine that was obviously highly suitable for a member of the aristocracy, since it consisted of shavings of emerald, sapphire, and pearl. Subsequently, three other more socially and professionally established physicians approved this prescription and ordered it to be administered again. Even so, when the child died shortly thereafter, the distraught father was ready to murder Cardano on the spot. However, while the count's friends held him back, the women of the household hustled Cardano away to safety. Cardano was sufficiently impressed by this sequence of events—which certainly provides an unnerving glimpse of the hazards for physician and patient of Renaissance medical practice among the aristocracy—to recount the whole story at least three times in different works.[2]

Reflection on the episode inspired him to begin writing his *Synesiorum somniorum libri*, the most substantial theoretical treatise about dreams composed during the Renaissance, which was finally published in 1562.[3] The story may also serve as an introduction to a consideration of how his theoretical ideas about, and actual use of, dreams fitted into his understanding of medical science and of the task of the physician. Medicine was only one of many contexts in which Cardano pondered dreams; the study of dreams penetrated and cross-fertilized his approaches to history, religion, occult sciences, and, of course, autobiography. To a possibly unique degree, he combined a learned, academic interest in dream interpretation with an intense commitment to meaningful and prophetic dreams that he believed he had experienced himself.

But even though Cardano's interest in dreams was unusually intense and took an unusually wide range of forms, the interest itself was not idiosyncratic. Sixteenth-century culture, elite and popular alike, gave large space to predictive experiences of various kinds: dreams, prophecies, portents, and visions. In a world charged with supernatural and religious meaning, prophecy and dreams touched on many spheres of life—including, as the careers of Nostradamus and Lucia de Léon in their different ways show, the dangerously political. In the medical world, attention to dreams may have been encouraged by the idea that prognosis was common to dream interpretation, astrology, and medicine. Perhaps as a result, learned interest in the ancient literature on dreams was, as I am not the first to note, especially flourishing in medical milieus.[4] In Cardano's case, not all the uses he found for dreams in medicine would necessarily have been approved by most of his medical colleagues. He related his theories about prophetic and guiding dreams to his own role as a medical practitioner and medical author, making only highly selective use of other traditions that linked dreams to health, disease, and medicine. But his ideas about dreams and medicine were nevertheless constructed from ancient sources and reflected the needs and constraints of his professional practice.

Cardano's treatment of dreams in the context of medicine shares objectives and methodology with his approach to the subject of dreams in general. Among these common features is his practice of recording, rewriting, and manipulating narratives of his own dreams for two different purposes. Cardano's two uses for his dreams can, I think, be distinguished even though a number of his dream narratives serve both ends simultaneously.

The first type of use was autobiographical. Cardano's interest in recording what he regarded as prophetic dreams relating to his medical career cannot be divorced from his autobiographical preoccupations. He habitually deployed prophetic dreams and their sequelae as structural elements in the story he constructed of his own life and recounted not only in *De propria vita* but also in various forms throughout his writings. His story of the case of the Borromeo child is a good example of this type of use, including the ultimate consequence that the dream induced him to write a book. It is only one of a number of instances in which a dream instructed or inspired this copious and eclectic author to write.[5] Cardano's use of dream narratives in an autobiographical context seems comparable to his similarly repetitive use of his own horoscope and the bibliography of his own writings. All were types of record, made at various times during his life; as such, they served to organize memory and provided a framework for self-expression. But in Cardano's hands horoscope, autobibliography, and dream narratives were all open to, indeed demanded, subsequent revision and reinterpretation of memory. He recast and reinterpreted horoscopes in the light of later events, most famously in the case of Edward VI of England, for whom he had predicted a long life before that monarch's death at the age of fifteen.[6] He published progressively expanded lists of his own writings over a period of thirty years. And he reflected on his "prophetic" dreams for decades after they occurred, continuing to revise and change the meaning he had attributed to them. Until the very end of his life, Cardano was still engaged in reinterpreting the details of a dream about his future that he had had in 1534. In 1562, he identified a twelve-year-old boy seen in that 1534 dream with a pupil who entered his household in 1558; in 1575, he interpreted the same boy as either his grandson (b. 1560) or a good spirit.[7] More remains to be said about repetition and self-reference in Cardano's autobiographical use of his dreams, his horoscope, and his autobibliography, but that is beyond the scope of this book.

Cardano's second use for dream narratives—this time placing his own dreams alongside those of a miscellany of historical personages, friends, and relatives—was as *exempla* to be employed in constructing a general theory of dreams. The last book of his treatise on dreams consists entirely of such examples. His dream theory, in turn, forms part of his endeavor to develop a natural philosophy and medicine that would somehow include, take account of, or explore uncertainty, randomness, particulars, idiosyncratic or individual characteristics, subtlety, and variety. Hence one of his most extended discussions of dream theory, apart from his treatise dedicated to the subject, occurs in the chapters on *mirabilia* of mankind and marvelous cures in *De rerum varietate*.[8] As Jean Céard has suggested, Cardano's interest in whether, and how, apparently random phenomena could be predicted is the unifying thread running through his involvement in subjects as diverse as astrology, physiognomy, games of chance—and dreams.[9]

In a more strictly medical context, his use of dreams can be connected with his self-presentation as critic and reformer of contemporary academic medicine. As has become apparent, his enthusiasm for *inventio* and *ingenium*, his attacks on medical colleagues, and his criticisms of Galen coexisted with his largely Aristotelian philosophy and in most respects Galenic medicine. Yet he was also simultaneously engaged in a search for alternative sources of authority in medicine. For Cardano, as for many of his contemporaries, the desire for reform was apt to be expressed and understood as a return to ancient authorities other than, and preferably even more ancient than, the standard school authors. In a variety of ways, Cardano's reading of alternative ancient authors or texts as guides to medical reform was focused on the problem of predictive knowledge. His call for reform of the Galenic doctrine of critical days by means of "the Hippocratic art of Ptolemy" required physicians to improve their technical command of astronomy and the calendar in order to achieve better understanding of supposedly recurrent cycles in illness.[10] Similarly, his view of the *Epidemics* treated the art of prognostication as central to Hippocratic medicine.[11] In this whole pattern of thought, ancient dream theories, too, might seem to promise ideas that could be given fresh emphasis in a renovated medicine. In his dream book Cardano insisted that medicine and dream interpretation together belonged in the category of "conjectural disciplines."[12] Drawing another parallel between them, he maintained that although dream interpretation in general was in no way an art, "there will be an art, and a science, pertaining to evident and perfect dreams of which the greatest part are destined to take effect, for most of these are true and there is some information about them; just as not all healing is a science, since many people are healed by chance: but there is some art and certain reasoning [*certa ratio*] about healing that is brought about by physicians."[13] These assertions classifying dream interpretation among useful practical arts, or even sciences, based on natural knowledge, placed it in respectable company. They made dream interpretation, as it were, innocent by association; but they joined medicine to a discipline or activity of more ambiguous status.

Renaissance dream theory had a rich and highly diversified store of sources on which to draw. Valuable recent work has been dedicated to clarifying these traditions in both their original form and their various subsequent reworkings.[14] Only a few salient points that seem especially relevant to Cardano's situation need be noted here. In the first place, even more than astrology (which, after all, had an irreducible technical and mathematical component), dream lore crossed the boundary between learned and popular culture. Dreams interested learned magi, cabalists, and physicians, Christian and Jewish alike; but dream interpretation also belonged to the vast repertoire of popular magical beliefs and practices.[15]

As Cardano frankly acknowledged, a principal source for large sections of his treatise on dreams was the dream book of Artemidorus (fl. second century A.D.).[16] This work was based on the assumption that some dream images contained disguised predictions of the future, which required interpretation by allegory or analogy. But the same image might have very different meanings for different dreamers, since the appropriate interpretation would vary according to the dreamer's age, sex, social status, occupation, and so on. Accordingly, Artemidorus's treatise consists chiefly of a directory of dream images considered to be significant, accompanied by multiple possible interpretations.[17] The work is among the ultimate sources of the medieval vernacular dream books; and fourteen of the eighteen sixteenth-century editions of Artemidorus are translations into vernacular languages. But the work also had a learned public. The Aldine Greek appeared in 1518, and a Latin translation—presumably itself the source for the vernacular versions just mentioned—went into three editions.[18] The Latin version, first published in 1539, was the work of the medical humanist Janus Cornarius. His preface shows very clearly that by that time learned men who wrote on dreams could feel a need to defend themselves against charges of frivolity and superstition. Cornarius was prepared for his translation to be denounced on the grounds that it communicated to Latin readers "fallacious and inane dreams that render minds frivolous and confusions that have already been exploded." He therefore reassured potential critics that in reality dream interpretation was a useful art; Christians should not condemn it as heathen and vain, but accept it as pious and desirable. However, the practice of this art needed to be restricted to those who were "weighty, prudent, and sober."[19] The critics Cornarius had in mind were his fellow Lutherans (and Luther was indeed deeply suspicious of his interest in pagan authors), but the attitudes of intellectuals to popular forms of divination were hardening in Counter-Reformation Europe too.[20] In this context, the presence, just noted, of a long discussion of natural causes of meaningful dreams in the chapter of *De varietate rerum* entitled "Superstitious Cure of Diseases" constitutes an implicit rebuttal of any accusation of superstition.

In fact, Cardano's fundamental understanding of the sensory and mental processes involved in dream formation rested on Aristotelian natural philosophy. Aristotle held that dreams resulted from fragmentary impressions left on the senses by previous waking experience and that they were affected by the condition of the body. His views provided a naturalistic explanation for the phenomena of dreaming, situated dreams at the boundary of body and mind, and legitimated academic discussion of the subject—perhaps as distinct from claims to interpret the dreams of patrons, clients, or patients—in the context of natural philosophy and the theoretical part of medicine, which was considered to be closely allied to natural philosophy.[21] Cardano, too, held that all dream images originated with the dreamer and were affected by the state of his or her mind and body. He maintained that most dreams reflected the dreamer's emotional state or recent experiences, or were induced by particular foods or the current state of the dreamer's humors (in which case they were useful for medical diagnosis).[22]

But whereas Aristotle had taken a rather dismissive attitude to prophetic dreams—implying that, while possible, they were rare and usually due to the dreamer's concentration of his waking thoughts on future action—prophetic dreams were central to Cardano's theory. He explained that such dreams occurred when the influence of the heavenly bodies affected the dreamer's *spiritus* and caused appropriate images to be drawn forth from the store already in the dreamer's memory.[23] Moreover, he emphasized that the most valuable kind of prophetic dreams, those directly caused by the power of the heavens, were more trustworthy even than astrological prognostication, since they resulted from a strong immediate impression made by the heavens rather than following occasionally fallible human calculations: "But [a dream] that enlightens is either established by the very order of fate, or results from the judgment of the dreamer himself (reached either through serious thought or with the help of a daimon), or comes from the heavens. But the dream from the heavens is nearest to truth; for the heavens are the cause of everything and astrologers predict many things, and in some things it is so and in others not. But the heavens impress something very strongly; since whatever they impress [on one in a dream], is really so."[24] The assertion obviously expressed a personal conviction. Nevertheless, Cardano was not the only leading sixteenth-century astrologer to give a place to dream interpretation. His astrological rival and critic Luca Gaurico included maxims from the text of the Hippocratic *Dreams* (*Regimen* 4) in his astrological handbook and was a believer in nonastrological as well as astrological predictions.[25] At least these two cases do not seem to bear out the thesis that in sixteenth-century Italian social practice learned astrology competed with, rather than encompassing, those forms of divination and prophecy, dream interpretation among them, that had a popular following.[26]

But enthusiasts for meaningful and especially for prophetic dreams—and certainly anyone who claimed to have personally experienced the latter—trod a potentially dangerous borderline as far as religious orthodoxy was concerned, since one possible source of such dreams was either divine or diabolical agency. An explanation that identified the heavenly bodies alone as the higher powers with which the soul of a person of pure life could be in touch through dreams was naturalistic. But Cardano's position on the source of prophetic dreams, including his own, may have been somewhat more ambiguous. A major source of his ideas about dreams, souls, and occult higher powers was the early-fifth-century Neoplatonic treatise of Synesius of Cyrene translated by Marsilio Ficino, after which Cardano named his dream book.[27] The higher powers to which Synesius refers seem something more than merely astral, and so Ficino—and perhaps Cardano—appears to have understood them.[28]

Cardano's overt position involved a prudent removal of supernaturally caused dreams from the scope of his discussion with the remark "I would not deny that in certain cases dream images [*idola*] of this kind are sent by the Gods, just as are medical cures of a defective part. . . . But these are miracles and outside the consideration of the art"; he cites the example of a dream in the New Testament.[29] And he protected his book on dreams with a dedicatory epistle addressed to Carlo Borromeo, recently appointed cardinal archbishop of Milan. (As already noted, the Borromeo family continued to be Cardano's patrons for most of his life, despite the unfortunate episode in 1536 that begins this chapter.) In this dedication, Cardano stressed that dream interpretation was one of the useful arts given to man by God.[30]

Nonetheless, from the standpoint of orthodoxy, some of Cardano's positions about dreams seem incautious, to say the least. For one thing, he had very little to say about the possibility that dreams might be inspired by evil demons.[31] In this one respect, he stands in sharp contrast to another learned medical writer on dreams among his contemporaries, the French royal physician and professor of medicine at the University of Toulouse Auger Ferrier, with whom he otherwise shared similar sources and Platonizing ideas. In Ferrier's treatise dreams caused by evil demons emerged as a major category. According to Ferrier, demons were responsible for erotic dreams that tempted the chaste (a type of dream ignored by Cardano) and dreams of luxury that tempted the sober.[32] Moreover, Cardano was ready to attribute a dream in the Old Testament to natural causes, maintaining that Pharaoh's dream of the fat and thin cattle was sent neither by God nor by demons.[33] And he described his father's dream of a large wingless angel dressed in blue who summoned Fazio Cardano to his death. (In the dream, Fazio escaped by hiding; next day he ordered his doors to be kept locked and took his special antiplague medicine, which enabled him to escape the plague even though a neighbor came in through a door left open by a careless maid and breathed "pestiferous contagion" on him.)[34] After his death, Fazio more than once appeared in his son's dreams and they had long conversations.[35] Stories of the return of deceased relatives as revenants to warn or advise their descendants were often told in Renaissance families; in popular accounts, such visitations might be regarded as inspiring fear, but also as edifying or helpful.[36] However, deliberate efforts to raise the dead fell into the category of necromancy and were severely condemned by ecclesiastical authorities. Possibly as a result of inquisitorial reaction to rumors about his chats with the deceased Fazio, Girolamo found it prudent to insert into his *Vita* an emphatic denial that he had ever tried to raise the dead.[37]

Not only popular oneiromancy and natural philosophy but also the discipline of medicine offered Cardano "a place for dreams."[38] Medical theory asserted a connection between dreams and the physiology of humors and temperaments. Although this doctrine had long been available via Rasis, Avicenna, and other medieval Arabo-Latin or Latin authors, direct access to the Hippocratic and Galenic texts that taught the importance of dreams in medicine became easier in Cardano's lifetime than ever before. By the 1540s, the Hippocratic *Dreams*, unknown in the Latin West before the 1470s, was readily available in print both in the original Greek and in several different Latin translations. It was, as already noted, part of *Regimen* (*De diaeta*), a work important to Cardano for philosophical as well as medical reasons.[39] The only Latin commentary on this work, by Cardano's adversary Julius Caesar Scaliger, was published in 1539.[40] Galen's *On Diagnosis from Dreams*, first translated into Latin in the early fourteenth century, was translated six more times between 1531 and 1562.[41] Hippocrates, Galen, and Synesius on dreams appeared all three together in an anthology edited by Ferrier in 1549.[42]

Both the Hippocratic and the Galenic treatise addressed dreams primarily as reflections of the patient's physical condition and asserted their diagnostic value, although *Dreams* also alluded to dreams of divine origin. The Hippocratic author explained that dreams were affected by the state of the body and therefore should be carefully considered by the physician. In general, pleasant dreams indicated a good state of physical health and disturbed dreams indicated poor health. Yet a Hippocratic physician was also supposed to pay attention to the detailed content of his patient's dreams. Thus dreams of springs and cisterns indicated bladder trouble and called for locally appropriate remedies.[43] Galen took up the same idea and situated it more firmly in the context of a systematic humoral physiology: "if someone dreams about a fire, he is troubled by yellow bile; if about smoke, fog, or deep shadows, by black bile; . . . and snow, hail, and ice [indicate] cold phlegm." Galen also provided actual examples of his own diagnostic use of his patients' dreams.[44]

Cardano certainly endorsed the ideas that dreams could be tools for medical diagnosis of physical conditions and that pleasant and untroubled dreams were a component of good physical health. He discussed foods and environments that he thought conducive, respectively, to sleep, to dreaming of any kind, and to pleasant dreams. Asserting that "it is no small thing to sleep enjoyably," for pleasant dreams he recommended the use of "foods that generate sweet blood," pleasant smelling plants, and certain gems and colors, especially an intense green (possibly a Ficinian echo?). By contrast, cabbage, chestnuts, onions, beans, and garlic would produce disturbing and frightening dreams.[45] A diet of these vegetables was, he thought, responsible for dreams which led witches to believe that they had traveled to distant places and had fantastic experiences. The qualifying comment that the witch ointment compounded from dead babies' fat and other unpleasant ingredients also helped to produce the illusion scarcely mitigates the stricture on the foods regarded as typical of an entire social class (Cardano proffered naturalistic explanations for night flights, the sabbath, etc., while maintaining that witches deserved execution for heresy and malice).[46] But since he was primarily interested in "true" dreams, rather than the insignificant kinds caused by the ingestion of particular foodstuffs, the state of the dreamer's humors, or residual fragments of memory and emotion, he laid special stress, following Synesius, on the need for abstinence and an appropriate diet on the part of those who sought to purify themselves in order to become receptive to "true" or prophetic dreams.[47]

Moreover, although he habitually incorporated anecdotes from his own extensive experience as a medical practitioner into his works, he did not, as far as I am aware, record any attempt on his part to diagnose a patient from the patient's dreams, or to regulate a patient's dreaming. As noted earlier, he devoted a whole book of his *Synesiorum somniorum libri* to examples of dreams—remarking with some justice that it was more fun to read (*"iucundior lectu"*) than the rest of the work[48]—but none of these examples appear to involve diagnosis by, or prescription for, dreams of a patient in his own medical practice. Many if not most of the examples are culled from Greek and Roman history and relate to politics or personal affairs. Indeed, he may have collected possibly predictive dreams ascribed to famous personages of antiquity as a historical enterprise paralleling his collection of horoscopes of notable figures of the past (even though a dream collection would not lend itself to the kind of historical analysis Cardano believed could be applied to horoscopes, as will become apparent in chapter 9). Some dreams by individuals known personally to Cardano, who were or may have been among his patients, are included, but these do not relate to health and disease. The few examples of diagnostic or medically significant dreams that are included are Cardano's own or reports from other physicians, among them a fifteenth-century author; most of them do not amount to much more than a dream warning of approaching death from illness for the dreamer or a member of the dreamer's family.[49]

Cardano's apparent failure to follow the program advocated in the Hippocratic *Dreams* is especially striking, given his interest in all the Hippocratic writings and comparisons of himself to Hippocrates. However, he classified *Dreams* among the least useful, though most enjoyable, of Hippocrates' works.[50] One reason for his reticence was doubtless the low intellectual and social status ascribed to popular oneiromantic practitioners. In any event, in the course of instructing medical practitioners how to interview a patient about his or her sleeping pattern, he advised, "[Ask] whether [there were] dreams and what they were like in general, but not specifically, lest you be taken for a dream interpreter but having inquired in particular how he or she felt on waking up."[51]

But there was surely also another reason why, when Cardano thought over his experiences with dreams in medicine, he paid little attention to the humorally caused dreams of his patients. His attention was focused elsewhere. His primary interest in dreams in a medical context lay in the true, prophetic dreaming of the gifted and virtuous physician, such as he believed—or hoped—himself to be. Hence his main interest in Hippocrates and Galen in this connection was less in the advice they had to give about patients' dreams than in the role dreams played in their own lives as physicians. And this role was a prominent one. For instance, Cardano garnered from the supposed letters of Hippocrates a long account of Hippocrates' dream when he was summoned to the philosopher Democritus, whom his fellow citizens believed to be mad; in this dream, the god Asclepius entrusts Hippocrates to the care of a goddess personifying Truth, thus ensuring his ability to form the right opinion.[52] The letter ends with the resounding assertion, put into the mouth of Hippocrates himself, that "Medicine and prophecy are related to each other, since Apollo is the author and father of both arts."[53]

The example of Galen was even more significant. Galen was an acknowledged model for self-expressive, autobiographical elements in Cardano's writings in two important respects: as the author of a book about his own books, and as a physician who included detailed analyses of his own cases in some of his works (see chapter 9). Galen's descriptions of the role dreams played in his career seem to have been equally influential. Moreover, in Galen's family as in Cardano's, the capacity for prophetic dreaming allegedly passed from father to son. Cardano carefully noted Galen's accounts of his dreams. He was particularly impressed by Galen's admission that his successful treatment of pain between his diaphragm and his liver by severing an artery in his hand had been suggested to him by Asclepius in a dream. "It is certainly a great example," he exclaimed admiringly, "that such a great man in medicine should put faith in a dream to the extent that he would use his own art to put his own life in danger. I also admire his probity, for what he could have claimed to have found out for himself through his fertility in *ingenium* he attributed to God, to whom he owed it. For this alone, the man is worthy of the immortality of his name and books."[54] (Galen's willingness to take personal risks and give credit where it was due similarly impressed an early reader of Cardano's dream book, who marked the passage carefully in the copy of the 1562 edition now at the New York Academy of Medicine.)

But the fundamental authority for Cardano's belief that proper attention to dreams was a key to interpreting one's own life was certainly Synesius. In his treatise, Synesius presented dreams as centrally important in the life of the soul. He explained that whereas in waking life we learn from human teachers, in dreams God instructs the soul directly. Because the important truths conveyed in dreams are in hidden form and mixed with uncertain things, they require interpretation by a form of divination. Since this divinatory art enables man to find out some of the things that God knows simply by virtue of his nature, it is the greatest of goods and an eminently praiseworthy subject of study. Of course, in a world that functions as one great harmonious organism, there are also innumerable other kinds of meaningful signs, but dreams are especially worthy of our attention. As Ficino's version of Synesius puts it, "This discipline ought to be studied more than the rest since this is from ourselves, and is intrinsic, and proper to each person's soul."[55] Headings added in Ficino's translation further emphasize not merely the validity but the superiority of knowledge drawn from dreams: "*Phantasia* is more perspicacious than the external senses," and "The *spiritus phantasticus* is the first vehicle of the soul."[56]

Synesius urged dream interpretation upon everyone. Cardano echoed this exhortation, emphasizing that everyone could and should examine dreams—men and women, old and young, rich and poor.[57] But Synesius had also stressed that, since each individual human composite of soul and body is different, dreaming was a highly individual matter; he dismissed with lofty contempt popular dream books that purported to provide rules for dream interpretation that could be applied to anyone.[58] A reader of Synesius would be likely to come away with the understanding that the best—perhaps the only—person to interpret dreams is the dreamer him or herself. And since proper Synesian dream interpretation required careful preparation of body, soul, and mind through abstemious diet, spiritual purity, and intelligent application to the subject, one could certainly conclude that some people would be better equipped to interpret their own dreams than others. One can also read in Synesius as rendered by Ficino that "God . . . made certain people sharers of the divine fruit and power in dreams," an idea that accords well with Cardano's notion of himself as the recipient of special natural gifts of awareness and understanding.[59] Furthermore, Synesius also suggested that just as a good daimon acted as preceptor to skillful discoverers of things during their waking hours, so too the wise man would be able to put his resting soul in touch with higher powers and more divine dreams.[60]

Synesian dream interpretation thus combines a pronounced element of self-examination with the belief that the ultimate source of true and useful dreams comes from above and is analogous to the guidance daimons may offer to inventive people. The probable appeal of these ideas to Cardano scarcely needs underlining. Moreover, as much as any of the compilers of the popular dream books he despised, Synesius taught that the truths conveyed in dreams were truths about the future. He alleged that according to credible reports, dreams had brought individuals divine advice or admonition, literary inspiration, warning of danger, and medical advice (Synesius's own experience was that dream advice had been very helpful in improving his literary style).[61] Synesius also advocated keeping records of dreams. He was perhaps thinking of public records for the guidance of future public action, since he seems to have regarded the idea as daring and impractical. Cardano echoed the advice for people in their private capacity.[62] He evidently followed it himself, when he kept notes on his own dreams and collected accounts of other people's both from histories and from the anecdotal reports of his friends and acquaintances.

Of course, by no means all the dreams of his own that Cardano found worth recording had anything to do with his practice of medicine. As he interpreted his dream life retrospectively, many dreams seemed to him to have foretold the tragedy of his son. Family relations in general also loomed large. Another group of dreams referred, he thought, to his medical career, but these do not have anything to do with the content of his medicine. For example, in 1538, he dreamed of a starry sky from which the planet Mercury was at first missing but then appeared among the most resplendent stars. He recognized the stars as the Milan College of Physicians, and Mercury as himself, at first excluded but soon to be admitted.[63] Moreover, not all the dreams that do relate to medical knowledge or therapeutic activity are in any way reminiscent of Synesius's theories or the dreams supposedly experienced by Hippocrates and Galen. Sometimes Cardano interpreted dreams about injuries to bodily organs with an arbitrary symbolism reminiscent of Artemidorus and other popular dream books. For example, when he dreamed that he saw his stomach full of food sitting outside his body, and on the next night that his fingers had been partially amputated, he decided that the partial amputation signified that the stomach would be replaced but would not function as effectively as before, and that the stomach signified the family.[64] Yet among his own dreams Cardano carefully recorded examples relating to his medical career in at least three of the four categories listed by Synesius—warning of danger, literary or scholarly inspiration, and medical advice. The extent to which he maintained that some of these dreams simultaneously belonged to the fourth category—that of dreams conveying divine guidance or admonition—is, as I hope to show, more problematic.

The dream included in the story of the Borromeo child provides a sufficient example of the category of dreams that warned of danger. Others, which need not be described in detail, refer to perils from disease or injury that threatened Cardano himself or members of his family (one such instance is, of course, the story of Fazio Cardano's visit from a blue angel in time of plague).

For all his self-presentation as primarily a gifted practitioner, medical authorship played a central part in Cardano's professional life. Here too his dreams did not fail him. For example, in 1557 when he woke up after dreaming of sweet music, he found that he understood why some people die of fevers and others do not, "which question I had been pondering for almost twenty-five years. Therefore . . . in the morning I immediately began to write that very beautiful book *Ars parva medendi* . . . in which almost the whole of medicine is contained. Thus from harmony divine wisdom was portended."[65] He thus managed to imitate Galen in modestly giving credit to a dream for something he could have claimed for himself, while simultaneously claiming a special, higher sanction for his own medical ideas.

The third category, that of dreams that give medical advice, is more complex. He recorded a number of dreams and sensations on awaking from sleep that seemed to him on subsequent reflection to have contained prophecy about his own health, advice about treatment, or inspiration for medical ideas. At the simplest level, he dreams that he suffers from a certain complaint, and subsequently does suffer from it, although with a slight variation in the symptoms. Dreams correctly foretell how to treat the disease and when it will go away.[66] But the remark about pondering—the verb is *incubo*, surely significantly in this context—the question about fever mortality for twenty-five years appears to suggest that he also deliberately tried to have dreams that would yield theoretical medical information. The story of the inspiration of his *Ars parva* also shows that he endeavored to maximize the extent to which his medical ideas depended on dreams by claiming dream inspiration, even in instances in which he did not recall any specific dream advice.

One of his fullest accounts of his procedure occurs in the chapter on diseases in his book *On the Usefulness That Can Be Drawn from Adversity*. Diseases, Cardano alleged, are useful because they are a guide to better regimen in future, they remind one to put one's affairs in order, and they test the sincerity of friends and the competence of physicians and pharmacists. As an example, he offered the following story.

On September 3, 1554, he fell ill with fever, which at first seemed mild; by the seventh day, however, the disease had affected his mouth and stomach to the point that he felt his heart and his powers weaken, and began to think that he had been poisoned. After treatment with medications he recovered but continued to feel slightly feverish in the evenings. The *medici* pronounced that he was suffering from double tertian fever, but Cardano the anxious patient was not convinced that the diagnosis was correct. Puzzled, he

> had recourse to the one I was accustomed to turn to, that is, God: whom with words of supplication I prayed that he would advise me in a dream what it was necessary to do. I slept at the sacred precincts of the temple that is dedicated to San Michele alla Chiusa, which is across the street from my house. Then having awakened earlier than usual before daybreak, I knew I had seen nothing in a dream, but on account of that unusual hour I believed that I had been woken up in order to be advised that I should consult for myself on my own behalf, which I did.[67]

Cardano ordered a servant to bring him the *Canon* of Avicenna "because I had no confidence that I could bear the labor of studying other books." (Even though that medieval Arabo-Latin tome was still widely used in the mid–sixteenth century, it requires some effort of imagination to envisage it as light reading for an invalid.) As he turned from body to book and back again, he found that he did not have any of the symptoms of tertian fever listed by Avicenna: not thirst, not vomiting, not a bitter taste in the mouth, not high fever, and not an outbreak of sweating as the bout of fever ended. He found instead that the condition of his pulse and urine and other unspecified symptoms exactly coincided with those described for ephemeral fever. Beginning to feel more hopeful, he next proceeded to look up what Avicenna—the author "as it were revealed to me from heaven [*authorem, quasi mihi divinitus oblatum*]"— and Galen recommended by way of diet and medication for ephemeral fever, and ordered that the appropriate light remedies be prepared.

In the course of the day, Cardano announced his conclusions to two physicians who attended him. One simply disagreed with the diagnosis on theoretical grounds, since he was committed to the view that there was no such thing as ephemeral fever. As Cardano saw it, this man preferred to put a friend's health in danger rather than respond to his arguments. The response of the other, described as a colleague and personal friend of long standing who owed him many favors, provides a rare glimpse of a spontaneous contemporary reaction to Cardano's claims to dream inspiration. This practitioner "was so far from receiving the news with a smile that he even added that I was insane and that this was one of what he called in his usual way figments of my imagination." The same man was equally dismissive both of Cardano's research and of medical learning in general, remarking with thoroughgoing medical fatalism that "the art [of medicine] does nothing to bring health to the sick, but whether [or not] someone knows the disease well or badly or even treats it rightly or wrongly, or prescribes one thing rather than another, it has [already] been decreed which patients will die and which be cured."[68]

Fortunately, the medications indicated by self-diagnosis produced immediate improvement and subsequent complete recovery. As for the opinions of Cardano's medical colleagues, they earned from him the comment that the obstinacy of physicians put patients in great danger, followed by the reflection: "if they treat me, whom they understand cannot be deceived, in this way, what happens to those wretched patients who are ignorant of the art [of medicine]?"[69]

But the most interesting feature of this story is surely the reference to prayer for medical enlightenment in a dream before sleeping in sacred precincts (even if the latter does turn out to mean only that Cardano slept in his own bed in his own house which happened to be near a church). If the choice of words is anything more than a rhetorical flourish, it seems to imply that his use of selected aspects of ancient dream theory extended to habitual attempts to undertake a Christian version of incubation, imitative of the practice associated in antiquity with the cult of Asclepius.

There is no doubt that Cardano was aware of the aspect of the cult of Asclepius that led supplicants to sleep in the god's temple in the expectation of receiving medical advice or cures from him in dreams. In a list of methods said to induce true—i.e., prophetic—dreams he included the brief but explicit remark: "in the temple of Aesculapius the sick were accustomed to have true dreams."[70] In this passage, he gave qualified endorsement to the idea that sleeping in a particular place might have some effect on dreams, although he laid much more emphasis on the right frame of mind and the right diet. He also included some warnings about the dangers of trying too hard to have meaningful dreams. He knew that Asclepius was credited with the dreams of Hippocrates and Galen already described, although these dreams did not, of course, involve temple incubation. Other specific references to temple incubation are hard to find in Cardano's works, so that it is difficult to determine how much he knew about the practice in detail.[71] One provocative, if brief, account was to be found in Auger Ferrier's treatise on dreams. After asserting that incubation had fallen into disuse, Ferrier allowed that "there are some superstitious men who select a certain place for themselves in which when they sleep after many and varied purifications, after certain religious prayers, they are advised about the affairs about which they desire to know."[72] Most likely Cardano also consulted Scaliger's exposition of the Hippocratic *Dreams*—the only available full commentary on that work—which cited ancient authors who provided information about the role of dreams in the cult of Asclepius.[73]

Among the authors named by Scaliger was Aelius Aristides, the second-century rhetorician whose *Sacred Discourses* contains a very full and personal account of the experience of incubation as well as extensive descriptions of the author's illnesses and self-treatment. One might expect that Cardano would have been attracted by such a work, but he seems to have made no use of it. Perhaps he was unwilling to read the untranslated Greek text of the *Sacred Discourses* in the 1517 edition of Aristides' orations.[74] A complete Latin translation of Aristides appeared in 1566, but most of Cardano's writings about dreams belong to an earlier time.[75] Alternatively, Aristides, intensely focused on his own ill health rather than on medical wisdom, quintessentially a patient and not a physician, may simply have seemed a less attractive model than Synesius, Hippocrates, and Galen.

But whatever the extent of Cardano's knowledge about ancient incubation in the cult of Asclepius, there seems to be a fundamental ambiguity in his application of his theory of prophetic dreams to his own experiences. On one hand, he insisted upon a naturalistic explanation that essentially presented the prophetic dreamer as a magus whose soul, while his body slept, was in touch with occult celestial, but natural and impersonal, powers in the universe. This explanation carefully and prudently excluded dreams sent by God. On the other hand, when Cardano prayed to God for medical enlightenment to be sent in a dream, he was presumably hoping that the Christian deity would do for him what Asclepius had done for Hippocrates and Galen. Moreover, he also strongly hinted that some of his own dreams were in fact supernatural in origin: "I will not indeed say [definitely] that the presence of a divine influence [*numen*] was at hand for me, but yet I am persuaded of it perhaps not absurdly, inasmuch as I was warned in advance so many times by dreams."[76]

Hostile medical reactions to his theory and practice of prophetic dreams came from several different standpoints. His colleague and friend at Milan simply dismissed Cardano's claims to divinatory dreams as crazy. Cardano's story of an entrapment scheme set up by opponents of his appointment to a professorial chair in medicine at the University of Bologna offers a glimpse of two other kinds of objection. According to this account, a group of senators and judges, who evidently believed that his naturalism implied dubious orthodoxy on the subject of demons, tried to lure him into agreeing to the proposition that demons did not exist and to signing petitions for the release of two women accused of witchcraft. The same group equated his prognostic arts with street prophecy and petty astrology, socially unworthy of a professor of medicine. As he indignantly put it, they asked him to interpret horoscopes "as if I were a soothsayer and prophet and not a professor of medicine."[77]

On an intellectual plane, his theories about divination from dreams elicited a lengthy repudiation and scathing denunciation from another philosopher-physician, namely, Francisco Sanches. According to Sanches, there was no such thing as divination by dreams, and if there were it would be useless. Either the future could not be changed, in which case there was no point in knowing it; or it could, in which case the prediction would not be true.[78] As far as prophetic dreams were concerned, Sanches was prepared to allow only Aristotle's idea that wise people who devoted much thought and imagination to their future actions might dream about them presciently.[79] Sanches's objections combined his own brand of Academic skepticism with Catholic fideism. But Sanches himself espoused a physiological theory of dreaming that he had derived from a medical source: the Hippocratic *Dreams*. According to Sanches, in dreams all the soul knows is the body's present state: in sleep, the soul, freed from distractions, experiences every nuance of the body's condition more acutely than in waking, so that movements of the humors stir up dream images in the *fantasia*.[80] It seems likely therefore that Sanches objected to Cardano's emphasis on divinatory dreams on medical as well as philosophical grounds, perceiving it as undermining the medical understanding and use of diagnostic dreams.

In important respects, Cardano's ideas about dreams were intimately connected with his medical profession and with his reading of ancient medical traditions and texts. He was deeply interested in renovating or improving systems for forecasting in medicine—aspects of his astrology and his endeavors to develop a systematic method of medical prognostication (including therapy choice) can both be seen in this light. Hippocratic prognostication and medical astrology were supposed to provide sets of rules, which could validly be applied in many different cases, presumably by any competent practitioner. In the case of these forms of prediction, Cardano presented himself as someone who had uncovered, recovered, or successfully adapted good Hippocratic or Ptolemaic rules, or even found new ones. At the same time, he frequently adverted to his unique gifts and insight. He seems to have conceived the interpretation of dreams in medicine in similar terms, as a form of prediction or prognostication in which both the reasoned application of rules and the understanding and power of the magus guided by dream inspiration exist in tension with one another. But he tipped the balance so far in favor of the individual gifts of the physician-dreamer that he failed to convince other physicians—the colleague who visited him when he was ill and Sanches—of the validity of his use of dreams. The method of the Hippocratic and Galenic treatises that provide rules for using the patient's dreams as a guide to medical diagnosis of physical conditions indeed bears a family resemblance to prognostication as understood in Renaissance medicine. Yet this was not the type of medical dream interpretation in which Cardano had much interest. Instead, he dwelt on the ability of the gifted physician—Hippocrates, Galen, himself—to have and correctly to interpret Synesian dreams that inspire with medical knowledge and protect from medical errors. But this ability, although involving rational interpretation, was conceived of as at once profoundly individual and dependent upon ultimately uncontrollable natural—or supernatural—forces. In fact, he believed that his own gift of dream inspiration deserted him in 1558, when "I seemed gradually to have been abandoned by that *numen*" and "some celestial power deserted me."[81]

PART FIVE

Medical Narratives

Chapter 9

HISTORIA, NARRATIVE, AND MEDICINE

FAMOUSLY, Cardano exemplifies the self-expressiveness of Renaissance culture, whether this is defined in nineteenth-century terms as individualism or in late-twentieth-century ones as self-fashioning. Indeed, his penchant for self-revelation struck his earliest biographer, Gabriel Naudé, as excessive; he would have been wiser and more decorous, Naudé thought, to be circumspect about his own difficulties and defects.[1] Cardano recounted his own history not only in the *Vita* but also scattered in fragments throughout his voluminous writings. In bibliographies of his own writings, in astrological treatises, in medical works, in his dream book, in moralistic treatises, he told and retold of his wretched childhood, his rejection by medical colleagues, his successes as a medical practitioner, mathematician, and astrologer, his prolific career as an author, his physical afflictions, the portents, dreams, and visions that came to him, and the tragedy of his elder son's execution.[2]

But this insistent recourse to narrative extended beyond the impulse to shape his own life history. In several of the disciplines to which he was most attracted, narrative plays a central or highly significant role: obviously, history itself falls into this category, but so too, in different ways, do astrology and the study of dreams, in both of which he collected or constructed narratives. He perhaps hoped to find in accumulated narratives of experience—his own and that of others—a tool for understanding both human society over time and in its physical environment and the health and fortunes of individuals.

Medicine, too, was a discipline in which from time to time he turned to narrative. The reader has by now encountered a number of examples of his medical stories. These stories are medical in one of several senses: a physician's description of a sick patient, a physician's summary of a patient's own story of his or her illness, or a physician's account of what he did for the patient. Medicine is, indeed, in fundamental ways a narrative discipline, although the form the narrative takes—and by whom it is told—has varied greatly over time.[3] Although Cardano's medical stories bear many signs of his characteristic combination of overconfidence and anxiety as well as of the breadth of his intellectual interests, they also belong to a larger pattern of development within Renaissance medicine. For a variety of reasons, Renaissance practitioners seem to have developed more interest than most of their scholastic forebears in recording narratives about individual patients and their diseases or injuries. No doubt both the new attention devoted to all forms of describing and collecting and a general shift toward more self-expressive writing apparent in many fields may have been partially responsible. But for the actual construction of their medical narratives, practitioners were able to draw not only on their professional experience but on a range of sources within medicine that provided a rich selection of ancient, medieval, and Renaissance models and genres.

Thus, from one point of view, Cardano's use of medical narrative looks like part of his constant endeavor, many times alluded to in the foregoing chapters, to understand the relation between particular instance and general rule. He often pursued this goal by way of retroactive analysis of narrated examples. This procedure is consonant with his entire approach to mastering knowledge and exactly parallels uses he made of two other narrative disciplines with which he was engaged, astrology and history. But he was also, simultaneously, participating in what may be thought of (not entirely accurately) as the Renaissance prehistory of the case history; his accounts, like those of other medical writers, both depend on sources and models within earlier traditions of medical narrative and reflect contemporary developments. This chapter will examine—and in some cases reexamine—his medical storytelling from both standpoints.

Cardano offered what he termed *historia* or *historiae* in medicine the high encomium of association with *antiqua tempora* and with Hippocrates. He declared that "in ancient times the medical art held *historiae* in the greatest esteem" and that among the chief merits of his own commentaries on the Hippocratic books was that they "give delight by *historia*."[4] Sixteenth-century writers of Latin commonly used *historia* in two senses, both of which preserved the ancient connotation of a narrative presenting the results of an inquiry exemplified respectively in the *Histories* of Herodotus and the *History of Animals* of Aristotle: the record of human experience and the description of nature. And the term might also be applied, as it had been by Galen and was by Cardano, to accounts of specific cases encountered in medical practice—a usage that addressed both human experience and natural phenomena.[5]

He himself was engaged by *historia* in all these meanings. He was the author of several short works on ancient history, the most noteworthy of which is an *Encomium of Nero*. In this he pointed out the prejudices and moral failings of Tacitus and Suetonius, the main sources for Nero's life, and observed that alienating the powerful, as Nero had done, was likely to result in lasting ill repute; he further alleged that Nero's recorded behavior was no worse than that of other less notorious rulers, drew attention to his various meritorious or constructive activities, and attributed any remaining failings to youthful exuberance and inexperience or the seductions of his mother, Agrippina.[6] This pioneering exercise in historical revisionism may show signs of the influence of Machiavelli in its love of paradox and occasional attempts to use ancient history to teach modern political lessons. Indeed, the parallel drawn by Machiavelli between the value of the collection and use of ancient *experimenta* in medicine and in political history[7] could well serve as a justification of the historical interests of Cardano the physician. In the *Encomium of Nero*, moreover, Cardano clearly showed an interest in analyzing how and on what basis historical judgments are arrived at. Although the ancient and medieval tradition that regarded history as a branch of rhetoric persisted in the sixteenth century, new and more analytic concepts were also emerging.[8] Nonetheless, for the most part the *Encomium of Nero* still seems to fall within the rhetorical tradition according to which human history was held to be more concerned with persuasion than with causation, and incapable of providing certain knowledge, or *scientia*.

Another view of human history, the product of his commitment to astrology and the Hippocratic environmental medicine of *Airs Waters Places*, presents itself in Cardano's astrological works.[9] In them he tried to develop a causal account, in which historical examples illustrated how the stars shaped human events. The content of his collections of horoscopes consists mostly of analysis of past lives—of famous historical personages, of his contemporaries, of members of his family, of himself—in the light of his interpretation of their respective nativities (horoscopes cast for the time of birth). In itself, there was nothing novel about casting and interpreting horoscopes retroactively.[10] Yet Cardano, who counted history among his major interests, clearly brought an exceptionally high level of interest to "historical" astrology. In his view, the evidence of past lives, properly interpreted, could be made to provide the strongest possible evidence for the validity of astrology in general. His interest in historical astrology must, I think, also be connected both with his attention, discussed in previous chapters, to medical prognosis (which linked past history with future outcome) and autopsy (which—supposedly—brought to light in the present hitherto hidden causes of phenomena in the past).

According to Cardano, Ptolemy's *Tetrabiblos* was "as useful for knowing the present and the past as the future."[11] Consequently, since he claimed to base his technique on the correct method of Ptolemy, the model astrologer, historical horoscopes also served as a device to make a methodological point.[12] The inclusion of celebrated historical figures would demonstrate that the known details of these completed lives confirmed the correctness of his techniques for casting the horoscope as well as demonstrating his skill in interpreting the various influences of the heavenly bodies. Thus many of the horoscopes in his *One Hundred Examples of Genitures* belong to major figures of recent history, among them Pope Julius II, Luther, Francesco Sforza, and Cosimo de' Medici. Used in this way, horoscopes, like autopsy, purportedly yielded manifest evidence, certain confirmation, and underlying reasons for conclusions that had previously been arrived at in a more impressionistic way. For example, analysis of the horoscope of Pope Julius II confirmed Cardano's unfavorable historical judgment of the pontiff's bellicose character.[13] The use of horoscopes as a tool of historical analysis at least had the merit of avoiding the perils of prediction, although when a prediction went wrong, Cardano, as always, stood ready to revise his views. Cardano's essay in self-criticism and self-exculpation for his failed prediction about Edward VI after it had been overtaken by events shares the characteristics of his entire approach to astrological history: the combination of laborious astrological computation with political and historical judgments already arrived at on other grounds.

An idea of his method can be gathered from his treatment of the question "Will spouses love one another?" in a work entitled *On [astrological] Interrogations*. "I subjoin a most admirable double, indeed a triple, example. In the first place it is necessary to narrate the history very briefly, then to gather the [astrological] reason for these events." The history turns out to be that of the marriage of Henri II of France and Catherine de' Medici. Cardano rated this as an example of marital harmony because of Henri's alleged refusal to divorce Catherine when she failed to have children for several years and her consequent good fortune: not of noble or royal blood, married to a second son, at one time apparently barren and threatened with divorce, she ended up a queen and the mother of kings. He evidently either did not know about or regarded as insignificant Henri's notorious devotion to Diane de Poitiers throughout most of his marriage to Catherine. And he also attributed indirect political consequences of this marriage to the stars: the marriage (arranged by Francis I in 1533) and hence the stars contributed to the continuing enmity between Francis I and Charles V.

In the example of the story of Henri II and Catherine de' Medici and elsewhere, Cardano used *historia* in connection with human affairs to mean not an extended sequential narrative but a brief story about a set of closely related events or a single individual or occurrence. This static view of the human past is apparent also in the *Encomium of Nero*, which analyzes Nero's government and character but does not provide a chronological narrative of the events of his reign. But although this episodic or exemplary approach to history remained widespread in the sixteenth century, it is characteristic neither of all Cardano's comments on the subject nor of all sixteenth-century historical writing. In some contexts and for some authors—for example, Guicciardini in practice and Bodin in theory—development over time was an essential component of the subject. Paolo Giovio both wrote narrative biographies of rulers and generals and sought to weave all the complex international politics and military affairs of his own time into the sweep of a single historical narrative. With his usual avidity for new books, Cardano seems to have read Giovio's *Lives of Illustrious Men* soon after it was published in 1551. Like many other contemporaries, he judged its author harshly, accusing him—unjustly—of pro-French bias and venality. Perhaps he was particularly incensed because he knew that Giovio was a fellow Lombard who like himself had trained in philosophy and medicine at the universities of Padua and Pavia (Giovio, who had a much more thorough humanistic and literary early education than Cardano, never regarded medicine as more than a means of making a living and left practice as early as possible in order to concentrate on a career as a historian and churchman). In his *Vita*, Cardano himself gloomily surveyed the fall of empires and dynasties that had led to the ridiculous (*ridicula*) result that the Roman Empire was now in Germany. He also noted the vast expansion of European knowledge of the world that had resulted from voyages to the Americas and east Asia, an enormous change that he expected to have long-term consequences in the shape of calamities, contempt for good arts, and the substitution of uncertainties for certainties. As far as the last of these three results is concerned, Cardano's claims to prophetic insight appear to have been made good.[14]

Nevertheless, in many contexts human history appeared as a series of episodes, whether these were treated as subjects for analysis, data from which rules could be constructed, or *exempla* on which to base rhetorical moralizing. Seen in this way, natural and human history were indeed closely associated. Natural histories (for example, Pliny's *Naturalis historia*, Aristotle's *Historia animalium*, and such contemporary contributions to the genre as Fuchs's *De historia stirpium* [1542]) were made up precisely of a multitude of separate short descriptions of different organisms, objects, or phenomena. Furthermore, a good many of the most impressive contributions of sixteenth-century botany, anatomy, and zoology rested upon a similar approach to nature.

In whatever other ways human and natural history might be linked, both rested on description. In his use of historical examples in astrological treatises, as in his natural philosophy and medicine more generally, Cardano seems to have been in search of a theoretical basis on which to build a science of nature and man that was both exact and genuinely descriptive, and in which particulars could somehow lead to certain knowledge. But, of course, he was also intensely aware—on the basis of his own experience both in his personal life and as a medical and astrological practitioner—of the random and apparently inexplicable nature of many occurrences, of the uncertainty of medical and astrological prognostication, and the difficulty, given the vast "variety of things" of distinguishing between the natural and the anomalous.[15] Hence he often seems to have turned to narrative when he especially wished to ponder the relation and relative preponderance of predictability and randomness, the normal and the anomalous in human experience.

All of the intellectual concerns outlined above can be traced in Cardano's use, and manipulation, of medical narrative. But his medical *historiae* were also shaped by medical tradition and the needs of his own professional career. As noted at the beginning of this book, the relation of the particulars of experience to theoretical knowledge of nature had a lengthy history as an epistemological issue within medicine. But whatever the theory, in practice Cardano and his contemporaries had access to a variety of models of narrative in medieval as well as ancient and contemporary medical texts. Medical writers provided descriptive accounts of the nature and course of diseases,[16] parts of the body (Vesalius speaks of the *historia* of the sacrum),[17] the spread of epidemics, and the cases of individual patients. Patients and other people who were not medical practitioners also produced accounts of illness—the author's or another's, individual or epidemic. Such "lay" narratives of illness occur in many different types of medieval and Renaissance writing: collections of miracles assembled at shrines or in the course of canonization processes, saints' lives, letters, chronicles or other historical works, and literary texts (of which the best known is presumably the prologue to the *Decameron*).

For present purposes, I shall confine "medical narrative" to accounts by medical practitioners of individual cases or patients. But it cannot be assumed that medical practitioners were unaware of or uninfluenced by nonprofessional forms of medical narrative. Patients told or tried to tell their stories to doctors, who reorganized and reinterpreted them according to the canons of medical knowledge; Taddeo Alderotti (d. 1295) was doubtless only one of many practitioners who worried over the extent to which patients' accounts of their own symptoms should be relied on.[18] Medical practitioners were as likely as anyone else in the general cultural context to be familiar with some of the accounts of miraculous healing that fill hagiographical material, and as little likely to reject them. And university-educated physicians were cultivated men, some of whom read widely in vernacular and Latin humanistic as well as professional literature. Moreover, all forms of medical narrative were stories that were put together, organized, and doubtless often improved upon for a purpose.[19] This is obviously likely to be the case in accounts of the illness and treatment of individual patients, which could easily be made to serve social, professional, or even religious purposes. But the same is true of medieval and Renaissance medical or physiological narratives that are wholly "scientific" in the sense that their authors had no discernible motivation other than to order data coherently and in accordance with accepted scientific principles. Accounts of disease tried to make sense of the relation of symptoms to processes going on inside the body that could not be directly investigated, to explain how medical theory (for example, of humors and temperament) related to perceived changes in bodily condition, or to hypothesize ways in which epidemics spread. The most rigorously descriptive anatomy that the medical renaissance of the sixteenth century afforded—Vesalius on the bones—involved narratives about the function of internal parts in the living body intended to accommodate Galenic physiological theory to new anatomical observations on the cadaver.[20]

The two chief genres of medical narrative about individual patients and their diseases employed by medieval and Renaissance medical practitioners were anecdotes embedded in general medical or surgical treatises and *consilia*, or letters of advice for individuals. Both emerged in the thirteenth century, apparently to a large extent independent of ancient antecedents. Some of the most important ancient examples of medical narrative about individuals were unknown or ignored in the medieval West. The stages in the reception of the Hippocratic *Epidemics* have already been noted in chapter 6. Galen's *On Prognosis* is largely given over to accounts of cases he had attended, but it was not translated into Latin until the fourteenth century and attracted little attention before the second half of the fifteenth.[21] Some case histories were included in two major Galenic works, the *Method of Healing*, Galen's principal book on therapeutics, and *On the Affected Places* on internal diseases, that were available in Latin from the twelfth century. Unquestionably, these books were esteemed and used by thirteenth- to fifteenth-century medical and surgical practitioners literate in Latin. But in the case of the *Method of Healing*, its great length and the variety of topics covered ensured that the work was not always read, or copied, in its entirety. The case histories are few in number, a single one being deployed by Galen as the starting point for discussion in each of several of the later books. However important in Galen's own design of his book, the narratives about individual patients may not have stood out for medieval readers as a major element in the work.[22]

Medieval medical narratives in the form of accounts of individual cases embedded in treatises are relatively rare and only a minor feature of the works in which they occur. Authors sometimes claimed that their purpose in including stories from their own practice was exemplary or pedagogical. So perhaps it was in some instances. But it often seems evident

that self-advertisement and the denigration of rivals were also motivations. Thus the late-thirteenth-century surgeon Lanfranco of Milan
made a point of relating how he had cured an abscess that one of his
own pupils had unsuccessfully tried to treat, and warned his readers
against consulting Anselmo of Genoa who had caused the deaths of
many people.[23] Characteristically, the stories emphasize the skill and success of the author's cures and lead up to a triumphantly successful outcome. In them, recipients of apparently fatal wounds, who have been
given up for dead by bystanders, family members, or rival practitioners,
are apt to make a complete recovery after being treated by the author
and then go on to father several children before departing on Crusade.[24]

Such anecdotes are indeed much more often found in books by surgical than by medical writers. The reasons for the discrepancy may be
practical. Some young physicians doubtless began to lecture and write in
an academic context before they had time to acquire much experience.
And it could be argued that surgeons were more likely than physicians
to have a few really dramatic successes—for example, successful treatment of large, visible wounds—to write about. But it is also conceivable
that some learned medical authors hesitated to include anecdotes about
individual cases in treatises and commentaries because of philosophical
reservations about the value of particulars, marking their sense of intellectual (and social) superiority to lesser members of the medical hierarchy in this as in many other ways. In the course of the fifteenth century,
however, physicians seem to have become somewhat readier than before
to introduce anecdotes from their own practice into written works.[25]

But *consilia* unquestionably constituted a recognized and reputable
genre of medical writing appropriate for learned physicians. The earliest
date from thirteenth-century Bologna and were perhaps modeled on
legal *consilia*. The popularity of the genre increased in the fifteenth century, when some physicians wrote them in large numbers.[26] In the sixteenth century, new collections continued to be produced and older
ones to be reprinted. Although this proliferation suggests increasing interest in collecting the results of experience, *consilia* were not designed
to provide complete histories of episodes of disease in individuals. Moreover, although some collections of *consilia* contain hundreds of cases,
their authors or editors never seem to have viewed them as a mechanism
for distinguishing the commonplace from the rare. They are essentially
records of consultations for which physicians received a fee; one of Cardano's notes a payment of four Hungarian gold coins.[27] Requests for advice came, often by letter, from patients, their local physicians, or their
family. All *consilia* provide recommendations for treatment; most identify the illness, although often very briefly. Some, but by no means all,
tell the story of an illness, describing the patient, his or her symptoms,

and the course of the disease up to the point when advice was sought. What the patient was paying for, however, was not descriptive narrative, but diagnosis, prognosis, and the prescription of remedies. Moreover, the consultant almost certainly had not attended the patient throughout the course of the illness (if so, there would have been no need of a written *consilium*) and, indeed, had not necessarily seen him or her at all.

The structure of some *consilia* that do describe illnesses reveals that the description was likely to be arrived at through the physician's asking a standard set of questions about the traditional sets of the naturals, the nonnaturals, and the contranaturals (that is, more or less, parts of the body, environmental and physiological conditions, and diseases) that, if adhered to rigidly, must have made it difficult for the patient freely to tell the story of his or her own illness, or for the physician to make observations outside established categories. Antonio Cermisone, a prolific fifteenth-century author of *consilia*, was praised for standardizing the format of his descriptions.[28] In the fifteenth century, some collections of *consilia* became highly formal and scholastic, replete with references to learned authorities and, in some instances, organized to follow the sequence of contents in learned works.[29] The point of making such a collection was presumably to provide medical students and practitioners with a conveniently arranged set of remedies endorsed by the reputation of a famous physician. Hence although the story of an individual's illness doubtless lies behind most *consilia*, it is seldom fully reflected in the written result.

Consilia, like surgeons' stories, if in less blatant ways, provided opportunities for a medical practitioner to paint a professional self-portrait in colors of his own choice. Examples by well-known physicians were assembled into collections, presumably by the authors or their pupils, and underwent some editing in the process.[30] In his *consilia* a physician could display his learning by including references to medical literature in support of the treatments he prescribed. He could identify by name any especially rich, noble, or otherwise distinguished patients. And since a *consilium* was essentially a record of a consultation, he was under no obligation to mention outcome.

Nevertheless, in *consilia*, the role of the physician-author usually remains relatively impersonal. For an early example of an entire collection of descriptive medical narratives that also incorporates substantial self-expression on the part of the author, one must turn to a work already familiar to the reader of this book, namely, Benivieni's collection of "hidden and wonderful causes of diseases and cures" discussed in chapter 7. Unlike the various collections of *consilia*, Benivieni's little book did not belong to any established genre of medical literature and found few direct imitators. But his approach to medical narrative reveals some emerging characteristics in Renaissance scientific writing. In the first place, the project of forming a whole collection of medical *mirabilia* was in itself an affirmation of the value of descriptive narrative—of telling stories about individual cases—in medicine. But the readiness of a physician to select cases from his own practice for classification as unusual, rare, or marvelous involved something more: it introduced a personal element, making the practitioner witness and judge in his own scientific narrative. Medieval medical literature has few precedents for the self-expression in Benivieni's collection, apart perhaps from Ugolino da Montecatini's (1345–1425) description of the benefits his patients had received from various mineral springs.[31] In that Ugolino attributed the efficacy of these springs to an occult property received through virtue of the stars, he, too, was to some extent engaged in making a collection of medical wonders. Furthermore, both these projects imply an awareness of a distinction between personal and reported observation that was still highly unusual in the fifteenth century. The numerous accounts of *experimenta* or experiences of all kinds in medieval and early Renaissance medical literature seldom attach any superior value to the writer's own experience. On the contrary, reports repeated many times would be likely to be accorded more weight. The contemporary value of ancient witnesses continued to be accepted throughout the sixteenth century (there are examples in one of the most noted products of Renaissance observational science, namely, the *Fabrica* of Vesalius).

But the most salient difference between Benivieni's collection and the genre of *consilia* is that *consilia* do not as a rule mention outcome, whereas outcome, whether fatal or not, provides the necessary closure for Benivieni's stories. It is unclear whether this aspect owes anything to classical case histories. A Greek manuscript of works of Hippocrates, including the as yet untranslated complete *Epidemics*, was present in Florence during Benivieni's lifetime. There is no evidence that he had access to this manuscript, although he knew Greek and moved in humanist and medical circles in which there was active interest in the translation of Hippocrates. If models are sought for this religiously oriented author's accounts of individuals and their diseases considered as brief, self-contained narratives, perhaps contemporary genres of storytelling outside medicine ought also to be considered: miracle stories among them.

The reception of the complete *Epidemics* in the early sixteenth century made readily available numerous examples of a type of case history that contrasts with all the varieties of narrative about individual patients or episodes of disease just described. Typically, histories in the *Epidemics* carefully follow the patient's progress over time, noting variations in his or her symptoms and general condition through days, sometimes months, of illness; they are minimally interventionist, in some instances mentioning no treatment of any kind; and they bleakly record frequent deaths. Whatever the motivation for noting down the information may have been, it was clearly neither self-advertisement on the part of the practitioner nor a request on the part of the patient. To take the example of the first case history in *Epidemics* 1, Philiscus who lived by the wall was ill with fever and upset bowels for six days; his active treatment consisted of the administration of a single suppository, the content of which is not mentioned; on the sixth day he died.

However, as Vivian Nutton has pointed out, it is hard to trace any direct influence of the reception of the *Epidemics* upon most of the stories about individual patients and their diseases told by sixteenth-century physicians and surgeons.[32] To take only two well-known instances, the "histories" included in the autobiographical *Apologie and Treatise* (1585) of Ambroise Paré are probative and exemplary defenses of his procedures; the lively and anecdotal "cures" compiled by William Clowes (ca. 1540–1604) into works on gunshot, surgery, syphilis, and struma to which Nutton has drawn attention are intended to instruct.[33] Both, of course, involve a very active presence of the author/practitioner in his narrative. Not coincidentally, both Paré and Clowes were surgeons, so that their narratives may be regarded, to some extent at least, as an amplification and enrichment of the centuries-old tradition of surgeons' stories. It is unclear to what extent the Hippocratic case histories influenced the actual practice in writing about patients of even Gianbattista Da Monte (d. 1551). In the last year of his life he lectured on *Epidemics* 1 with special reference to the case histories and is said to have urged on his students at Padua the importance of writing descriptions of cases. But to whatever extent the Hippocratic histories may have influenced his own descriptions of hospital patients, these descriptions survive interspersed among his more numerous conventional *consilia*.[34]

As compared to their scholastic predecessors, however, leading sixteenth-century academic physicians seem notably more self-expressive and more involved in self-presentation. Others besides Cardano, though much less frequently, deployed their own unhappy experiences as cautionary examples: Argenterio used a moving account of his young wife's death to illustrate the weakness of Galenic diagnosis.[35] Others besides Cardano, though less extravagantly, adverted to their own extraordinary qualities: Vesalius made sure his readers knew not only of his youth when he wrote the *Fabrica* but also that he had been born with a caul (carefully preserved by his mother), traditionally a sign of remarkable powers.[36] On a more general level, the vogue for humanistic medical *epistolae*, of which a number of collections were published, in some cases involved a more personal style of written communication among physicians (though many items were simply *consilia* under another name). In a period of much conscious appropriation and *imitatio* of ancient culture, not only were ancient texts the indispensable substratum of scientific knowledge, but the ancients themselves—and even their fictional creations—served as models for scientific personality and activity. Attention has recently been drawn, for example, to Ulisse Aldrovandi's rhetorical identification, in autobiographical narrative and iconography, of himself and his travels in search of knowledge with his Homeric namesake.[37] Similarly, it has been suggested that Fabrizio of Acquapendente's interest in comparative anatomy was a less fanciful imitation of Aristotelian zoology.[38] Yet the most obvious ancient model for ambitious physicians was Galen. If one may judge by the number of translations, sixteenth-century interest in Galen's *On Prognosis*, which consists almost entirely of accounts of his own successful cases, was no less than in the Hippocratic *Epidemics*. Fresh interest in the *Method of Healing* stimulated by Renaissance concern with method may also have engendered greater appreciation of Galen's use in some books of that work of a case history as the starting point for a detailed analysis of diagnosis and treatment.[39] Galen's use of his own cases for exemplary exposition, autobiographical presence in his medical works, assumption of moral superiority, denunciation of opposing views, and insistence on the importance of anatomy carried many resonances for Renaissance medical culture. Falloppia was perhaps not far off the mark when he accused Vesalius of wanting to be as infallible as Galen.[40]

But Cardano, as we have seen, had a special commitment to the *Epidemics* and to the image of Hippocrates. That image included the author of the *Epidemics* as a model narrator of medical *historiae*. The reader will indeed recall from chapter 6 Cardano's insistence that he had learned a method of prognosis for himself by repeatedly reading over the Hippocratic case histories. The idea that reasoned analysis of Hippocratic case histories would yield rules of prognosis both has obvious parallels with Cardano's interest as an astrologer in analyzing the horoscopes of historical personages and also recalls Galenic case analysis. If there is substance to his allegation that as a young man he had kept his own case-book modeled on the *Epidemics*, it presumably predated by some fifty years the personal notes and casebook loosely modeled on the *Epidemics* kept by Guillaume de Baillou at Paris in the 1570s, to which attention has been drawn as a pioneering effort.[41] Cardano also thought the Hippocratic case histories should be used as models by others, explaining that the purpose of his analysis of twenty-two of the case histories from *Epidemics* 1 and 3 was "not only so that I might declare these twenty-two *exempla* of Hippocrates or teach the *historia*, and thence the cure, of diseases and causes, . . . but . . . so that anyone with similar observations from the art of medicine will be able to augment that art, which in our times can be done so much more easily and better to the extent that our age is more distinguished in the art of dissecting human bodies."[42]

Nevertheless, where medical narrative was concerned, Cardano's claim that his own practice was comparable to that of Hippocrates involved him in one of his many contradictions. For one thing, the norms of medical practice led him to write wholly conventional *consilia*. There seems little to distinguish most of them from the productions of his thirteenth- to fifteenth-century predecessors, except for the presence of cases of *morbus gallicus* and perhaps somewhat more attention to the factor of development of disease over time. The reader is evidently meant to infer favorable outcome, since by far the longest *consilium* describes the illness and prescribes the treatment of the Scottish archbishop, whose cure was a high point of Cardano's career.[43]

In other works, moreover, his confessional urge, professional difficulties, and claims to mastery of medicine as of so many other sciences impelled him to recount many *historiae* about his own practice that—in marked contrast to the histories in the *Epidemics*—were rich in autobiographical detail and strongly emphasized success. Here he had an ancient model: that model was not Hippocrates but Galen, who incorporated autobiography into his medical works, wrote a bibliography of his own books, and included in his treatises anecdotes about his practice designed to illustrate his own therapeutic successes.[44] In Cardano's case, the influence of the Galenic model of self-expressiveness in scientific treatises was exceptionally powerful. It affected not only the medical writings under immediate consideration here but also his astrological and natural philosophical works, just as these in turn probably helped to pass on the same model to other scientific writers.

Cardano avowedly assembled the collection of his own "wonderful cures and prognostications" discussed in chapter 7 in imitation of Galen's *On Prognosis*; he made the Galenic parallel even more overt when he published the collection as a section of the work to which he gave the Galenic title *Methodus medendi*. Presented in this setting, these short narratives—which provide less description of pathology than Benivieni and fewer details of remedies than some *consilia*—serve a double purpose. In the first place, they constitute a set of examples or experiences appended to a general work, an organizing principle to which Cardano repeatedly had recourse when writing about disciplines that he regarded as holding keys to natural knowledge but also as in some sense uncertain or conjectural. He used exactly the same kind of structure in his writings on astrology and dreams; undoubtedly it reflects his constant endeavor to make sense of particulars in all their multitude and diversity.[45]

Second, more than merely containing elements of the personal, the stories are put together in a way that is genuinely autobiographical. Although divided into separate "cures" and "prognostications," they present a continuous narrative covering the years 1534–61 in which any departures from chronological order are duly noted, and which includes characterization, lively dialogue, and self-justification and -interpretation. The story they have to tell is, of course, of the author's start in practice in Milan, poor and without friends or patrons, and of his gradual acquisition of respectful and grateful patients, despite the continued hostility of arrogant medical colleagues in positions of influence.

The heightened drama, rich social context, and polemical tone of some of the accounts may have been inspired by Galen's descriptions of his own cures in *On Prognosis*.[46] Perhaps both Galen's example and Cardano's sense of his own special gifts combined to give the story of the cure of Gaspare Roulla, recounted in chapter 7, its very different thrust from the self-congratulatory anecdotes recorded by medieval surgeons. Those stories, however exaggerated and conventional, are straightforward advertisements of the author's skill and knowledge. Their atmosphere is pragmatic and technical, rather than marvelous. Similarly, the claim that the author's treatments succeed where those of medical colleagues fail is a topos of medieval surgeons' stories and frequently found in Benivieni. But in Cardano's version, senior colleagues are harshly denounced for greed as well as incompetence. Fairly typical is his story of a nobleman who for five years had suffered from *morbus gallicus*, accompanied by two kinds of fever, creeping ulcers in his head, wasting, and swellings in his thighs. This unfortunate patient had been butchered and exploited by various physicians on whom he had spent more than a thousand gold crowns. But in a mere eighty days, at a cost of a mere eighty crowns, Cardano had cured him completely by administering a potion consisting of guiac (the New World wood in which many sixteenth-century physicians reposed confidence) and other herbs.[47] Yet whatever his self-promoting rhetoric owed to Galen's example, Cardano presented himself not merely as more skilled and morally superior to— because less avaricious than—the other physicians of Milan, but also as Galen's rival rather than his disciple. He explicitly claimed to have cured more patients of desperate diseases than Galen himself (and, elsewhere, than Hippocrates).[48]

Moreover, there are also un-Galenic elements in the stories in the *Wonderful Cures*. Galenic rationality as well as Hippocratic wisdom is undercut, not only by the possible allusions to Cardano's sense of his occult powers previously discussed, but also by remarkably frank acknowledgment of the role of social contacts, patronage, and luck in fostering or hindering a medical career. The story of his relations with the pharmacist Donato Lanza, already briefly alluded to, is particularly rich in revealing details. Cardano chanced to become acquainted with Lanza, an upright man, through a common interest in music. His temporarily successful treatment of Lanza for *phthoe* led to subsequent treatment of another member of Lanza's family. Perhaps Cardano and Lanza entered into an arrangement then common among physicians and pharmacists whereby the pharmacist recommended the physician's services and the physician prescribed the pharmacist's remedies. In any event, "on account of both his own benefit and [my] treatment of his relative and others, Donato Lanza worked hard to ensure that my name would be known to everyone and that I might shine in the city." Then Lanza left his pharmacy and entered the service of Francesco Sfondrati. When Sfondrati's small son fell ill, Lanza saw to it that Cardano was summoned. Two other more famous physicians were at a loss. Cardano saw the child's neck contorted backward, demonstrated that it could not be straightened, and pronounced his diagnosis: "*opisthotonos*" (tetanic spasm). Only the most distinguished of the other physicians even knew what the word meant. "Impelled by divine inspiration," he handsomely acknowledged Cardano's skill in diagnosis. "Therefore," Cardano concluded, "in this part I had propitious fortune and I cured the boy, and fairly quickly. . . . Therefore from that hour so much glory accrued to me that if Sfondrati had remained in Milan for an entire year all the citizens would have flowed to me, and so in a short time I would have obtained first place among all the *medici* of our city." But, alas, Sfondrati left Milan, and Cardano's booster Donato Lanza, while fleeing the police (*praetoris familia*) (his probity having presumably temporarily deserted him), jumped out of a window and hid for a long time in a water tank; this adventure taxed his already weakened constitution and he died four years after Cardano first treated him for *phthoe*.[49]

Yet in a few narratives scattered through his medical works one can, I think, detect traces of Cardano's interest in the case histories in the *Epidemics* and perhaps of the method of analysis he claimed to have learned from them at the beginning of his career. Occasional accounts record the entire course of a patient's illness over time together with the outcome, up to and including death. Yet even these cases do not, in reality, read very like the *Epidemics*. The description serves as a jumping-off point for explicit causal analysis of the illness and explanation of the reasons for the preferred method of treatment, a method more reminiscent of Galen in *Methodus medendi* than of Hippocrates. Moreover, the physician-narrator's presence and intervention are much more assertive than in the *Epidemics*. Professional colleagues and competitors also often enter the story. The patient dies, but not before Cardano has reported his own repeated interventions and his reflections during the course of treatment. And although failure in therapy is admitted, success in diagnosis and prognosis is invariably claimed. Such is his description of the illness and death of

> Vicenzo Cospo of Bologna, a senator and a friend of mine, fifty years old, of tall stature, thick body, thin thighs, bad color, excessively timid, carrying a *fons* in his arm already for many years, exerting himself a lot, and afterward resting; he devoured many different coarse, bad foods, such as chestnuts, *itria* [?], vegetables, and cheese, with other things too, at one meal. This year he used to eat three or four watermelons in one day. On October 21, 1569, he was seized by a double tertian fever; but there was rigor on Friday, and with it vomiting and dark feces; he was not sweating: the fever was ending. Having been called the fifth day, around evening, I knew of no other symptoms. In the morning he seemed to be more or less all right: but he had already taken food, bread cooked with liquid; however, he also drank water for the accession [of fever] was threatening. In the evening when I came back, I noticed his pulse was weak. He was cheerful, lying on his left side so that he could receive (I believe) visitors. Where I kept on trying to feel the pulse, I did not find it, and I was wondering if this happened because of me, that is, on account of my stupidity [*ne id mihi causa mea contingeret, scilicet ob stuporem*]. I undertook to touch him again; I noticed I had not been deceived, for indeed I found the pulse, but it was very languid, small, not very fast but rather frequent. Certain therefore about his condition and having warned the other physician, I prescribed him a little bit of diluted wine for supper, along with a dish of egg yolk. The following morning we gave him theriac and fomented his belly with absinth and even anointed the heart. Fever followed, without vomiting or defecation. A sufficiently robust pulse, and as usual, large, rapid, and frequent. Copious sweating followed, since he had also sweated the previous night. When the seventh day had gone past, we were afraid of the circuit [of critical days]; the remedies of the previous day were applied. When I came about the sixteenth hour (but he had already taken food), I found him feverish, since the accession had not yet supervened (but it was exacerbated on even days and took place later). When the accession [of fever] and a little rigor came, his forces collapsed but he defecated a little, as on the sixth day, and he vomited nothing. Before sunset, he died.[50]

On the basis of exhaustive consideration of every symptom and its timing, Cardano's analysis of this narrative eliminated diagnoses of poisoning (the corpse did not swell up or putrefy immediately), an internal abscess (the fever was not acute and continuous), and plague (there was no plague in the city) and settled on double tertian fever, even though the symptoms were, in his view, abnormal for that complaint. Careful observation in conjunction with an endeavor to explain the phenomena in terms of established disease theory yielded but a second *historia* put together by Cardano, that of the internal bodily processes; and this second story could be linked to the original narrative of illness only in what seems—given the range of diseases considered—a highly arbitrary manner.

If one may judge by the advice he gave others, Cardano would have constructed his account of the illness and death of Vicenzo Cospo from the results of questioning patient and attendants, combined with his own observation and physical examination of the patient. The methodology was standard, although Cardano's recommendations for physical examination seem relatively elaborate: he advised observing whether the patient could turn his or her head freely, taking the pulse, palpating the abdomen for swelling, pain, hardness, and tension, watching out for abnormal respiration and signs of mental confusion, and examining all the excreta. His interrogation, too, was in detail—the physician should ask not only whether the patient slept and whether he or she dreamed but also whether he or she slept in a canopied bed with a mattress. With critical days in mind, he insisted on careful inquiry into the duration of the illness, the time of day when the patient fell ill, and the frequency and severity of attacks of fever. He noted that at Milan, unlike Bologna, it was the practice to keep a day-by-day record of a patient's illness in order to follow the "critical days."[51] The practice doubtless appealed to him both because of his interest in *historia* and because of his conviction of the importance of critical days and his own correct interpretation of them according to "the Hippocratic art of Ptolemy."[52] The amount of detail in the finished narrative about Cospo would certainly seem to suggest that it is based on notes or memoranda made at or soon after the time.

In his account of the case of another friend, his colleague Gianbattista Pellegrini, Cardano brought together in a single *historia* most of the characteristics that have emerged from the separate examples discussed above. He told the story to illustrate the usefulness of autopsy (see chapter 5). In the narrative of Pellegrini's illness, he combined autobiography, case history, and self-advertisement—as a diagnostician and anatomist if not as a therapist—with a carefully observed and vividly recounted story of the fatal illness of a patient; and, for once, this physician's story also incorporates recognizable echoes of the patient's own account of his sensations.

> But I will tell an outstanding example that happened, so that I might see it today, while I am writing these things, that is, on September 7, 1566, and so that physicians may understand how much they fail in diagnosis of diseases of the internal parts, which Hippocrates also testifies, and how use-

ful is dissection of the bodies of those who die of disease, and how much good the best treatment can do. Gianbattista Pellegrini of Bologna, professor of arts and medicine, was already ill for some months. He was a most studious and very upright man of forty-eight, of completely melancholy habit, timid, slow, dark, emaciated, a small eater and moderate in drink, having the somewhat younger wife whom his temperament and cares needed, with five children. He had a scanty domestic establishment and many difficulties. Initially, therefore, his belly swelled; he called a celebrated medicus who having judged it to be dropsy, as it was, applied many hot fomentations externally. . . . Then, as it were spontaneously after several months, exactly a year ago, that is, on September 6, 1565 (for he died yesterday) he began to excrete crude humors and much water in his feces for many days and so the swollen belly went down; he got up and through the winter was walking about, but with a cane and only in his house, there seemed to be a hard tumor in the right hypochondrium and he could not straighten himself, he was dragged down as if by a chain within, and he breathed with difficulty. But in the spring his breathing deteriorated and the tension of the place increased; he used to feel while he turned over as if a weight in the parts around the heart was transferred from the right to the left, and the fever intensified, and again he was compelled to go to bed and to resort to those hot remedies and softening unguents, and so through the whole summer he was treated while declining from bad to worse. [Another physician arrives, carries on with the prior treatment and accomplishes nothing.] When I chanced to carry some commentaries to him [Pellegrini], in order that I might seek [some in] exchange, I found him burning with continuous fever, with a very rapid and frequent pulse, now hard, now sufficiently soft; the fever attacked him about midday sometimes—that is, on alternate days—with coldness; at other times it was very much exacerbated, with almost no sleep, constant appetite for food, great difficulty in breathing; the parts about the heart were palpitating and the right [side] was sufficiently tense. That other physician was treating him as for hectic fever. . . . I said . . . I did not believe it to be hectic fever, but after forty days, and it was about the middle of August (for he lived about twenty days from this opinion), I said openly that it was not in any way a hard tumor in the liver, nor in any of the digestive or reproductive organs, but the whole disease was almost principally in the lungs: and was edema and it was going to suffocate him. Therefore I undertook treatment, but achieved nothing, but a little while afterward he choked to death [*strangulatus*].[53]

Despite the vividness and particularity of some of his descriptions, Cardano's accounts of his own cases, like those of any single practitioner, provide only a limited point of entry into the history of the case history. We can as yet draw no general picture of the Renaissance prehistory of the early modern case history based on clinical and pathological observation—to the development of which Sydenham (1624–89) and Morgagni (1682–1771), respectively, were leading contributors. In particular, satisfactory general assessment has yet to be reached of the relative importance of, and the interaction between, the growing readiness of fifteenth-century practitioners to record details about their own cases within traditional medieval genres of medical writing and the sixteenth-century study and imitation of newly edited, translated, or printed ancient examples and interpretations of case histories.

The variety of Cardano's medical narratives and the diverse uses to which he put them exhibit the fluidity and, sometimes, confusion characteristic not only of their author but more generally of Renaissance reworkings of ancient scientific authorities and traditional epistemologies. Yet these narratives are informative about his concepts of good method in medicine as well as revealing of connections among his roles as astrologer, historian, and physician. They exemplify his desire for a natural and human history based on the record of particular experiences and guaranteed by the exactitude of mathematical astrology or autopsy. They also show, once again, the way he read his ancient authors for current usefulness. His *imitatio* of Hippocrates included emphasis on the value of the case histories in the *Epidemics* and the belief that he had learned prognostic method from them. But whatever his supposedly Hippocratic casebook may have been like, his surviving stories about his patients reveal only occasonal traces of the influence of the impersonal and often noninterventionist Hippocratic case histories. Instead, Galenic self-presentation and Galenic case analysis inspired him to *imitatio* of—or perhaps rivalry with—Galen. But equally clear is his pragmatic, and lucrative, professional attachment to the medieval genre of the *consilium*. And if some of his stories are aggressively self-promotional, others embody his recognition of the role of social factors and chance in medical reputations, including his own.

Chapter 10

THE PHYSICIAN AS PATIENT

THE PATIENT whose health Cardano monitored most closely was, of course, himself. Given the time and energy his multiple interests, activities, and writings must have demanded, one has no difficulty in believing his boast that from the age of seven until his early fifties he was sick enough to go to bed on only two occasions for a total of less than a week. Nevertheless, he came to perceive himself as a person who had always had a weak constitution and who had suffered lifelong poor health. Moreover, his fascination—or obsession—with every aspect of his own experience extended to the details of his health history. As a result he told the story or stories of his own health a number of times, both in the form of summaries of his entire history and in that of accounts of particular episodes. If the experience was that of Cardano the patient, the organization, scientific assumptions, and interpretations in these accounts were those of Cardano the physician and man of learning. They therefore present a series of rich, albeit complex and idiosyncratic, examples of Renaissance medical narrative.

Once he reached middle age, Cardano seems to have undertaken a practice of conducting a review of his entire life about every decade. In the mid-1540s, 1550s, and 1560s the framework for his investigation was astrological; he reexamined and reinterpreted his horoscope in the light of further meditation on his present and past. In the mid-1570s the last of these self-examinations produced the famous autobiography. Although health was only one of many areas of life to be recorded, remembered, and interpreted in these narratives, it was a prominent category in all of them. Thus Cardano surveyed the entire history of his health to date on four different occasions: in an interpretation of his own horoscope written in 1545, in an interpretation of his recast horoscope in 1554, in an updating of the 1554 interpretation written probably in 1564, and in a chapter of his *Vita* (1575).[1] Repetition, reworking, and self-reference are salient features of these narratives about health and disease as of Cardano's various presentations of his life in general. Both horoscopes and dreams provided him with tools for interpreting the past as well as foretelling the future. But in using either to study the way in which the heavenly influences worked themselves out over the course of an individual life, it was necessary constantly to readjust interpretation and deepen understanding against the changing pattern of apparently random events. For this endeavor the life he knew most intimately—his own—constituted the best possible case study.

The narrative accompanying the horoscope cast in 1545, when Cardano was forty-four, is divided in the traditional manner into sections on life, parents, wife, brothers, sons, wealth, profession, fame and power, habits, bodily form, and death. Of these, only "life" is relevant here. It is entirely given over to ill health. Cardano interpreted every episode of illness in the light of both the horoscope for his nativity and the heavenly positions at the time he fell ill. Malign celestial influences at various points in his life ensured that he was born apparently dead, suffered from pestilence as a newborn, had dropsy and perhaps other diseases in early childhood, nearly died of diarrhea or dysentery at the age of eight, had pestilence again at the age of twenty-one, ran a high fever for seven days at the age of twenty-seven, had catarrh for seven months on end at the age of twenty-nine, and was continuously afflicted with excessive urination from the age of thirty-six.[2] Nevertheless, on the whole, the tone is positive and optimistic. The various illnesses are presented as dangerous but brief and in all instances except the last followed by complete recovery. If unfavorable astral influences had brought on his diseases, other, favorable, ones had always arrived just in time to save him. When he had diarrhea at the age of eight and all the *medici* gave him up for lost, he recovered "by the divine nod, yet nature was also robust, because the moon was powerful and illuminated by rays of Jupiter and Mars. . . ."[3] Moreover, Cardano explicitly stressed that these were the only illnesses he had suffered, and that of those he had had as an adult, only two had kept him in bed, and those for a total of only six days between them. In this account, too, only an exclusive relation between the heavenly bodies and Cardano's body is taken into consideration; despite the mention of pestilence, there is no allusion to other deaths or to epidemics.

The idea of chronic affliction emerges only in the story of his copious urination, and only in decidedly mild and reassuring form. Although in that year the situation of the heavens was so dangerous that Cardano thought he must be going to die, "I did not get an illness that kept me in bed, but only copious urination . . . which obliged me to get up four times every night and it was without burning." Happily, too, his own medical skill combined with more favorable skies soon ameliorated the condition: "understanding the cause, I was helped by hot remedies and the copiousness immediately diminished to the point that I was no longer obliged to get up at night." Yet Cardano knew that he would never be completely free of this condition "because my father died with a flow of urine."[4] Thus the elder Cardano's powerful influence throughout his son's life extended not only to posthumous appearances in his dreams but also, in the younger man's view, to determining many aspects of his physical and mental constitution.

But only a decade later, in the much more elaborate horoscope of 1554, Cardano's health is painted in darker colors. For the new version, he recast the actual horoscope of his nativity, using an improved method of dividing the houses, and amplified the accompanying astrological data.[5] He also completely revised and considerably expanded the narrative analysis. The material on health and illness is now divided among a general introduction, a survey of his life, and sections on "form and temperament of the body" and "diseases [morbi] and defects [vitia] of the body."[6] The introduction is still in the main positive in tone. Once again the reader learns that Cardano had scarcely ever been confined to bed by illness since the age of eight. The introductory portion further asserts that he was stronger in his fifties than he had ever been as a child, and adduces as further evidence of improvement in health over time his recovery at the age of thirty from the decade of impotence. However, it also introduces for the first time the claim that for forty-four years between the ages of eight and fifty-two he had never "passed even a single day firm in health and without pain."[7]

The survey of his life runs through almost the same set of illnesses as the previous horoscope, with the addition of one episode in the intervening period, namely, forty days of fever at the age of fifty-three. There is, however, a new emphasis on family illness and epidemic disease. Three older stepsiblings, thirteen-year-old Tommaso, eight-year-old Caterina, and three-year-old Ambrosio, died in the outbreak of pestilence that attacked the infant Cardano. The dysentery he suffered from at the age of eight was the result of an epidemic in which all the remaining descendants of his maternal grandfather other than Cardano himself, sixteen of them, died. His mother, in addition to three of her four children, lost all her brothers, sisters, nephews, and nieces to epidemic disease.[8] Moreover, even acute diseases are now perceived as capable of turning into other, chronic, diseases or defects, and thus in some sense never going away. The dysentery at eight left him with night sweats that lasted until the age of thirty-six, and these in turn were transformed into the excessive urination. This, as we have seen, he expected to last a lifetime; he now described it as an abnormal condition that had become "almost natural" to him.[9]

Hence chronic conditions, defects, or disabilities are the new focus of attention. The role of family predisposition has become more obtrusive: Cardano has never been good-looking or physically strong because he was born of elderly parents (at the time of his conception his father was fifty-six and his mother thirty-seven).[10] His short stature is also determined by his short parents, although, more favorably, he has inherited sharp eyesight from his father. The specific problems enumerated are all either permanent or of many years' duration. He now recorded the astral reasons why he suffered from a chronic flow of phlegm from the brain to the stomach, the twenty-eight years of night sweats and decade of impotence mentioned above, skin disease (*scabies*) from the age of twenty-four to fifty-one, hemorrhoids up to the age of twenty-eight and after that from time to time, heart palpitations until age twenty-seven, severe gout beginning at the age of forty-four, weakness of the eyes, a speech defect, and tearing in the left eye resulting from an injury. Ominously, moreover, several of these conditions were an unavoidable legacy from his parents: the flow of phlegm to the stomach he believed he had inherited from both; the palpitations of the heart and the speech defect were inherited from his father. When Cardano reviewed his health again in the 1560s, he had only minor changes and additions to make. For example, in even longer retrospect, he upped the number of maternal kin who had died in the plague epidemic to more than twenty; and he noted that, as he had predicted a decade earlier, he had acquired "varicose veins or the stone," and recorded a slight accident injuring his face in 1564.[11]

Considered as a record of experience, this litany of chronic or long-lasting complaints may suggest the Renaissance world of physical malaise and decay described by Piero Camporesi.[12] But what is chiefly of interest for present purposes is Cardano's own increasing emphasis on this aspect of his health, or rather ill health, as he moved from his mid-forties to his mid-fifties. The change of emphasis can be read in several ways, none of them mutually exclusive. The new version could simply exemplify the growing awareness of physical imperfection and fragility that is likely to accompany advancing age in anyone. Such an interpretation is questionable, given that several years after writing the horoscope narrative of 1554, Cardano felt capable of asserting before a live audience, "as you can see, old age has obviously not sapped my energies, does not afflict me [*(ut vos videtis) non plane me enervavit, non afflixit senectus*]."[13] It seems more as if there was a significant reevaluation or shift in his memory of his past when he wrote the revised narrative; what came to his mind were not only problems that might be attributed to aging (for example, gout) but also long-past sufferings that he had not mentioned before. Strikingly, no further shift in his view of his health reflects the mood of despair that followed the great tragedy of his life, his son's execution in 1560. Other sections of the revised horoscope narrative of about 1564 contain much about the younger Cardano's death, but the material on Girolamo's own health is very little changed from ten years earlier.

But the reorganization of the narrative about his health that he undertook in 1554 also provides a more sophisticated and attentive medical description. The introduction of the separate category of *vitia* appears to respond to contemporary interest in rethinking traditional ways of describing and classifying illness. In particular, the proper use of the word *morbus* was intensely debated. Thus, for example, Da Monte in lectures delivered at Padua in the 1540s objected to its use for conditions such as renal calculus or for anatomical anomalies.[14]

In the *Vita* the opening chapters on Cardano's family and his horoscope at the time of nativity provide the governing framework for both book and life. As far as physical health is concerned, these chapters provide the crucial information that the Cardano family was always exceptionally long-lived, while the heavens had ensured that Girolamo as an individual would be "destitute of bodily powers."[15] Accordingly, the seventy-four-year-old author opened the separate chapter that he devoted to the history of his health with the words "I was a man with an infirm state of body in several ways, by nature, by chance, and by symptoms."[16] The narrative about Cardano's health in this chapter is purely medical, not astrological. Nevertheless, it takes up and refines yet further the same story told in the horoscope narratives. In this final version, as the opening sentence just quoted indicates, the structure is elaborated into a triple division of types of infirmity. Instead of the two categories of "diseases" and "defects" (*morbi* and *vitia*), the reader is now presented with three separate lists: infirmities that are somehow inherent in Cardano's physical makeup; illnesses resulting from chance; and an ambiguous third category of "symptoms" (*symptomata*).

The afflictions listed under the first two categories correspond more or less closely to those identified respectively as *vitia* and *morbi* in the second horoscope. The infirmities that belong to Cardano "by nature" encompass most of the "defects" of the second horoscope, some described with elaborations. New items chiefly relate to advancing age: loss of teeth beginning in his sixties, indigestion after the age of seventy-two, and, most likely, the week of sleeplessness at every change of season and permanent skin disease or itching. But cure does not necessarily remove an item from this list: Cardano included hemorrhoids, gout, and hereditary heart palpitations among the infirmities to which he was subjected "by nature," even though he simultaneously claimed to have been completely cured of all of them. Moreover, he evidently believed that for infirmities "by nature" medical treatment might do more harm than good. A double hernia—hereditary from his father, as he believed—that became troublesome in his fifties spontaneously disappeared on the left side, on which it was untreated, but the right side, vigorously treated with ligatures and other means, only got worse. Others who were afflicted with excessive urination at the same time as he and who had sought out the help of physicians had long since died; he, however, had survived with this condition for forty years.[17]

The significance attached to "nature" in this passage is worth pondering. The term may refer to Cardano's individual physical makeup, that is, presumably his temperament or complexion (*krasis*) in the terminology of Galenic physiological theory. Nor would this interpretation rule out the possibility that he thought himself among the fortunate few actually endowed with perfection of temperament. The reader may recall that in his theoretical discussion of the subject in the *Contradictiones* (analyzed in chapter 3), he had been careful to emphasize that a perfectly balanced temperament involved not freedom from all disease but rather the ability to resist or overcome it (*"necesse est et cuiusque viventis morbos sentire, at omnibus resistit temperatura aequalis"*).[18] Alternatively, since such conditions as, for example, loss of teeth in old age must have been in the sixteenth century effectively a universal experience, what is signified, at least in the case of some conditions, may be nature in a broader sense: general human nature or even Nature herself. Yet Galenic medicine taught the perfection of nature and regarded disease and disability of all kinds as essentially *un*natural. This notion runs through the system of ideas at every level, from Galen's lengthy and scientifically sophisticated teleological demonstration of Nature's perfect design of the human body in *De usu partium* to the commonplace that the physician works with nature in bringing about cure. In the standard classification of "things natural, nonnaturals, and contranaturals" all forms of disease and disability fell under the last category; according to this definition gout, hemorrhoids, and most of the other items on Cardano's list are specifically *against* nature. Indeed, *podagra* (gout) is listed as an example of the contranaturals in the standard medieval handbook of Galenic medical theory known as the *Isagoge* of Johannitius. Cardano's willingness to consider these infirmities his "by nature" may thus be yet another instance of his interest in the boundaries of the natural and the limits of natural diversity.

The illnesses that came "by chance" are more or less the same list of short-term, acute diseases already familiar from the two horoscopes. One or two have dropped out, or been added, or are remembered somewhat differently. But the main innovation is the idea that, after all, these diseases may have happened to him "by chance." Across the successive accounts of his own acute illnesses the balance shifts from an initial emphasis on the predisposing, if not wholly determining, role of the stars toward progressively greater emphasis on random, nonpredetermined, factors. The first horoscope apparently attributed both attacks of illness and recovery from them to astral influences focused on Cardano as an individual. The second horoscope allowed for interactions among astrological influences on the individual, family predisposition, and the influences (presumably also ultimately astrological, but not excluding more proximate causes) responsible for epidemics. The chapter in the *Vita* puts chance or random factors in first place, leaving the reader to infer an interaction with the individual horoscope and family history that frames the *Vita* as a whole. Presumably, the chance factors in question include exposure to epidemics, unwholesome air, and so on.

The basis on which particular phenomena were selected for assignment to the third category, that of symptoms, is not readily apparent. "Symptoms" include several phenomena of Cardano's childhood and early youth that he had previously passed over without notice (night terrors, difficulty breathing outdoors in a cold wind, cold feet in bed at night); one of the conditions counted under "defects" in the second horoscope (night sweats); two and perhaps three of the illnesses previously listed as "diseases" or "caused by chance"; and a heterogeneous collection of other problems, most notably acrophobia, fear of mad dogs, and bouts of *amor hereos* (lovesickness), some of them so severe that he contemplated suicide.[19] The proper understanding of the distinctions among disease, symptom, and sign was in fact yet another problematic area of medical debate in Cardano's day. Argenterio acquired his notoriety as a "neoteric" chiefly because he sharply attacked Galen's usage of the terms in question as inconsistent and confused.[20] In fact, neither Argenterio nor any of his contemporaries was in a position to move beyond semantic criticisms. Cardano's heterogeneous assemblage of "symptoms"—including his repetition of conditions described as "diseases" earlier in the same chapter—is an indication of the confused and shifting state of terminology at a time in which the need to define traditional categories more precisely was clearer than the means by which the task could be accomplished.

Cardano's progressive exploration of his health throughout his lifetime seems an innovative enterprise. With the possible exception of occasional *consilia* that briefly sketched the patient's past history, none of the models of medical narrative considered in chapter 9 followed the entire health history of an individual through a lifetime. His four narratives yield a rare chronological record of the illnesses and infirmities of one long sixteenth-century life from its beginning almost until its end. They incorporate changing evaluations and shifts of memory that are as interesting from the standpoint of the history of the psychology of aging as from that of memory, the self, and autobiographical writing. And they reveal his intellect and professional knowledge constantly at work, analyzing his own health history in the light of his astrological theories and current debates in learned medicine.

But the chronological and analytical surveys in the horoscopes and *Vita* do not yield much detail about the experience of ill health or injury. He reserved that subject for the moral treatise *On the Uses of Adversity*, Book 2 of which is devoted to physical handicaps—deformity, disease, pain, old age, blindness, deafness, mutism, weakness or loss of memory (*oblivio*), impotence, lameness, paralysis, falling in love, and death. Cardano explicitly used his own experiences as examples of four of the conditions on this list: impotence, disease (the forty days of fever he suffered in 1554), old age, and weakness of memory. A fifth, falling in love, seems written with enough feeling to be the fruit of personal experience. The inclusion of love among physical disabilities is in line with a long tradition of medical literature. But Cardano's exposition ignored the topic of the lover's physical malaise, manifested in pallor, sighing, and the like, favored by medieval medical writers on *amor hereos*. His chapter combined an appreciative tribute to both family affection and the pleasures of love with an agonized appraisal of the fear and shame involved in loving boys.[21]

In the accounts of his problems with memory and of his first awareness of the forthcoming onset of old age, the emphasis is on his power to manage or ameliorate the situation. Industry and God's help enabled him to improve the naturally weak memory with which he had been born. When he recognized in his late fifties that his physical strength was beginning to lessen, he decided to exchange the demands of medical practice for a return to teaching and writing and prescribed himself medication to help his voice while lecturing.

By contrast, the story of his years of impotence throughout his twenties, "a calamity, an insult of nature [*calamitas, ludibrium naturae*]," seems a heartfelt account of psychological suffering.

> This incredible evil happened to me in my twenty-first year. Then . . . I first began habitually to lie with a girl, and was already as it seemed to me sufficiently strong and ready for sex. But the thing ended otherwise. For being obliged to return home [*in patriam*], from that time until my thirty-first year was completed, that is, for a whole decade, it was never permitted to me to lie with a woman. For even though I took many to bed with me, especially in the year in which I was rector [of the student] University [of Arts and Medicine] of Padua, when I was carefree, at the most flourishing age, and had strong forces for everything else—in the case of foods, I used abstinence and enjoyment with equal industry—yet I left them all dry. So that as since I often did the same thing with tedium, shame, and despair I decided totally to desist from this experience. For indeed sometimes I had little women with me for three whole nights and I could not do anything. Frankly, I think this one thing was to me the worst of ills. Not servitude to my father, not poverty, not illnesses, not enmities, quarrels, injuries from citizens, rejection by the medical profession, false calumnies, and that infinite heap of troubles could drive me to despair, hatred of life, contempt of pleasures and perpetual sadness; this one thing certainly could.[22]

As Cardano well knew, impotence was widely regarded as a condition especially susceptible of being induced by charms or spells. In its most extreme and lurid form (as set forth, for example, by the authors of the

Malleus maleficarum in 1484) this belief involved the idea that causing impotence in men was one of the main objectives and activities of the Devil and his agents the witches. Cardano believed in the existence and evil intentions of witches, but not that they had all the powers attributed to them. For all his despair over an affliction that blighted his young manhood, he did not attribute impotence in himself or any other man to witchcraft, demons, magical ligatures, or evil spells cast by women. As noted previously, in his professional capacity he explicitly denied that impotence could be either cause or removed by magic, attributing it instead either to the patient's own *imaginatio* or to a natural physical cause (imbalance in the patient's humors). When it came to his own case, in the work just quoted he offered no explanation of the cause of his suffering. It was finally relieved, as unaccountably as it had afflicted him, by the onset of another disease. Perhaps, he thought, God had chosen this strange method of liberating him as a way of showing Cardano that he owed everything to God. Elsewhere, however, in horoscopic narratives, he attributed both his affliction and his recovery from it more comprehensibly and more reassuringly to the stars.

But the illness with which he chose to illustrate the chapter on disease is described in much less emotional terms. Here, the dramatic emphasis is less on his suffering than on the combination of dream wisdom and medical skill with which, as recounted in chapter 8, he succeeded in curing himself. In addition, the experience led him to adopt an improved regimen, provided an opportunity to nag his sons into attending to their studies, obliged him to give up gambling, and left him free to work on two books: "Therefore by this treatment, together with the purgation of the body in the disease that I had just had and with the measures I had taken on account of it, I not only lived in good health . . . but although I was indeed growing older as if carried by a river flowing against me, yet I had improving health."[23] This last claim obviously illustrates the moral point of the treatise in which the story is included. But it also describes an illness that took place in the same year in which Cardano elaborated his horoscopic narrative into a picture of chronic ill health. Possibly, this is just another instance of his indifference to consistency. It seems more likely that the remark is a striking testimonial to the way in which one sixteenth-century physician-patient weighed the relative significance of acute disease and chronic infirmities in his own life.

In historical hindsight, acute diseases in the form of lethal epidemics appear a salient feature of early modern urban life. But the lasting impact of epidemics upon the survivors might well be less than that of other, chronic forms of morbidity. The life of Chiara Micheri was no doubt altered forever by the outbreaks of pestilence that swept away three of her children and almost all her other relatives (to whom she might often have needed to turn, given the elder Cardano's long delay in marrying her). But for her only surviving son, Girolamo, the epidemics he had survived in childhood could have been scarcely more than an oft-repeated family story. When his reminiscences turned to his personal experience of acute disease, his memory called forth only infrequent and in most instances brief episodes. They seemed to him important chiefly because his recovery from them guaranteed that he had thrown off the effects of a sickly childhood to become a fairly healthy middle-aged adult. Although Cardano's memories of his childhood illnesses were presumably colored by his mother's description (she used to insist that he would not live long),[24] there is little reason to doubt the accuracy in essentials of his recollections of subsequent acute illnesses. His habitual note taking for autobiography, astrology, medical prognostication, and oneiromancy all ensured that he would record his illnesses. Moreover, such a relatively benign history of acute disease was, no doubt, by no means unusual among privileged sectors of the population. Whatever the hazards of medical practice, and whatever his relative poverty compared to colleagues or social superiors, Cardano did not share the circumstances of the poor among whom epidemic diseases chiefly flourished in sixteenth-century cities. Thus chronic, debilitating, but nonlethal disabilities, not acute diseases, formed for him the picture of ill health. As he came to focus more and more upon such disabilities, whether because of his own aging, or for psychological reasons, or because of issues in current medical debate, or a combination of all three, he came more and more to regard himself as a person "of infirm state of body."

Although the sixteenth century was a period rich in the production of medical narrative of one kind or another, autobiographical narrative by patients was still relatively rare. The exceptions are illustrious and of great value from the standpoint of the history of writing about the self—Montaigne and Von Hutten come to mind—but hardly representative of "normal" lay perceptions of health and disease. Cardano, too, is an anomalous case. Many contemporaries in relatively privileged sectors of Italian city life may have had physically similar medical histories, in which occasional encounters with acute disease were interspersed among litanies of chronic but relatively minor infirmities. But Cardano's self-presentation as a patient, in several senses—as an individual on whom influences from his family, from the stars, from chance all converge—is perpetually informed by his stance as a physician and his use of astrology to structure and analyze history. Furthermore, the medical ideas that he brought to bear on his own health, although in general Galenic, were also interpenetrated by his eclectic learning, his beliefs about

EPILOGUE

ON FEBRUARY 18, 1571, the Inquisitor of Bologna, Antonio Baldinucci, handed down the sentence of the Congregation of the Holy Office on Cardano. He had already voluntarily renounced teaching, in a futile attempt to satisfy the Inquisition. Subsequently, he had been first imprisoned and then held under house arrest for several months. He was now condemned to abjure *coram congregationem*, that is, in a private inquisitorial ceremony rather than a humiliating public one. Having done so, he further committed himself, in a letter to Pius V, never to teach again in the Papal States and to publish no more books.[1] At the age of nearly seventy he had lost his job, suffered damage to his reputation, and been forbidden his lifelong intellectual pursuit. By inquisitorial standards the punishment was a light one.

Following the advice of his old friend and patron Cardinal Morone, he moved to Rome. There, Morone ultimately succeeded in securing a papal pension for Cardano when Gregory XIII—a former professor at Bologna and a Catholic reformer of milder temperament than his austere predecessor—acceded to the papacy in 1573. And there, in most accounts, the story more or less ends. The only activity of the last few years of Cardano's life that has attracted much attention is the composition of the famous autobiography. In some versions of the Cardano myth that began to emerge soon after his death and flourishes still, he is depicted as a broken-down, pathetic figure. But Cardano seems to have rallied from the latest blows just as he had from so many others. In the years at Rome, he was busily engaged in the same two activities that had filled so much of his time since the long-ago days at Sacco: writing and the practice of medicine.

If the pace of his activities at Rome was less frantic than it had been at Milan twenty years earlier, it was still brisk enough to do credit to a man twenty years younger. Apart from his autobiography, Cardano wrote one other nonmedical work at Rome. In 1574, evidently hoping to get permission to publish, he sent an appeal to the pope via the Congregation of the Index of Prohibited Books. In it, Cardano requested leave to write a set of retractions of the errors in his own works. Such an apologia would, he predicted, be more useful to the Holy See than his errors had been damaging to it. He endeavored to strengthen his case by emphasizing that the errors in his works were just that, errors, never heresies, and that neither he nor anyone in his household had ever been stained with heresy either through their associations, in ordinary social conversation, or in the course of lecturing or disputing ("*né in conversatione, né in compagnia né legendo né disputando*").[2] Both assertions may be true, at least in intention; as Ian Maclean has pointed out, Cardano may not necessarily have been aware of the Protestant affiliations of some of his publishers. Nevertheless, the suspicion generated by his unconventional philosophical ideas, complex attitude to the supernatural, and perhaps some of his social and professional contacts (in Italy as well as with northerners) had evidently not been completely allayed, despite the resolution of the inquisitorial proceedings against him.[3] Cardano did not obtain permission to publish his own corrections of his work.

He had in fact been at work on a set of *Castigationes* of his own books since shortly after his trial in Bologna. He completed it in 1573, the year before he wrote the appeal referred to in the previous paragraph.[4] Most of it is devoted to *De varietate rerum*, although *De subtilitate*, the commentary on Ptolemy, his dream book, and his philosophical works are also included. Cardano's notion of castigations included the correction of typographical errors, the addition of a few more hits at his old enemy Julius Caesar Scaliger (3r, 5v, 16r), and the accretion of yet more particulars about the variety of things in the world, from the small but very strong-smelling mushrooms of Ruthenia to Cardinal Ascanio's parrot that could recite the Lord's Prayer (5v, 9r). On dangerous theological topics he offered either a clear retraction or an exculpatory plea: he expunged the horoscope of Christ and insisted that he had discussed the immortality of the soul purely from a philosophical standpoint (23v, 24v). By contrast, on the more ambiguous subjects of astral influences, divination, miracles, dreams, and demons, he amplified his explanations in a way that seems intended to justify his views. He defended the proposition that the celestial bodies exerted an influence other than and in addition to their light and heat, explained that the physical portents in his body were entirely natural (*totum naturale*), asserted the reality and usefulness of divination, insisted that the proposition that some apparently miraculous happenings were either natural or fraudulent did not negate true supernatural miracles performed by God, and defended the reality and value of warning dreams and the superior sensitivity of some people as dream interpreters (3v, 10v, 16r, 19v, 24r). On these topics, his concession to the idea of castigation was to add cautions: primarily that it was important not to invoke demons in connection with any of these occult or prognostic arts, "for no one can know how worthy he or she is of his or her *genius* [*nemo scire potest quam dignus sit suo genio*

(16v)]." In short, in Rome as before, Cardano retained confidence in his stars, his dreams, and perhaps his *genius*.

But most of the writing he did in Rome was medical. He continued to work on his Hippocrates project from the time he arrived in Rome until shortly before his death. He completed two substantial medical books and at least one shorter treatise there.[5] The absence in the *Castigationes* of any reference to works on medicine probably indicates that they were never included in the ban on publication; medical works were certainly excluded from the works put on the Index in 1580.[6] Thus the commentary on *Aliment*, the last of the series based on his lectures at Bologna, was published in Rome in 1574. The other major medical work of his Roman years, the massive exposition of his views on diet in *De sanitate tuenda*, was a new undertaking. It too was published in Rome, four years after the author's death, having been seen through the press by his pupil Rodolfo Silvestri. As Cardano had planned, it was dedicated to Gregory XIII, who sponsored—and paid for—publication.[7]

At Rome as elsewhere, we are in the dark about the nature and extent of Cardano's medical practice. His own description of it was as enthusiastic as ever, if not more so. In 1573, he endeavored to persuade the city authorities of Bologna to get the ban on his teaching in the Papal States rescinded and either restore his professorship or grant him a pension. As an inducement, he wrote to a Bolognese official that "here at Rome I have performed so many marvelous cures that I never did a quarter as many at Pavia or at Bologna or at Milan or in England, and the whole reason is that my mind is sincerely concentrated on nothing else but practicing medicine well."[8] The letter did not produce the desired result.

But Cardano the physician clearly continued to inspire confidence in both civic authorities and some patients of high ecclesiastical rank. He was one of a group of physicians and a surgeon ordered by the governor of the city to conduct an autopsy on the corpse of the French ambassador to the Holy See.[9] He wrote *consilia* for members of the College of Cardinals.[10] There is also striking independent testimony to Cardano's high standing among medical colleagues at Rome. On September 13, 1574, the city's College of Physicians admitted Cardano; he succeeded to the seat of one of its most distinguished members, the recently deceased anatomist Bartolomeo Eustachi. Cardano's power to impress was evidently undiminished. The members of the college greeted their new colleague with a respect that bordered on awe. The minutes of the meeting at which he was enrolled refer to him as "the most excellent and extremely famous doctor of arts and medicine Dominus Girolamo Cardano of Milan," and declare that he was accepted unanimously and *multum alacriter* as wonderfully (*mirabiliter*) deserving of admission. "On account of the eminence and high merit of his excellence both of doctrine and conduct [*propter suae excellentiae tum doctrinae tum morum eminentiam et excelsivitatem*]," he was given the extraordinary privilege of addressing the college at once and in Italian, rather than remaining silent until after his third meeting and then speaking Latin, as the college statutes required. He was also made a permanent *promotor* of the college, entitled to present other candidates for membership.[11] Cardano continued to attend meetings of the college regularly until June 1576, three months before his death. On November 24, the college admitted his student Rodolfo Silvestri, in his place.[12]

But whatever ecclesiastical authorities may have supposed, Cardano's medicine could never be isolated from his intellectual universe as a whole. For Cardano, medicine encompassed every aspect of human knowledge, power, and technique as more circumscribed approaches to nature—exemplified for him by the collecting and depicting characteristic of the nascent discipline of natural history—never could. As he put it, in words that simultaneously illuminate his own career, reflect his deepest convictions, and recall the most vibrant aspects of contemporary medical culture:

> The physician asks whether diseases and cures are sent by God, just as Hippocrates did. And directing his mind upward, he becomes a theologian. He asks what the soul is, and whether it is mortal or immortal. He asks what power the stars have, and whether disease and cures depend on them. . . . Thus considering the motion of the stars, and their risings and settings, and also the returning times of genitures [i.e., "revolutions," a major category of astrological interpretation], he treats most of astrology. Thence he turns to the winds, constitutions of the year, rains, clear or cloudy skies, cold and heat, so you will say he learns perfect meteorology. . . . Again, when he considers the structure and convenience of houses, he is a most skilled architect. . . . I set aside the art of cooking, which it is certainly appropriate for him to know. . . . I will add only those things that so much pertain to the physician that they are proper to him, the knowledge of which is indeed so wonderful that one physician seems to know more things than all other craftsmen and philosophers combined. For what can be said or thought to be greater among mortals than that one man should not only know all plants and fruits and stones, metals, fish, birds, serpents, quadrupeds and all their parts, but also their generation and that of insects? . . . And what is greatest of all, that he should also know forces and secrets, powers and miracles. As if in this respect the physician is compared to the philosopher, the philosopher indeed seems small compared to the physician. Does not the physician alone depict herbs, trees, fruit, seeds, flowers? Does not he alone know their powers? And the same goes for everything that the

earth produces. What shall I say then of that marvelous ability to dissect our bodies and of the knowledge of the function of every part? The physician alone knows the power of the elements: he teaches also how to heal disturbances of mores; do not these things (let us frankly confess the obvious) approach divinity? What shall I say about the most subtle and marvelous knowledge of pulses and urines . . . in which he seems to want to strive with nature itself, with the very Maker of things . . . ? What shall I say about the divine oracles of prognostication of the expert physician who knows the time and manner of death or cure better than any prophet?[13]

NOTES

CHAPTER 1
INTRODUCTION

1. "Habeat studiosus horologium, et speculum semper parata: horologium, quoniam in tanta rerum confusione, ac mole necesse est, ut horas digerere sciat, eoque magis professor sit, aut doceat pueros, aut scribat. Speculum ut dignoscat habitum corporis, ut ante morbos occurrere malo corporis habitui possit" (Cardano, *De sanitate tuenda* 4.16, *Opera* 6:267). Werner Friedrich Kümmel, "Der Homo litteratus und die Kunst, gesund zu leben. Zur Entfaltung eines Zweiges der Diätetik im Humanismus," *Humanismus und Medizin*, ed. Rudolf Schmitz and Gundolf Keil (Bonn, 1984), p. 83, notes the same passage and calls attention to other, symbolic and moralizing, uses of these images in the Renaissance. Although the term *horologium* was used for a variety of timekeeping devices in the sixteenth century, there can be no doubt that Cardano had a mechanical clock in mind. His mathematical and mechanical interests—and love of all kinds of gadgets, devices, and rarities—combined to give him a keen interest in clocks and clockmaking. See Cardano, *De rerum varietate* 9.47, *Opera* 187–88, and Philip McNair, "Poliziano's Horoscope," in *Cultural Aspects of the Italian Renaissance: Essays in Honour of Paul Oskar Kristeller*, ed. Cecil H. Clough (Manchester and New York, 1976), pp. 261–75, at p. 269.

2. "usque adeo vetus medicina a pristino decore ante plures annos descivit. Porro quum illa iam pridem in tanta huius seculi . . . foelicitate cum omnibus studiis ita reviviscere, atque a profundissimis tenebris caput suum erigere coepisset, ut veterem candorem citra controversiam in nonullis Academiis propemodum recuperasse videretur" (Andreas Vesalius, *De humani corporis fabrica libri septem* [Basel, 1543], praefatio, fol. *3r). There are, however, precedents for assertions of the revival of medicine or its subdisciplines extending back to the thirteenth century. For some affirmations of thirteenth-century surgeons, see Chiara Crisciani, "History, Novelty, and Progress in Scholastic Medicine," *Osiris* 6 (1990): 118–39, at pp. 131–34; some examples of assertions of this type about medicine by fifteenth-century literary humanists are collected in Nancy G. Siraisi, "The Physician's Task: Medical Reputations in Humanist Collective Biographies," in *The Rational Arts of Living*, ed. A. C. Crombie and Nancy G. Siraisi, Smith College Studies in History, vol. 50 (Northampton, Mass., 1987), pp. 105–33.

3. Antonio Riccobono, *De gymnasio patavino commentaria* (Padua, 1598), fol. 71r.

4. VP is a main but not the only source for Cardano's biography. The account given here follows the concise but thorough summary in G. Gliozzi, "Cardano, Gerolamo," *Dizionario biografico degli italiani* 19 (1975): 759–63. Mario Gliozzi, "Cardano, Girolamo," *Dictionary of Scientific Biography* 3 (New York, 1971): 64–67, provides a shorter biography but a fuller account of Cardano's

mathematics. I make no attempt to list here the extensive older secondary literature on Cardano; very full bibliographies are provided in Gliozzi, "Cardano," p. 763, and in Ingegno, pp. 21–31. A comprehensive bibliography of the older literature is also found in James Eckman, *Jerome Cardan, Supplements to the Bulletin of the History of Medicine*, no. 7 (Baltimore, 1946), pp. 90–112.

5. Here and throughout the term "university" is used in its modern English sense, in preference to the more technically correct *studium*, for the academic institution as a whole. "University" (*universitas*) is occasionally also used in its historical sense to denote separate associations within medieval and Renaissance *studia*, e.g., the university of students of arts and medicine as distinct from the university of students of law.

6. *Artis magnae, sive de regulis algebraicis, liber unus* (Nuremberg, 1545); *In Cl. Ptolemaei Pelusiensis IIII de astrorum iudiciis aut ut vulgo vocant quadripartitae constructionis libros* [= *Tetrabiblos*] *commentaria* (Basel, 1554, 1578; Lyon, 1555); *De consolatione libri tres* (Venice, 1542); *De subtilitate libri XXI* (Lyon, 1550), reissued many times in Latin, as well as being translated into French and German in the author's lifetime; *De rerum varietate libri XVII* (Basel, 1557), also reissued a number of times. See IA, pp. 512–23, and Ian Maclean, "Cardano and His Publishers, 1534–1663," Kessler, pp. 309–38.

7. Cardano's *Opera omnia* were edited by Charles Spon, professor of medicine at Montpellier. The edition is not, in fact, complete. The medical works occupy vols. 6, 7, 8, and 9, and a large part of vol. 10.

8. *De subtilitate* 1.1., *Opera* 3:357–58. On Cardano as a scientific popularizer, see Ian Maclean, "The Interpretation of Natural Signs: Cardano's *De subtilitate* versus Scaliger's *Exercitationes*," in *Occult and Scientific Mentalities in the Renaissance*, ed. Brian Vickers (Cambridge, 1984), pp. 231–52. On the concept of subtlety, see ibid., pp. 238–39, and Ingegno, pp. 209–20.

9. Largely as a result of the work of Frances Yates, whose *Giordano Bruno and the Hermetic Tradition* (London, 1964) and "The Hermetic Tradition in Renaissance Science," in *Art, Science, and History in the Renaissance*, ed. Charles Singleton (Baltimore, 1967), pp. 255–74, sparked a generation of contentious scholarship. Few historians would now completely endorse Yates's views of the influence of Renaissance hermetism, or occultism, on the future development of science, but her work made a contribution of great value by opening up scholarly investigation into an important and previously neglected area of sixteenth-century culture.

10. In inventories of books belonging to sixty-six Paris physicians from the early sixteenth century until 1665, Cardano is the sixteenth- or seventeenth-century author most frequently named; works listed include his writings on regimen and Hippocratic commentaries (see chaps. 4 and 6); see Françoise Lehoux, *Le cadre de vie des médecins parisiens aux XVIe et XVIIe siècles* (Paris, 1976), p. 478.

11. "Itaque jure merito haec commentaria omnibus nostris operibus praestant" (LP 1557, *Opera* 1:70).

12. His first list of his own books was printed with his *Practica arithmetice* (Milan, 1539); it is edited in Maclean, "Cardano and His Publishers," pp. 337–38. Subsequent, successively enlarged versions of his bibliography were published in 1544, 1557, and 1562 (LP 1544, LP 1557, LP 1562). On Cardano's

use of his own dreams and his own horoscope in various of his works, see further chaps. 8 and 10, below. In addition, autobiographical meditations, anecdotes, or reminiscences are scattered throughout his work. VP (*Opera* 1:1–54) was first published by Gabriel Naudé (Paris, 1643).

13. After recounting his early difficulties in finding a satisfactory publisher, Cardano continued " . . . continuo enim eo opere impresso, coeperunt omnia commutari. Nam adieceram Catalogum qualemcunque librorum nostrorum, quos vel scripseram, vel coeperam scribere: et liberis [*sic*] distrahi coepit in Galliis atque Germaniis. Itaque cum tunc esset Andreas Osiander Norimbergae, vir Latinae, Graecae, Hebraeicaeque linguae peritus, tum typographus Ioannes Petreius, bonis literis, si quis alius, favens, inito consilio totis viribus mecum agere coeperunt, ut aliquod opus illis traderem ut imprimerent. Atque ita initium gloriae nostrae, si qua deinceps fuit, hinc ortum habuit" (LP 1562, *Opera* 1:104). See also Maclean, "Cardano and His Publishers."

14. "Imitatus sum in hoc scribendi genere Galenum et Erasmum, qui ambo catalogum librorum suorum scripserunt" (LP 1562, *Opera* 1:106). Elsewhere, he expanded the list of his autobiographical models to include Caesar, Cicero, and Marcus Aurelius (ibid., p. 96). The authenticity of the autobiographical sketch attributed to Erasmus has been questioned. Erasmus's catalog of his works, like Cardano's repeatedly updated (by Erasmus himself and, after his death, by his publisher), was published in successively more expanded separate editions in Basel (1523, 1524, and 1537), and in the front matter to the 1540 Basel edition of his *Opera omnia*. See Erika Rummel, *The Erasmus Reader* (Toronto, 1990), p. 21.

15. Carlo Gregori, "Rappresentazione e difesa: Osservazioni sul *De vita propria* di Gerolamo Cardano," *Quaderni storici* 73 (1990): 225–34; idem, "L'elogio del silenzio e la simulazione come modelli di comportamento in Gerolamo Cardano," in *Sapere e/è potere. Discipline, dispute e professioni nell'università medievale e moderna. Il caso bolognese a confronto*, vol. 3, *Dalle discipline ai ruoli sociali*, ed. Angela De Benedictis (Bologna, 1990), pp. 73–84.

16. Andrea Cesalpino, *Peripateticarum quaestionum libri V* (Venice, 1571, and several other early editions); Gianbattista Da Monte, *In primam fen libri primi Canonis Avicennae explanatio* (Venice, 1554), fols. 23v–54r; for discussion of Da Monte's commentary see Nancy G. Siraisi, *Avicenna in Renaissance Italy* (Princeton, 1987), pp. 248–54. Giancarlo Zanier, *Ricerche sulla diffusione e fortuna del "De incantationibus" di Pomponazzi* (Florence, 1975), 1–16, draws attention to the numerous examples of cures discussed by Pomponazzi in his work on incantations, namely, Pietro Pomponazzi, *De naturalium effectuum admirandorum causis et de incantationibus liber*, which I have consulted in his *Opera* (Basel, 1567). Pomponazzi (1462–1525) held a doctorate in medicine from Padua (see Charles H. Lohr, *Latin Aristotle Commentaries*, vol. 2, *Renaissance Authors* [Florence, 1988], p. 347).

17. Georgius Agricola (1494–1555), *De re metallica*, trans. H. C. and L. H. Hoover (reprint, New York, 1950), p. vii; Bruno Accordi, "Michele Mercati (1541–93) e la Metallotheca," *Geologia Romana* 19 (1980): 1–50; on Rondelet (1507–66), Karen Reeds, *Botany in Medieval and Renaissance Universities* (New York, 1991), pp. 55–72.

18. LP 1544, *Opera* 1:57.

19. Carlo Cipolla, *Public Health and the Medical Profession in the Renaissance* (Cambridge, 1976), pp. 77–83, notes the low social status in late-sixteenth-century Italy of university-trained physicians without publications or current university connections or membership in a city college of medicine, and he documents the large numbers of such men who were practicing in smaller centers in Tuscany in 1630.

20. For a summary comparative account of the origins and development of some of the principal medieval university faculties of medicine, see Nancy G. Siraisi, "The Faculty of Medicine," in *A History of the University in Europe*, vol. 1, *Universities in the Middle Ages*, ed. Hilde de Ridder-Symoens (Cambridge, 1992), pp. 360–87. On Pavia, see Tiziana Pesenti, "Le origini dell'insegnamento medico a Pavia," *Storia di Pavia*, vol. 3, pt. 2 (Milan, 1990), pp. 454–74.

21. Jerome J. Bylebyl, "The School of Padua: Humanistic Medicine in the Sixteenth Century," in *Health, Medicine and Mortality in the Sixteenth Century*, ed. Charles Webster (Cambridge, 1979), pp. 335–70, at pp. 352–53; Siraisi, *Avicenna*.

22. No single study gives a comprehensive account of the phenomenon of medical humanism. However, see Bylebyl, "School of Padua"; Daniela Mugnai Carrara, *La biblioteca di Nicolò Leoniceno* (Florence, 1991); and the numerous articles of Vivian Nutton. The last are, in fact, too numerous to be listed here, and I note only his monograph, *John Caius and the Manuscripts of Galen*, supplementary vol. no. 13, Cambridge Philological Society (1987), and "The Changing Languages of Medicine, 1450–1550," in *Vocabulary of Teaching and Research between Middle Ages and Renaissance*, ed. Olga Weijers (Turnhout, 1995), pp. 183–98. For discussion of various ways in which ancient texts were read, see Anthony Grafton, "Renaissance Readers and Ancient Texts," in his *Defenders of the Text: The Traditions of Scholarship in an Age of Science, 1450–1800* (Cambridge, Mass., 1991), pp. 23–46. For a contribution to the continuing debate over the impact of humanism on science in general, taking a judiciously favorably view of humanism, see idem, "Humanism, Magic, and Science," in *The Impact of Humanism on Western Europe*, ed. Anthony Goodman and Angus MacKay (London and New York, 1990), pp. 99–117.

23. See Charles B. Schmitt, "The Faculty of Arts at Pisa in the Time of Galileo," no. 9 in his *Studies in Renaissance Philosophy and Science* (London, 1981), pp. 243–72, at pp. 248–51; Bylebyl, "School of Padua," pp. 344–46; Pietro Vaccari, *Storia della Università di Pavia*, 2d ed. (Pavia, 1957), pp. 97–98, and *Statuti e ordinamenti per l'Università di Pavia dall'anno 1361 al 1859* (Pavia, 1925), p. 155. Richard L. Kagan, "Universities in Italy 1500–1700," in *Les universités européennes du XVIe au XVIIIe siècle: Histoire sociale des populations étudiantes*, vol. 1, ed. Dominique Julia, Jacques Revel, and Roger Chartier (Paris, 1986), pp. 153–185, provides a comparative overview of the social history of early modern Italian universities.

24. Much information about these varieties of medical practice is to be found in William Eamon, *Science and the Secrets of Nature: Books of Secrets in Medieval and Early Modern Culture* (Princeton, 1994).

25. *Proxeneta seu de prudentia civili, Opera* 1:355–474; for analysis see Gregori, "L'elogio del silenzio."

26. See the perceptive introduction to Gerolamo Cardano, *Della mia vita,* ed. Alfonso Ingegno (Milan, 1982).

27. VP, chap. 18, *Opera* 1:14; *De subtilitate* bk. 17, *Opera* 3:626.

28. A thought-provoking analysis is found in Ian Maclean, "Montaigne, Cardano: The Reading of Subtlety / The Subtlety of Reading," *French Studies* 37 (1983): 143–56.

29. An excellent recent study of this aspect of Renaissance scientific culture is Paula Findlen, *Possessing Nature: Museums, Collecting, and Scientific Culture in Early Modern Italy* (Berkeley and Los Angeles, 1994).

30. For these issues the study by Katharine Park and Lorraine Daston, *Wonders and the Order of Nature, 1150–1750* (New York: Zone Books, forthcoming, 1997), offers fresh insights and much information.

31. Jackie Pigeaud, "L'Hippocratisme de Cardan: Etude sur le Commentaire d'AEL par Cardan," *Res publica litterarum* 8 (1975): 219–29. A few specific contributions to medical knowledge allegedly made by Cardano have been noted by older historians of medicine; see nn. 22 and 78 to chap. 2.

32. See earlier notes to this chapter and bibliography.

33. Germana Ernst, " 'Veritatis amor dulcissimus.' Aspetti dell'astrologia in Cardano," in Kessler; Anthony Grafton, *Cardano's Cosmos: The Three Worlds of a Renaissance Magus* (Cambridge: Harvard University Press, forthcoming, 1997). See also idem, *Girolamo Cardano and the Tradition of Classical Astrology,* Rothschild Lecture, 1995, Department of the History of Science, Harvard University (Cambridge, 1996), and "From Apotheosis to Analysis: Some Late Renaissance Histories of Classical Astronomy," in *History and the Disciplines,* ed. Donald E. Kelley (Rochester, N.Y.: Rochester University Press, forthcoming, 1997).

CHAPTER 2

PRACTITIONER AND PATIENTS

1. "Cum in hac urbe, invidia laboraremus, nec lucrum suppeditaret impensis, multa ut nova inveniremus, tentavimus in arte: nam extra artem nihil non cessit. Tandem phthisis (quam phthoen vocant) multis seculis curam deploratam excogitavi, sanavique multos, qui nunc supervivunt: nec difficilius quam Gallicum morbum" (Cardano, *De sapientia libri V,* 5, *Opera* 1:578). The work was first published in Nuremberg, in 1544 (IA *132. 049).

2. (1) Cardano, *Liber de libris propriis* (Lyon, 1557; IA *132. 073), with title, p. 3, *Hieronymi Cardani Mediolanensis medici liber De libris propriis, eorumque ordine, et usu, ac de mirabilibus operibus in arte medica per ipsum factis* . . . , with the cures on pp. 121–91; this = *Opera,* 1:60–95, with the cures on pp. 82–94.

(2) Cardano, *De curationibus et praedictionibus admirandis,* printed with his *Somniorum synesiorum . . . libri IIII* (Basel, 1562; IA *132. 083), pp. 118–37 (second series of pagination).

(3) Cardano, *De methodo medendi sectiones quatuor* (Paris, 1565; IA *132. 098), sectio 3, *De admirandis curationibus, et praedictionibus morborum*, pp. 211–56 (= *Opera* 7:253–64).

The text is the same in nos. (2) and (3); inc. "Hunc librum in catalogum caeterorum non solum ob parvitatem ascribere neglexi, sed quod antea pars fuerit libri de libris propriis. Nunc postquam eam tractationem ab illa seiunxi, visum est, ut breviter, quae mihi in arte contigerunt mira, enarrem: Galeni exemplo, in libro de Praedictione ad Posthumum fretus, imo illum potius imitatus."

In addition, he included a chapter on his "felicitas in curando" in the autobiography first printed many years after his death; see VP 40, *Opera* 1:31–34.

3. "Nec mireris, o Lector, nec mentiri suspiceris, haec omnia ita se habent, et huiusmodi contigerunt, et maiora, et longe plura: numerum non teneo, sed existimo ad clxxx accedere, et plus ultra: nec tamen inaniter gloriari suspiceris, aut cupere, vel sperare me praeferri Hippocrati" (VP 40, *Opera* 1:34).

4. Cardano's principal works on practical aspects of medicine include:

De malo recentiorum medicorum usu libellus. . . . Eiusdem libellus de simplicium medicinarum noxa (Venice, 1536, 1545; IA *132. 044, 053). The first edition contains only chaps. 1–72. The second edition, which added new chapters to bring the number up to one hundred, was subsequently incorporated into *De methodo medendi*.

Quaedam opuscula, artem medicam exercentibus utilissima, ut sunt, de aqua et aethere, de cyna radice. . . . (Basel, 1559; IA *132. 077; *Opera* 2:570–614; 7:266–70).

. . . De venenorum differentiis, viribus et adversus ea remediorum praesidiis ac praesertim De pestis generibus omnibus praeservatione et cura libri III (Basel, 1564; IA. *132. 093; Padua, 1653; *Opera* 7:275–355).

Ars curandi parva quae est absolutissimus medendi methodos. . . . (Basel, 1564, 1566; IA *132. 094, 100; *Opera* 7:143–99).

De methodo medendi sectiones quatuor (Paris, 1565; IA *132. 098), a compilation consisting of the first two treatises listed above, namely, (1) the contents (without the title) of the second edition of *De malo recentiorum medicorum usu*, and (2) *De simplicium medicinarum noxa*; (3) *De admirandis curationibus* (see n. 2 above); (4) a number of *consilia*. *Opera* 7:199–264 contains sections 1–3.

De causis, signis, et locis morborum, liber unus (Bologna, 1569; IA *132. 107; *Opera* 7:65–108).

Opus novum cunctis de sanitate tuenda ac vita producenda studiosis apprime necessarium (Rome, 1580, 1582; IA *132. 118, 121; *Opera* 6:8–294).

Opuscula medica senilia (*De dentibus, De rationali curandi ratione, De facultatibus medicamentorum, De morbo regio*) (Lyon, 1638; *Opera* 9:247–407).

De usu ciborum liber, Opera 7:1–64.

De urinis liber, Opera 7:109–42.

Consilia medica ad varios partium morbos spectantia, Opera 9:47–246 (a number of these *consilia* were published in Cardano's lifetime in conjunction with various of his other works).

De morbis articularibus, Opera 9:407–52.

5. Many of the same cases recur in the accounts of his cures in LP 1557, CA, and VP 40 (as in n. 2, above), but each of the last two works adds more names. The section on his cures in LP 1557 names more than seventy patients treated between 1534 and the explicit date 1554; there are also references to the "children" of a family and to "many" others. CA adds about a dozen new names, presumably treated between 1554 and 1561, the date of the last case in this collection. VP adds ten new names of patients treated after 1561. These are the names of people Cardano believed he had treated successfully, not a roster of all his patients. Some but not all of his fifty-seven *consilia* (*Opera* 9:47–246) appear to have been intended for patients named in one of the foregoing lists. Names of other individual patients crop up from time to time in his Hippocratic commentaries and prescriptive works on medical practice.

6. Useful studies of health and mortality in fifteenth- and sixteenth-century northern Italy include Giuliana Albini, *Guerra, fame, peste: Crisi di mortalità e sistema sanitario nella Lombardia tardomedioevale* (Bologna, 1982); Ann Carmichael, "The Health Status of Florentines in the Fifteenth Century," in *Life and Death in Fifteenth-Century Florence*, ed. Marcel Tetel, Ronald G. Witt, and Rona Goffen (Durham, N.C., 1989), pp. 28–45 (despite its title, this essay contains information directly relating to Milan at the beginning of the sixteenth century); Anna Maria Nada Patrone, *Il cibo del ricco ed il cibo del povero. Contributo alla storia qualitativa dell'alimentazione: L'area pedemontana negli ultimi secoli del Medio Evo* (Turin, 1981); Dante Zanetti, "La morte a Milano nei secoli XVI–XVIII: Appunti per una ricerca," *Rivista storica italiana* 88 (1976): 803–51. The very extensive Milan death registers have not so far been completely studied for the middle decades of the sixteenth century. Much information about the social context of patients and practitioners in sixteenth-century Bologna is to be found in Gianna Pomata, *La promessa di guarigione. Malati e curatori in antico regime: Bologna XVI–XVIII secolo* (Rome, 1994). Lehoux, *Le cadre de vie*, provides interesting comparisons.

7. See chap. 9 (and also the passages quoted in nn. 2 and 3, above).

8. Cipolla, *Public Health*, pp. 67–124, esp. pp. 72–78 (with reference to Tuscany in the early seventeenth century); Eamon, *Science and the Secrets of Nature*, esp. pp. 168–93 and 235–50. In late-sixteenth-century London, about half those practicing some form of medicine were unlicensed; see Charles Webster and Margaret Pelling, "Medical Practitioners," in *Health, Medicine and Mortality in the Sixteenth Century*, ed. Charles Webster (Cambridge, 1979), pp. 165–235, esp. pp. 182–88. According to Cipolla, *Public Health*, p. 70, in Tuscany in the same period licensing regulations were considerably more effective.

9. As for example, the pressure brought to bear upon the physicians attending Don Carlos, son of Philip II, for his head injury in 1562, to allow a Morisco medical practitioner to treat the prince with secret unguents. See Dionisio Daza Chacon (1510–96), *Practica y teorica de Cirugia* (Madrid, 1678), 2:195. Daza Chacon's description of the illness and treatment of Don Carlos is translated in C. D. O'Malley, *Andreas Vesalius of Brussels, 1514–1564* (Berkeley and Los Angeles, 1964), pp. 407–19, with the passage cited at p. 412.

10. Pomata, *La promessa di guarigione*, pp. 102–7.

11. See, for example, Bylebyl, "School of Padua," p. 351.

12. "Et ego alioqui in medendo fortunatissimus, tum primum etiam intentus in re maxime, et auxilio libelli a me conscripti nuper, quem Artem medendi parvam appellaveram, adeo profeceram, ut neque Galenum aetate sua, nec aliorum quemquam, qui post floruerunt, adeo felicem in artis operibus, seu sanando seu producendo vitam eorum, qui sanari non possent, seu praedicendo, fuisse, existimaverim" (UC 2.4, *Opera* 2:50).

13. ACP, *Opera* 7:143–98. Regarding the dream inspiration of this work, see SS 4.4, *Opera* 5:726, and discussion in chap. 8, below.

"Duo sat sunt in hoc opere admiranda: unum quod quae ab Hippocratis aetate ad hanc usque diem ignota manserunt, tum etiam ex Galeno in lucem revocavimus: alterum, ut qui librum hunc [sc. ACP] teneat, quae intus quasi in superficie posita sint, teneat, ac spectare sibi videatur, ac de futuris tanquam praesentibus pronunciare possit. Scio incredibilia videri: sed qui legerit et intellexerit, non audebit negare: est enim e Dialecticae fructibus. Scriptus est autem plus quam vicies, insumpto in anagnostas talento: ordinatus, si quis alius liber, subtilitate et structura: librum refert Artis magnae in Arithmetica, illiusque vices in medicina gerit: unde ex hoc ad magnam evectus sum, non quidem sapientiae sed operum apud vulgum, scientiae autem apud praecipuos amicos, qui librum illum viderunt, opinionem. Quapropter infinita in laudem meam conscripta sunt, tum carmine, tum soluta oratione . . ." (LP 1562, *Opera* 1:114).

14. "Contra naturam pugnat anima Mundi, seu illius vis, quae nos multis modis affligit, nam reluctantes ex altis locis praecipites agit: et dum languemus, noxiam materiam impellit contra membra regia ac spiritus urgetque illa" (ACP, *Opera* 7:148).

15. "Nuper (cum ego alias quosdam Galeni errores adnotassem, et ex trecentis forsan triginta in cuiusdam manus incidissent, nec cur damnarem adiectum foret) ausus est tamen ille edito libello medicinae heresiarcham me appellare, qui totis viribus Galenum duodecim editis contradicentium medicorum libris tuear. Atque ille ob id Galenicum se posse dici sperat. Alii cum aegros queri ex longitudine morbi videant, et haeredes tristes illis mortuis hos laetos, illos nihil queri: malunt occidere tentando adversus artis praecepta, quam protrahendo ex arte sanare. Atque ob id quaeri solent homines nunquam alias fuisse plus medicorum quam nunc, nec unquam tamen minus in arte excitatorum: ob haec igitur hunc librum ad levandos labores, et ex methodo tamen quam brevissima medendum [*sic*] in publicum edo, et responsum simul ad criminationem illius falsam quam brevissimum, et dialecticam. In qua praeter id quod ordinatim quicquid est ab Aristotele ea in disciplina conscriptum quam brevissime contineatur, etiam Hippocratis et Galeni tum etiam Euclidis ac Ptolomaei [*sic*] dialecticam adieci. Quod si per fata licuisset et peculiarem Plotini annectere potuissem, perlibenter facturus eram ne quid ad ornatum deesset. . . . Tum vero cum summam malorum nostrorum in contemptu religionis, et falsa de his quae post mortem sunt opinione esse animadverterem, quod totum a philosophorum placitis aut non recte sententium aut non recte intellectorum proficisceretur, cum non plus ego dubitarem de animorum immortalitate etiam citra religionis nostrae constantissimam auctoritatem, quam quod ovum ovum esset, quae de rerum ipsarum principiis inveneram, huic proposito congruentia, in unum collegi libellum velut senectutis solamen (nam totam hanc tractationem in quarto et quinto Theonoston diffuse

conscripseram) quem utilitatis communis causa edere volo cum caeteris" (ibid., *Opera* 7:143–44). In the Basel editions of 1564 and 1566, *Ars curandi parva* was published as part of a two-volume set, the second volume of which included Cardano's *Apologia ad Andream Camutium.*

16. The copy is now in the Rare Book Room of the New York Academy of Medicine, along with a substantial part of the rest of the large alchemical and medical library collected by Winthrop (1605/6–76). A few of the books in the Winthrop collection were, however, acquired by later members of the family.

17. "Sed pro Inventione, Ratio dux erit. Experimentum autem, magister" (Cardano, *De sapientia* 5, *Opera* 1:578).

18. VP 44, *Opera* 1:40.

19. See Crisciani, "History, Novelty, and Progress," p. 123.

20. Rome, Biblioteca Nazionale Centrale, MS S. Francesca a Ripa 4, 99 fols., Cardanus [*Experimenta*], 7r, "De usu huius libri." The *experimenta* are medicinal recipes; the manuscript is very incomplete; after the formal proem explaining the method it consists largely of blank pages headed by titles of *experimenta.*

21. VP 44, *Opera* 1:40.

22. *De malo usu* 36, has been credited by some medical historians with containing an early description of typhus; see Eckman, *Jerome Cardan*, pp. 67–68, for sources and discussion.

23. "Quod raro et oscitanter administrationem exercent anatomicam" (MM, sectio 1 [= *De malo usu*], 89, *Opera* 7:238). For discussion, see chap. 5.

24. "Vigesimus tertius abusus est, cum omnes eas aegritudines ad curam suam pertinere negant, quae sunt manifestae, in quibus accusari possunt: eas autem omnes profitentur, quae sunt difficillimae, accusarique nequeunt, decorationem igitur et infantium morbos mulierculis; dentium dolores, tonsoribus; vulnera, ulcera, collectiones, chirurgicis; oculorum vitia circunforaneis herbariis; ramicem et herniam, circulatoribus; puerperarum dolores, obstetricibus; gallicam luem impostoribus; luxatos fractosque articulos, restauratoribus relinquunt" (MM, sectio 1 [= *De malo usu*], 23, *Opera* 7:210).

25. N. 4, above.

26. Leonhart Fuchs, *Errata recentiorum medicorum LX numero, adiectis eorundem confutationibus* (Hagenau, 1530).

27. MM, sectio 1 (= *De malo usu*), 16, 23, 100, *Opera* 7:208, 210, 245–46.

28. LP 1562, *Opera* 1:145.

29. N. 4, above.

30. N. 2, above, and for further discussion chap. 9.

31. VP 40, *Opera* 1:33.

32. Ibid., and ibid., chap. 17, p. 13.

33. The entire journey, including the time spent in Scotland, took 310 days. See LP 1557, *Opera* 1:93.

34. See n. 2, above. Cardano's publication strategies and his use of northern European publishers are well analyzed in Ian Maclean, "Cardano and His Publishers," Kessler, pp. 309–38.

35. The first printed set of statutes, issued in 1517, raised the admission requirements by stipulating legitimacy and noble birth and extending the university studies required; previously, four years' academic study of medicine had been

called for; see A. Bottero, "I più antichi statuti del collegio dei medici di Milano," *Archivio storico lombardo*, n.s., 8 (1943): 77, 89.

36. Roger French, "Berengario da Carpi and the Use of Commentary in Anatomical Teaching," in *The Medical Renaissance of the Sixteenth Century*, ed. Andrew Wear, Roger French, and I. M. Lonie (Cambridge, 1985), p. 45; Nancy G. Siraisi, "Giovanni Argenterio and Sixteenth-Century Medical Innovation: Between Princely Patronage and Academic Controversy," *Osiris* 6 (1990): 165.

37. ". . . multi invidi dicerent me literas medicinae nescire quod totus mathematicis viderer intentus" (LP 1544, *Opera* 1:57).

38. "Quare non video, cur mihi Cina sit experimento in phthoe cura tentanda: tum magis, quod generosi quidam medici nostri voluerunt in cura illius Thesaurario Martino illam exhibire, conspiratione eripientes illum e manibus meis" (Cardano, *Consilia medica ad varios partium morbos spectantia*, no. 27, *Opera* 9:168); this *consilium* is identical with the brief treatise *De radice cina*, *Opera* 7:265–66.

39. "Unde quosdam experieris alioquin tibi iure magis infensos, mitiores, quod eruditionis sint participes, quod ego etiam hic Mediolani experior . . . nam neque rite latine loqui norunt, neque philosophiae partem ullam attigere, neque rationem artis intelligunt, nec praecepta medendi. Sed finxerunt sibi quaedam commenta, quibus illudant plebeculae" (Cardano, *De oxymelitis usu in pleuritide. Ad Thaddaeum Dunum medicum epistola*, *Opera* 7:272). The whole correspondence is published in *Thaddaei Duni Locarniensis medici et Francisci Cigalini, Ioannisque Pauli Turriani medicorum Novocomensium clarissimorum, item Hieronymi Cardani medici et philosophi celeberrimi disputationum per epistolas liber unus* (Zurich, n.d., preface dated 1555). Cardano's contribution was the single letter quoted (no. 8, pp. 64–85, with date on p. 85); no. 9, pp. 85–105 is Duno's defensive reply. Duno (1523–1613) published medical works at Zurich and Strasbourg; see Richard J. Durling, *A Catalogue of Sixteenth Century Printed Books in the National Library of Medicine* (Bethesda, 1967), nos. 1320–24.

40. Kristian Jensen, "Cardanus and His Readers in the Sixteenth Century," Kessler, pp. 256–308, at pp. 293–308.

41. Cardano, *De oxymelitis usu in pleuritide*, *Opera* 7:273.

42. VP 14, *Opera* 1:12; *Liber de exemplis centum geniturarum*, no. 14, *Opera* 5:466, first published Cardano, *Libelli quinque. . . . V. de exemplis centum geniturarum* (Nuremberg, 1547; IA *132. 054); *Theonoston* bk. 2, *Opera* 2:381 (on this work, written after 1558 and not published in the author's lifetime, see further chap. 4). On Corti (1475–1544), see Vivian Nutton, " 'Qui magni Galeni doctrinam in re medica primus revocavit': Matteo Corti und der Galenismus im medizinischen Unterricht der Renaissance," in *Der Humanismus und die oberen Facultäten*, ed. Gundolf Keil (Weinheim, 1987), pp. 173–84, and A. De Ferrari, "Corti (Curti, Curzio, de Curte, de Corte), Matteo," *Dizionario biografico degli italiani* 29 (Rome, 1983): 795–97. I give the death date as corrected by Nutton.

43. *De oxymelitis usu in pleuritide*, *Opera* 7:273–74. Most of the works of Da Monte (1489–1551)—and all his major works—were published posthumously.

Writing in 1551, Cardano might have been referring to either Gianbattista Da Monte, *Metaphrasis summaria eorum quae ad medicamentorum doctrinam attinent excerpta ab accuratis auditoribus ex quotidianis praelectionibus in Patavino gymnasio publice explicatis . . . anno salutis 1549* (Padua, 1550) (Durling, *Catalogue*, no. 3277), or idem, *De differentiis medicamentorum et causis diversarum virium ac facultatum in medicamentis tractatus pulcherrimus exceptus ex ore enarrantis quartam partem primi libri Avicennae* (Wittenberg, 1551) (Durling, *Catalogue*, no. 3278). Both are brief works based on lecture notes taken down by Da Monte's auditors. On Fernel and Cardano, see further chap. 7; Fernel's *De naturali parte medicinae*, later incorporated into his *Medicina*, or *Universa medicina*, reached Padua ca. 1546 ("ante viginti octo annos"), according to an epistle by Johannes Crato von Krafftheim, dated 1574, prefaced to Jean Fernel, *Universa medicina* (Lyon, 1581) and other editions of that work; see also Siraisi, *Avicenna*, pp. 102–3. On Cardano and Fernel, see further chapter 7.

44. *De oxymelitis usu in pleuritide, Opera* 7:273. Advice that the physician should study mathematics is given in Letter 22 of Hippocrates, *Pseudepigraphic Writings*, ed. Wesley D. Smith (Leiden, 1990), p. 101.

45. "Multum igitur debere nos sentimus Fuchsio, qui etiam praeter eruditionem leporem addidit et brevitatem, ut viventium scripta cum voluptate legi coeperint" (*De oxymelitis usu in pleuritide, Opera* 7:273).

46. "Habet linguam latinam satis politam, graecas literas callet, brevis est et minime nugax, et clarus ac ordinatus, Galeni libros saepius revolvit, multam habet simplicium medicamentorum cognitionem, multa scripsit, docet libenter quae novit, laboriosus homo certe et eruditus" (ibid.).

47. Eamon, *Science and the Secrets of Nature*, pp. 168–93.

48. That is, if we are to assume that the recommendations in chap. 65 of *De malo usu* represent Cardano's practice: "Sexagesimusquintus error est, quia in empicis et phthisicis perdiderunt curam veram: et est, quod si sanies sit alba, iuvat incidere ac exurere secundum pectus in loco in quo velocius petia exiccatur. Et licet Albucasis capite 31, partis primae, videatur hoc quasi ignorasse: attamen invenimus nos Hippocratem super hoc convenienter ausum, et ratio testificatur super hoc, quandoquidem nulla alia salutis spes invenitur, et quod sit in exterioribus licet periculosius, necessario tamen magis fit in interioribus: et hoc est primum in quo plurimi moriuntur, qui sanari integre possent" (MM, sectio 1 [= *De malo usu*], 65, *Opera* 7:226). There follow recipes for potions and plasters headed "Ad Phthisim, remedia Authoris optima" and instructions for listening to the patient's chest to determine where purulent matter had collected: "Cum quis purulenta spuit, tunc aegrum in sede ponito ieiunum, ac alius eum humeris concutiat, movendo fortiter et velociter, ac aurem admove pectori, qua part sonitus exauditur, ea pus collectum est."

49. Mario Biagioli, "The Social Status of Italian Mathematicians, 1450–1600," *History of Science* 27 (1989): 41–95, at p. 55.

50. " 'Ego ex tot, tantisque immensi laboris scriptis, quorum in libello de libris propriis catalogum recenses, solum vidi libros de Sapientia, et de subtilitate, et de consolatione, qui una cum libris de sapienta annexi sunt. . . . Me vero plurimum delectavit quod librum de Sapientia quintum evolvens, viderim quod

tibi iure vendicas experimentum, ubi inter caetera sic scribis. . . . "Cum in hac urbe invidia diu laboremus . . . [etc.]" ' " (letter of Guilielmus Casanatus, physician to Archbishop Hamilton, included in LP 1557, *Opera* 1:89).

51. ". . . ut phthisicus haberetur: siquidem et tabidus et cum maxima ima tussi, et febre lenta obierat" (Cardano, *De causis, signis, ac locis morborum, Opera* 7:94).

52. Carmichael, "The Health Status of Florentines in the Fifteenth Century," pp. 38–42. According to Carmichael, "The pattern of mortality from chronic respiratory disease in Milan around 1500 is, I argue, indistinguishable from that three hundred years later when tuberculosis 'threaten[ed] the very survival of the European race' " (ibid., p. 41). "Sempre [in 1616] diffusi soni i sintomi che fanno risalire la morte ad affezioni delle vie respiratorie" (Zanetti, "La morte a Milano nei secoli XVI–XVIII," p. 833; see also p. 831). The Milanese death registers began to be kept in 1452; members of the College of Physicians were obliged to certify the cause of death for all individuals over the age of two.

53. Cardano, "Historia morbi validissimi," appended to his *Consilia, Opera* 9:245–46.

54. LP 1557, *Opera* 1:83–84; CA, *curationes* 5 and 10, *Opera* 7:254, 255.

55. "medici dicebant eum non vera phthoe laborasse, tantum potest invidia ut mentiri non pudeat, . . . ; namque cum plures sanassem eiusmodi, adeo ut ausus sim scribere me pthisicos et difficultate spirandi sanasse, in phthisicis et medici ipsi et ego mendaces fuimus: sed ego bona fide haec scripseram deceptusque fui spe mea. . . . Post quinque annos hic quem sanatum sperabam. . . . reiecto pulmone more aliorum phthisicorum mortuus est. Cum vero interrogarem post obitum uxorem, reperi tussim nunquam ex toto sublatum; ex quo apparet siccatum ulcus distulisse interitum, non quod verus phthisicus non esset" (LP 1557, *Opera* 1:82–83 [for the date of composition, see n. 5, above]).

56. Gabriel Naudé, *Vita Cardani*, in Cardano, *Opera* 1:i2r.

57. CA, *curationes* 4, 5, 8–10, *Opera* 7:254 (first published in 1562; see n. 2, above). He also continued to believe that he had completely cured one patient with *phthoe exquisita*; see ibid., *curatio* 5, p. 254.

58. The contest was held in 1548, Cardano being represented by his pupil Lodovico Ferrari. The affair and the disputes leading up to it are known chiefly from Tartaglia's accounts. A detailed narrative of the entire quarrel between Cardano and Tartaglia (largely justifying Cardano) is contained in Oystein Ore, *Cardano, the Gambling Scholar* (Princeton, 1953), pp. 61–107. On the relative social status of Cardano and Tartaglia, see Biagioli, "Social Status of Italian Mathematicians," p. 50.

59. Eamon, *Science and the Secrets of Nature*, p. 179. VP 40, *Opera* 1:33.

60. Cardano cast a posthumous horoscope for Sfondrati; it included a brief biography, which characterized his life, with justice, as remarkable and unusual (Cardano, *Liber duodecim geniturarum, genitura* 7, *Opera* 5:515–16. See also *Enciclopedia italiana di scienze, lettere ed arti*, 31 (Rome, 1949), p. 571.

61. For an evaluation of the relative availability of patronage in the different states of the Italian peninsula in the sixteenth and seventeenth centuries, see Findlen, *Possessing Nature*, pp. 349–51.

62. On the Gadi, LP 1557, *Opera* 1:82; CA, *curatio* 1, *Opera* 7:253; VP 40,

Opera 1:32 and n. 67, below. On the Borromeo, treatment of the young son of Count Camillo Borromeo: LP 1557, *Opera* 1:65; SS 4, *Opera* 5:723–24; VP 33, *Opera* 1:25 (for discussion, see chap. 9, below); attendance on Margherita de' Medici, wife of Giberto Borromeo (Margherita and Giberto were the parents of San Carlo Borromeo): VP 17, *Opera* 1:13. For the family relationships, see the family tree on the verso of the frontispiece in Ede Ginex Palmiere, *San Carlo Borromeo: L'uomo e la sua epoca* (Milan, 1984), and *Dizionario Biografici degli Italiani*, s.v. Borromeo, Camillo.

63. LP 1557, *Opera* 1:83; CA, *curatio* 15, *Opera* 7:256–57; VP 40, *Opera* 1:31–32, and n. 54, above.

64. See Margaret L. King, *The Death of the Child Valerio Marcello* (Chicago, 1994), and Katharine Park, "The Criminal and the Saintly Body: Autopsy and Dissection in Renaissance Italy," *Renaissance Quarterly* 47 (1994): 1–33, at pp. 8–10.

65. On court medicine in the early modern period, see Vivian Nutton, ed., *Medicine at the Courts of Europe* (London, 1990).

66. Alfonso d'Avalos, governor 1538–46 (VP 4, *Opera* 1:4); Ferrante Gonzaga and Gonzalo Fernandez (see n. 67, below).

67. Cardano, *Practica aritmeticae* (Milan, 1530; IA *132. 046), *Opera* 4:13, and n. 62, above; *De subtilitate libri XXI* (Basel, 1560; IA *132. 081), fol. a3r, *Opera* 3:353, and VP 40, *Opera* 1:33. Gonzalo Fernandez was governor 1558–60. The first edition (Lyon, 1550; IA *132. 056) was dedicated to Ferrante Gonzaga, governor 1546–55.

68. VP 32, *Opera* 1:24.

69. Ibid. 40, *Opera* 1:33; *Liber XII geniturarum*, *Opera* 5:524.

70. *Liber XII geniturarum*, *Opera* 5:507

71. "Vel si potior curandi via periculosa sit: vel inusitata, vel difficilis, vel longior, vel si desunt necessaria vel aeger princeps est, vel si unicus sit filius patri aut matri: vel si consanguinei illius viri violenti sint: aut ipse aeger iracundus . . ." (ACP, *Opera* 7:197).

72. Another example, extreme though in this instance benign, of the emotional investment a noble father could have in the health of a son is provided in King, *Death of the Child Valerio Marcello*.

73. LP 1557, *Opera* 1:85, 86, 60. Sicco was also the dedicatee of LP 1562.

74. VP 4, *Opera* 1:4; VP 15, *Opera* 1:12.

75. N. 62, above. Carlo Borromeo spent much of the reign of his maternal uncle, Pope Pius IV (1559–65), at the Curia; during this period his duties concerned the administration of the Papal States, of which Bologna formed part.

76. Cardinal Morone (1509–80) was already among Cardano's patrons in 1546 (VP 4, *Opera* 1:4). For Cardano's trip from Bologna to Modena to attend Morone (which must therefore have taken place between 1564, the beginning of Morone's second period as bishop of Modena, and 1570, when Cardano left Bologna), see n. 69, above. Cardano, *Consilia medica ad varios partium morbos spectantia*, no. 53, "Victus regimen pro illustrissimo Cardinali Morono," *Opera* 9:230–31 (see further chap. 4); VP 17, *Opera* 1:13–14; VP 15, *Opera* 1:12; Gliozzi, "Cardano, Gerolamo," pp. 760–61. On Morone, see Massimo Firpo, *Inquisizione romana e Controriforma: Studi sul cardinal Giovanni Morone e il suo*

processo d'eresia (Bologna, 1992), and Susanna Peyronal Rambaldi, *Speranza e crisi nel Cinquecento modenese: Tensioni religiose e vita cittadina ai tempi di Giovanni Morone* (Milan, 1979). Peyronal Rambaldi notes that Giovanni Morone's father was in the service of Francisco II Sforza (ibid., pp. 69-70). The records of Morone's trial are edited in Massimo Firpo, ed., *Il processo inquisitoriale del cardinale Giovanni Morone*, 6 vols. in 7 (Rome, 1981-95). Whatever the unorthodoxy of his views, Cardano was not in any way involved in Morone's trial, if one may judge by the absence of his name from the indexes of the first six volumes of this set (I have been unable to secure access to the last volume).

77. ". . . sendo gli animi nostri e di tutta questa città molto alieni da esso Cardano, nelle cui mani non ci seria persona nè nobile nè popolare che confidasse mettere la salute et vita sua" (letter of the Quaranta [civic officials], November 29, 1561, edited in Alessandro Simili, "Gerolamo Cardano lettore e medico a Bologna. Nota I: La condotta di G. Cardano," *Atti e Memorie dell'Accademia di Storia dell'Arte Sanitaria* 39 [1940]: 39); for the condotta of of 1563, see Emilio Costa, "Gerolamo Cardano allo Studio di Bologna," *Archivio storico italiano*, 5th ser., 35 (1905): 425-36, at p. 431; "censentes operam Excellentissimi philosophi et Medici D. Hieronimi Cardani Mediolanensis, qui aliquot iam annos in hac civitate et Academia Bononiense egregi colitur et celebratur, eidi (sic) civitati et scholastico ordine peraeque honorificam et frugiferam fore . . ." (Cardano's condotta of 1570, edited in Alessandro Simili, "Gerolamo Cardano lettore e medico a Bologna. Nota III: Le accuse e la partenza," *Atti e Memorie dell'Accademia di Storia dell'Arte Sanitaria*, 2d ser., 32 [1966]: 2); "per leggere . . . non riesce ne satisfà al studio, ne anco alla Città nel medicare, et che ciò sia vero, si conosce che non viene scolare alcuno al studio particolarmente tirato dalla fama et nome di Lui, et nelle infirmità anco qui nella Città poco è chiamato, onde si può dire ch'egli sia inutile, et per consequenza, che sia gettata una spesa tanto grossa" (letter of the Conservatori dello Studio, January 20, 1571, ibid., p. 3). See also n. 10, above.

78. Eckman, *Jerome Cardan*, pp. 67-73, collects a number of examples of the latter approach. See also G. Bellagarda, "Quattro studi su G. Cardano. II. Il 'De dentibus' di G. Cardano," *Minerva stomatologica* 14 (1965): 563-67; idem, "G. Cardano e la scoperta dell'infezione focale," *Minerva stomatologica* 15 (1966): 563-66; idem, "Quattro studi su G. Cardano. IV. G. Cardano e l'odontoiatria," *Minerva stomatologica* 15 (1966): 695-99.

CHAPTER 3

ARGUMENT AND EXPERIENCE

1. "Scripsi enim mihi Collectanea quaedam e diversis auctoribus satis magna, quorum usus nullus mihi prope est" (LP 1562, *Opera* 1:97); "Scripsi et Epidemia, orsus ab anno MDXXVI usque ad annum MDXXXIII, quorum initium est, Anno MDXXVI die xxiv Septembris, quae mihi natalis fuit, contuli me in Saccense oppidum . . . " (LP 1557, *Opera* 1:62).

2. On the publication history of the *Contradictiones*, see further below. The only other medical works by Cardano published in the 1540s and 1550s were two small volumes on practice, namely, the second edition of *De malo usu*

(1545) and *Quaedam opuscula* (1559). See n. 4 to chap. 2. On the role of the Senate of Milan, put in charge of the university and given the power of nominating professors by the edict of Charles V known as the *Constitutiones domini mediolanensis* of 1541 (1.3), see chap. 1, n. 23.

3. The *Contradictiones* (of which more may have been lost) occupy *Opera* 6:295–923; cf. *De rerum varietate, Opera* 3:1–351; *De subtilitate*, ibid. 352–672. These are double-columned folio volumes.

4. Ingegno, pp. 209–376, contains a penetrating analysis of aspects of the *Contradictiones* in relation to Cardano's philosophy of nature in a series of long notes in the chapter on natural philosophy.

5. On epistemological problems and discussions in thirteenth- to fifteenth-century medicine, see Jole Agrimi and Chiara Crisciani, *Edocere medicos* (Naples, 1988), passim; eaedem, "Medicina e logica in maestri bolognesi tra Due e Trecento: Problemi e temi di ricerca," in *L'insegnamento della logica a Bologna nel XIV secolo*, ed. Dino Buzzetti et al. (Bologna, 1992), pp. 187–239; Michael R. McVaugh, "The Nature and Limits of Medical Certitude at Early Fourteenth-Century Montpellier," *Osiris* 6 (1990): 62–84; Per-Gunnar Ottosson, *Scholastic Medicine and Philosophy* (Naples, 1984), pp. 65–126.

6. See Jole Agrimi and Chiara Crisciani, *Les consilia médicaux*, Typologie des sources du Moyen Age Occidental, fasc. 69 (Turnhout, 1994); Danielle Jacquart, "Theory, Everyday Practice, and Three Fifteenth-Century Physicians," *Osiris* 6 (1990): 161–80; Tiziana Pesenti, "Michele Savonarola a Padova: L'ambiente, le opere, la cultura medica, " *Quaderni per la storia dell'Università di Padova 9/10* (1977): 45–101. See further chap. 9, below.

7. LP 1562, *Opera* 1:97, makes it clear that the collection of epidemics made at Sacco was modeled on the Hippocratic *Epidemics*. See further chap. 6, below.

8. LP 1544, *Opera* 1:56; LP 1557, *Opera* 1:61; LP 1562, *Opera* 1:97.

9. According to LP 1557, *Opera* 1:61, Cardano had already begun collecting medical *contradictiones* while still a student at Pavia (that is, before 1523). "Moris autem fuit nobis, ut quoscunque qui in arte aliqua scripsissent, prius legerem, quam in eadem quicquam componerem. Per idem ferme tempus et ad annum usque XXXI duos libros magnos composui: alterum Aetii magnitudine, de medicinae regulis in quatuor distributum. . . . Reliquum in quo medicinae sententias contrarias, quotquot invenire potui, una collegi Graecorum, Arabum, Latinorum; hae autem ferme quadringentae magnitudo libri ut Conciliatoris" (LP 1544, *Opera* 1:56). He transferred to Padua in 1524. For the state of the work in 1543, see LP 1544, *Opera* 1:59.

10. *Contradicentium medicorum liber continens contradictiones centum octo* (Venice, 1545; IA *132. 052); *Contradicentium medicorum liber primus [-secundus] continens contradictiones centum et octo* (Lyon, 1548; IA *132. 055). "Nuper hoc Martio mense, anni ut dixi MDXLVI . . ." (*Contradictiones* 2.5.9, *Opera* 6:564). There were three subsequent editions of bks. 1 and 2: Paris, 1564–65 (IA *132. 096); Paris, 1565 (IA *132. 097); and Marburg, 1607 (British Library 1169 c. 6). I have not seen the last of these editions.

11. Two books appear to be lost (and may never have existed in more than fragmentary form). In bks. 3–10 there are references to Cardano's *De subtilitate*, first published in 1550 (*Contradictiones* 4.5, *Opera* 6:688), *Theonoston*, begun

under another title in 1555 (LP 1562, *Opera* 1:112; *Contradictiones* 3.6, p. 658), and the critique of Vesalius in Falloppia's *Observationes anatomicae*, first published in 1561 (*Contradictiones* 4.17, p. 696). But bks. 3–10 were presumably complete in something like their present form by 1563, since *Contradictiones* 10.26 is referred to in Cardano's commentary on part of bk. 1 of the *Canon* of Avicenna, which bears a preface dated in that year; see *Opera* 9:458, 490. The single *contradictio* printed in the collection *De balneis omnia quae extant apud Graecos, Latinos, et Arabas, tam medicos quam quoscunque caeterarum artium probatos scriptores* ... (Venice 1553), fol. 226v, and headed "Ex Hieronymi Gardani [*sic*] Contradictionibus, Contradictione III. Articulari morbo, an balneum competat" is actually *Contradictiones* 1.4.3 (*Opera* 6:366).

12. "Verum qui ante nos fuere, quam leviter atque oscitanter haec tractaverint, praeter unum Conciliatorem, ac in dissectione Vesalium, in paucisque admodum aliis Fuchsium, cum Ferrariensibus, non est cur recitem ..." (*Contradictiones*, dedicatory letter to the Senate of Milan, *Opera* 6:297).

13. I used Pietro d'Abano, *Conciliator: Ristampa fotomeccanica dell'edizione Venetiis apud Iuntas 1565*, ed. Ezio Riondato and Luigi Olivieri (Padua, 1985). For the horoscope of religions, see *differentia* 9, fol. 15r. A recent general study of Pietro d'Abano is Eugenia Paschetto, *Pietro d'Abano, medico e filosofo* ([Florence, 1984]). On astrology and the rise of religions, se J. D. North, "Astrology and the Fortunes of Churches," *Centaurus* 24 (1980): 181–211.

14. See n. 9, above.

15. In his comm. *Tetrabiblos*, *Opera* 5:221–22. As Gabriel Naudé pointed out in his life of Cardano prefaced to the collected edition of the latter's works, Cardano was not the first to do this (Naudé, *Vita Cardani*, *Opera* 1:i[4]r–v.

16. Siraisi, *Avicenna* (esp. pp. 64–65 as regards early-sixteenth-century printed editions of scholastic commentaries).

17. In 1548, 1554, and 1565. *Conciliator*, ed. Riondato and Olivieri, includes a "nota bibliografica" by L. Olivieri (pp. ix–xi) giving further details about Renaissance editions of the work.

18. "Arabum sententiam, rationes, experimentaque non sprevi. An decuit eruditissimos viros, optimosque Philosophos, ob solam vel linguae asperitatem, vel rudes interpretes aspernari? Quosdam Graece obgannientes, nec Philosophiae, nec medicinae gnaros, solum nomen Galeni, tamque illud Hebraeorum ineffabile Dei quod septuaginta duobus elementis constare affirmant, iactantes amplecti, tum maxime quod rationes negligere se praeferunt, vere autem fugiunt. Fateor Iacobum, & Ugonem, turbamque illam quam Gentilis excitat chimericis idolis plenam, parum ad medicinam conferre. Sed in uno Conciliatore, Avicenna, Raseque, quid habes praeter linguam, quae regionis aut aetatis fuit calamitas, quod impar tuis sit egregiis inventis. Quid cum subtilitate Averrois, cum iudicio Avicennae, cum gravitate Rasis, cum doctrina Conciliatoris conferri potest?" (*Contradictiones* [Lyon, 1548], epistle *ad lectorem* at end of bk. 2, pp. 464–65).

19. Ingegno, pp. 257–67; also Alfonso Ingegno, "Il perfetto e il furioso," *Il piccolo Hans: Rivista di analisi materialistica* 75/76 (Autumn–Winter 1992–93): 11–31.

20. Galen, *De temperamentis* 1.5, 1.6, 1.9, Kühn 1:534–51; 559–71; *De op-*

tima corporis constitutione, Kühn 4:737–49; Aristotle, *De partibus animalium* 2.2, 653a26–36.

21. *Conciliator, differentia* 18, fols. 27v–29v. Galen mentioned the canon of Polykleitos in *De temperamentis* 1.9, Kühn 1:566; also *De placitis Hippocratis et Platonis* 5.3, ed. and trans. Phillip De Lacy (Berlin, 1981), 1:309, and *De usu partium* 17.1, trans. Margaret T. May (*Galen on the Usefulness of the Parts of the Body*) (Ithaca, 1968), 2:726–7. Only the first of these passages is likely to have been known to Pietro d'Abano. For Vesalius, see Vesalius, *Fabrica* (1543) 5.19, p. 548, and Jackie Pigeaud, "Formes et normes dans le *De fabrica* de Vésale," in *Le corps à la Renaissance. Actes du XXXe Colloque de Tours 1987*, ed. Jean Céard, Marie Madeleine Fontaine, and Jean-Claude Margolin (Paris, 1990), pp. 399–421, at 413–18, and idem, "Les problèmes de la création chez Galien," in *Galen und das hellenistische Erbe*, ed. Jutta Kollesch and Diethard Nickel, *Sudhoffs Archiv*, Beiheft 32 (Stuttgart, 1993), pp. 87–103.

22. *Contradictiones* 1.6.9, *Opera* 6:411–13; 2.6.14, pp. 633–37.

23. "Addit vero ibi de Christo multa, non solum impia, sed absurda: et dum Philosophum agit more quorundam, qui optimum argumentum existimant Philosophi impietatem, et in leges [1548; *Opera*: legis] iacta probra: et medici maledicere de Arabibus, cum hi Galenum solo nomine salutaverint, illi vero in lege quidem superstitiosi, in philosophia autem inanes sint et fatui, nam Philosophus non haec acta diceret ut postmodum in causas reduceret naturales, quemadmodum Conciliator, et Pomponatius facere nituntur, fabulosis absurdissimisque imaginationibus" (ibid. 1.6.9, *Opera* 6:412).

24. "ingenio superet Archimedem, eloquentia naturali Ciceronem, multaque alia innumera efficiat, quae singula pro miraculo haberi soleant: his omnibus in unum collectis, palam est eum qui tali temperie [1548; *Opera*: temberie] praeditus sit admirationem maximam populis praebiturum, proque divino homine habendum, ac quasi Deum inter mortales cohabitaturum" (ibid. 2.6.14, *Opera* 6:636).

25. Ingegno, pp. 263–66; idem, "Il perfetto e il furioso." On Cardano's views on longevity and his own health, see further chaps. 4 and 10, below.

26. *Conciliator, differentia* 3, fol. 7r; see also Nancy G. Siraisi, "Medicine, Physiology, and Anatomy in Early Sixteenth-Century Critiques of the Arts and Sciences," in *New Perspectives on Renaissance Thought*, ed. John Henry and Sarah Hutton (London, 1990), pp. 214–29, at pp. 219–20, and sources cited in n. 5, above.

27. *Contradictiones* 1.3.1, *Opera* 6:336–37; 1.5.4, pp. 380–81; 1.6.10, pp. 414–15.

28. See Adriano Carugo, "Giuseppe Moleto: Mathematics and the Aristotelian Theory of Science at Padua in the Second Half of the Sixteenth Century," in *Aristotelismo veneto e scienza moderna* (Padua, 1983), pp. 509–16.

29. "Omnes enim artifices, qui cum hoc etiam sunt scientes, ut musici, et geometrae, etiam percipiunt rem prout est, et indivisibile, quia tale indivisibile puta diapason, potest esse firmum et non fluens: quia non est in materia generabili, et corruptibili ut sic. Ille etiam astrologus qui considerat luminarium coniunctionem, quae est momentanea, quamvis non maneat, considerat tamen, quia nihil vult operari circa illam. Cum igitur medicus sit sciens, et non purus artifex,

et habeat operari circa subiectum suum, et subiectum non constet unquam sub uno affectu propter materiam: cogitur medicus solus inter omnes scientes diiudicare ex sensu, non ex rei veritate" (*Contradictiones* 1.6.10, *Opera* 6:415). Cf. *Contradictiones* 1.3.10, *Opera* 6:360, and "Verum cum ad nostri intellectus imbecillitatem respicimus non illarum [scientiarum] natura, sed nostra vitio fit ut res pene contrario modo se habeat: Nam relicta mathematica, certissima omnium est medicina, inde philosophia naturalis, post astrologia, ultima omnium est theologia" (comm. *Tetrabiblos* 2.9.51, *Opera* 5:206).

30. *Contradictiones* 1.3.1, pp. 336–37.

31. On the development of scholastic *quaestiones* in medicine and their connections both with procedures developed in scholastic theology and with natural questions and problem literature, see Danielle Jacquart, "La question disputée dans les facultés de médecine," in Bernardo C. Bàzan, John F. Wippel, Gérard Fransen, and Danielle Jacquart, *Les questions disputées et les questions quodlibétiques dans les facultés de théologie, de droit et de médecine*, Typologie des sources du Moyen Age occidental, fasc. 44–45 (Turnhout, 1983), pp. 281–313; Brian Lawn, *The Salernitan Questions: An Introduction to the History of Medieval and Renaissance Problem Literature* (Oxford, 1963); and idem, *The Rise and Decline of the Scholastic "Quaestio Disputata" with Special Emphasis on Its Use in the Teaching of Medicine and Science* (Leiden, 1993).

32. *Contradictiones* 2.1.4., *Opera* 6:442–46.

33. "Conscripsi igitur revocatus ab eo exercitationis impetu, duos libros Floridorum, id est medicarum disputationum. . . . Proprius usus libri maximaque utilitas est difficillimas medicinae quaestiones simplici oratione edocere. Ordinem quoque et facilitatem secuti sumus, ut si ad subiectam materiam respicias, adeo necessaria sit, ut sine horum cognitione medicus esse non possit: sin ad facilitatem, quemlibet possit invitare ad legendum: si ad ordinem, et facile invenire possis, et inventa memoriae commendare" (LP 1557, *Opera* 1:65–66). In the seventeenth-century *Opera* the title *Floridorum libri* was given (possibly by the editor) to Cardano's commentary on part of the *Canon* of Avicenna, which is evidently not the work referred to here.

34. "Fuerunt hi libri necessarii, nedum utiles, ut multorum simul autorum memoria coleretur: et ne dubitaremus quinam libri fide digni essent, vel qui apocryphi, vel et minus celebris scriptoris: et ut sciremus quibus in casibus haec aut illa convenirent" (LP 1562, *Opera* 1:106). But here, although the title, date of publication, and names of the publishers of the first two editions match the *Contradictiones*, Cardano gave a different incipit and said the work was in eight books. Presumably memory failed him at this point.

35. Fourteenth- and fifteenth-century scholastic medical writers are cited fairly often in the *Contradictiones*, by no means always in disagreement; e.g., *Contradictiones* 1.3.17, *Opera* 6:397 (Giacomo da Forlì, Ugo Benzi, Turisanus); 1.6.10, p. 414 (Gentile da Foligno, Dino del Garbo [d. 1327], Taddeo Alderotti [d. 1295]).

36. See chap. 6, below.

37. LP 1544, *Opera* 1:59.

38. "Proprium autem gravis viri est, statim ad rem properare. Et ad hoc, opus est multa lectione, toto triduo ingens volumen devorantes: indicio [*sic*; iudicio]

opus est, pertrita vel parum utilia praetereundo, obscurorum expectare occasionem, obelisco signando" (VP 39, *Opera* 1:31).

39. Frances Yates, *The Art of Memory* (Chicago, 1966); Anthony Grafton, "L'umanista come lettore," in *Storia della lettura nel mondo occidentale*, ed. Guglielmo Cavallo and Roger Chartier (Rome and Bari, 1995), pp. 199–242; Ann Blair, "Humanist Methods in Natural Philosophy: The Commonplace Book," *Journal of the History of Ideas* 53 (1992): 541–51.

40. Richard J. Durling, "An Early Manual for the Medical Student and the Newly-Fledged Practitioner: Martin Stainpeis' *Liber de modo studendi seu legendi in medicina* ([Vienna] 1520)," *Clio Medica* 3 (1970): 5–33, at p. 22.

41. "unus praecipue Gymnasiarcha noster Integerrimus non modo me rogavit, ut statuta mihi iuxta consuetudinem disputandi die, contra tua de elementis paradoxa argumentarer . . ." (*Andreae Camutii disputationes, quibus Hieronymi Cardani magni nominis viri Conclusiones infirmantur, Galenus ab eiusdem iniuria vindicatur, Hippocratis praeterea aliquot loca diligentius multo, quam unquam alias, explicantur . . .* [Pavia, 1563], fol. 72r).

42. According to Guglielmo da Saliceto (d. 1276/80), "inhonestum est et indecens est coram infirmo et laicis de causis infirmitatis et operationibus disputando determinare . . . melius et decentius videtur ut omnis inquisitio cum altero et socio fiat in secreto . . . quia laici semper detrahunt sapientibus" (Guglielmo da Saliceto, *Summa conservationis et curationis* [Venice, 1489], proem, sig. a2r).

43. Daza Chacon, *Practica y teorica de Cirugia*, 2:200; the translation is O'Malley's (*Andreas Vesalius*, p. 418). It was possible to overdo it; on one of these occasions Philip II asked Daza Chacon not to quote quite so many texts (ibid.).

44. VP 40, *Opera* 1:31–32 (Cardano also recounted this story in other contexts—see further chap. 9).

45. "Aponensis, qui ante nos medicas controversias dirimere agressus" (*Controversiarum medicarum et philosophicarum Francisci Vallesii* [Frankfurt, 1590], p. 240). The preface takes a strongly pro-Galenic stand. On Valles (1524–92) and the *Controversiae*, see José Maria López Piñero, *Los temas polémicos de la medicina renacentista: Las Controversias (1556), de Francisco Valles* (Madrid, 1988). See also Giancarlo Zanier, *Medicina e filosofia tra '500 e '600* (Milan, 1983), pp. 20–38.

46. "qui ante nos quaestiones medicas, barbare illi quidem omnes scripserunt. Quoniam vero in quovis opere nihil contingere potest legentibus, aut iocundius, aut utilius ordine: delectationi et memoriae eorum, qui in hunc librum inciderint, consulentes, in decem libros totum opus censuimus distribuendum . . ." (Valles, *Controversiae*, p. 2); similarly, and with more detail about scholastic "barbarism," ibid., p. 55.

47. López Piñero, *Los temas polémicos*, pp. 10–16, 63–65.

48. *Contradictiones*, preface *ad lectorem*, *Opera* 6:299.

49. For subjects taught and professors between the 1530s and the 1560s, see *Memorie e documenti per la storia dell'Università di Pavia e degli uomini più illustri che v'insegnavano* (Pavia, 1875), pp. 122–28; regarding the proposal to build an anatomy theater, Giacomo Parodi, *Elenchus privilegiorum, et actuum*

publice Ticinensis Studii a seculo nono ad nostra tempora (Pavia, 1753), p. 66. Anna Giulia Cavagna, *Libri e tipografi a Pavia nel Cinquecento: Note per la storia dell'Università e della cultura* (Milan, 1981), throws much light on the sixteenth-century university by tracing the ups and downs of publishing in Pavia during that period.

50. The most famous example of which is Hermann Boerhaave, *Institutiones medicae* (Leiden, 1707). On the development of this genre and its relation to the earlier methods of teaching of medical theory and the emergence of early textbooks of physiology, see Lester S. King, *The Road to Medical Enlightenment, 1650–1695* (London, 1970), pp. 16, 181–83, and Siraisi, *Avicenna*, pp. 101–3.

51. *Contradictiones* 1.5.6–7, *Opera* 6:381–87.

52. Ibid. 2.2.7, *Opera* 6:467–86 (see further chap. 7). Pietro d'Abano also discussed this question, but a good deal more concisely.

53. "De signis calidi [1548; *Opera*: calidis] cerebri" (*Contradictiones* 2.1.13, *Opera* 6:457); "An signa posita a Galeno de cerebro, in secundo Artis medicae, sint intelligenda, humoribus aequalibus existentibus" (ibid. 2.1.14, p. 457); "An cerebrum expurget superflua per nares, oculos, et aures" (ibid. 2.1.15, pp. 457–58).

54. See Massimo Luigi Bianchi, "Scholastische Motive im ersten und zweiten Buch des *De subtilitate* Girolamo Cardanos," Kessler, pp. 115–30.

55. Cardano complained bitterly about Scotus, comparing him very unfavorably to publishers outside Italy (LP 1562, *Opera* 1:103–4). Bks. 3–10 published in the posthumous *Opera* betray no traces of the arrangement claimed in the preface *ad lectorem*, other than the occasional occurrence of some topical clusters. But there is, of course, no way of knowing whether these books represent Cardano's intended arrangement.

56. See, for example, Anthony Grafton, "On the Scholarship of Politian and Its Context," *Journal of the Warburg and Courtauld Institutes* 40 (1977): 157–58; also Donald Frame, *Montaigne's Essais: A Study* (Englewood Cliffs, N.J., 1969), pp. 72–85, on Montaigne's self-conscious use of random and miscellaneous topics.

57. "Contradictiones quoque ad scholia et castigationes quasi pertinent" (LP 1562, *Opera* 1:145).

58. "Et quamquam longe facilius, quorundam more, antiquorum opinionibus acquiescendo, hunc, tum caeteros libros absoluissem: quia tamen seriam nimis rem agimus, et in qua vita hominum periclitatur, non philosophorum nugae aut praecepta oratoria, diligentius in singulis, cum res id postulat, rationem evidentem requirimus" (*Contradictiones*, dedicatory letter to the Senate of Milan, *Opera* 6:297).

59. "quae dubia visa sunt, rationibus subijcere tentavimus. . . . in cunctis ratione duce praeter etiam autoritatem usus sum: ut si ea cum illorum sententia consentiret, firmius esset iudicium: si repugnaret, nostra opinione recitata, integram lectoribus eligendi quae magis placeret facultatem relinquerem" (ibid., p. 298).

60. "unica igitur in Galeni iudicio spes relinquebatur; sed huius etiam maxima operum pars, antiquitate intercidit: et quae supersunt saepe evariant: et ipse, ut existimo, cum medendo plurimum occuparetur, ac multa scribere vellet, non

satis sibi constat. . . . Sed vel sic tamen, poterat nobis omnis litis esse voluntarius iudex, si non in dissectionibus liquido apparuisset, constanter illum tanquam visa, contradicendi studio affirmare, quae nec vidisset omnino, nec vera essent: ut iam nos non Vesalio credentes, sed oculis nostris, non de iudicio, quod saepe contigerat, sed de fide dubitaremus" (ibid., p. 297).

61. ". . . laudavi Andream Vesaliam ob virtutem: nam hominem nondum e facie novi: & mihi hoc certe commune est cum illo, ut pro veritate ipsa quandoque Galeno adversatus sim" (*Contradictiones* [Lyon, 1548], epistle *ad lectorem* at the end of bk. 2, p. 463).

62. "Sed, en [*sic*] impium est Galeno adversari? Heu stulte, ac miser, an non ille homo fuit? an non solum omnibus suis praedecessoribus, uno excepto Hippocrate, contradixit? sed etiam eos, per quos profecerat, magistros ignorantiae arguit? En, audi quid dicat, dum medicamenta ad singulos morbos conscribit. At vero Archigenes, ut si quis alius, quae ad medicam speculationem attinent, diligenter ediscere studuit, atque ob id quam plurima scripta memoratu digna reliquit. Non tamen in omnibus sane quae tradidit irreprehensibilis mihi videtur: verum velut & ipse pleraque eorum virorum, a quibus adiutus evasit optimus, reprehendit: sic par est ipsum delinquentem a nobis posteris redargui. Difficile enim est, ut qui homo sit, non in multis peccet: Quaedam videlicet penitus ignorando, quaedam male iudicando, quaedam tandem negligentius scriptis tradendo. Sic nos rationem ac experimentum praeponentes, in reliquis Galeno, ut par est, plusquam caeteris aliis omnibus tribuimus. At qui omnia illa tribuunt, non tam illius esse studiosi videntur, quam reliqua omnia ignorare. Quod si modicae pecuniae causa siliquam Indam, manna, saccharum, rhabarbarumque Galeni medicamentis, et Hippocratis relictis amplectuntur: quaenam, rogo impietas est, ubi error Galeni multorum hominum morte pensatur, ubive experimento ipsi contradicit, illum vel infensis astris tueri velle? Ergo illa ex toto, et reliqua Galeno ignota relinque medicamenta, tuncque prorsus te credam esse Galenicum. Verum, dicis non adeo foeliciter mihi res in medendo succedunt, relinquentque me homines. Itaque non te Galeni amor detinet, sed praeceps inverecundia. Quid enim prohibet si in manifestis multa Galenus ignoravit, in occultioribus longe plure nescivisset? At dices, singulares rerum species ignorare potuit, medica ars praeceptis generalibus constat: quae ille non solum scivit sed etiam tradidit. Sed si tradidit, non pervenerunt: qua autem non pervenerant, sunt ac si non tradita nobis fuissent. Cum enim multa, imo plusquam dimidium scriptorum suorum perierint, si non illa repetit ac frustra scripsit, necesse est nos omnibus his indigere. Deinde si per generalem rationem regulam illam intelligis, quae docet, contraria contrariis curari: ego sane fateor omnia tradidisse Galenum: sed et ante eum Hippocratem, nulloque huius causa libro indigemus. Sed si singulorum morborum signa, modos, causas, symptomata, auxilia: tum corporis partium numerum, situm, utilitatem, qualitatemque intelligimus, necesse est etiam in scriptis Galeni multa, velut inter illius medicamenta, ac maxime necessaria deesse. Quamobrem nec his duobus libris tantum, sed decem aliis ista sum prosecutus" (ibid., pp. 463–64).

63. For example, "His ergo intellectis, ad conciliandum haec dicta veniamus . . ." (*Contradictiones* 1.3.8, *Opera* 6:349); "Ad id, quod quaeritur, an [cerebrum] humidius sit quam frigidius, eadem ferme convenit responsio. Nam per se

sumptum frigidius est, cum utroque elemento frigido participet iuxta Aristotelis sententiam. Galenus vero, arbitratur humidius esse: quam quam si quis velit, illum cum Aristotele possit concordare . . ." (ibid. 2.1.5, *Opera* 6:447). On this point, see also Ingegno, p. 232.

64. On the general problem of the status ascribed to particulars in the sixteenth and seventeenth centuries, see Lorraine Daston, "Marvelous Facts and Miraculous Evidence in Early Modern Europe," *Critical Inquiry* 18 (1991): 93–124.

65. *Contradictiones* 2.2.6, *Opera* 6:467.

66. Ibid. 1.1.12, *Opera* 6:309–10; 1.1.16, p. 311; 1.3.14, p. 355; 1.3.24, p. 362.

67. ". . . librum de Vita nostra scribere aggredimur. Testati nihil adiectum iactantiae, aut ornandae rei causa. Sed quantum licuit collectis eventibus, quibus interfuerunt discipuli . . . tum a nobis conscriptae historiae partibus, librum conflasse" (VP, proem, *Opera* 1:1). On the narrative aspects of his medicine, see Part 5, below.

68. "Supersunt et duo consilia conscripta pro Archiepiscopo S. Andreae in metropoli Scotiae: multa quoque et sine numero consilia scripta pro Anglis, Scotis, Gallis, Germanis, Italis, Hispanis, Cimbris, Blandis, aliisque non ex harum numero gentium hominibus. . . . Eodem tempore [1545] coepi librum Experimentorum, colligens quae alias scripseram, quem perpetuo auxi" (LP 1562, *Opera* 1:107–8). Cardano's *consilia* survive in some numbers, if not in the profusion this remark suggests; a selection of fifty-seven is printed in *Opera* 9:47–246. At least two manuscripts of Cardano's *experimenta* survive, namely, Rome, Biblioteca Nazionale Centrale, MSS S. Francesca a Ripa 2 and 4, both of which may be partially autograph. The former (MS S. Francesca a Ripa 2, headed on p. 1 in a later hand "Experimenta Cardani," 95 fols.) is a disordered notebook with crossings out. A list of 297 numbered *experimenta* at the beginning does not completely correspond with the actual contents. For MS S. Francesca a Ripa 4, see n. 20 to chap. 2. In both, the *experimenta* are medicinal recipes.

69. See, for example, Ann Blair, *The Theater of Nature: Jean Bodin and Renaissance Science* (Princeton: Princeton University Press, forthcoming, 1997).

70. "Quo fit, ut denuo ad accusandum hos descendam, qui adeo omnium Arabum sententiam, etiam in experimentis floccifaciunt, ut nihil illis tribuere velint. Nam Fuchsius ipse in suo libro de simplicibus, de ea agit, ac si solum calida vel frigida, sed sicca tamen temperie prorsus sit. Sed vide absurditatem, cum Graecos tantum sequantur, quid attinet Plinium immiscere, quo nemo in rebus medicis, aut inconstantior, aut magis fallax vel rudis. Ergo et istud pene impium, deserere Avicennam, Rasim, Averroem, Avenzoar, totque clarissimi ingenii viros medicos ac philosophos. . . . Ergo grammatici grammaticos sequantur, nos cum medicis erimus. . . . Videmus singulis diebus qui Galenum imitantur non leves errores admittere, experimentisque Arabum inferiores esse" (*Contradictiones* 2.3.15, *Opera* 6:514).

71. Ibid. 2.5.9, *Opera* 6:561–66.

72. Ibid., pp. 562–64.

73. The demand for works on this subject is suggested by the fact that Pietro

d'Abano's *De venenis* was printed at least six times during the sixteenth century; see Durling, *Catalogue*, nos. 7–12, 242. See also Lynn Thorndike, *A History of Magic and Experimental Science*, vol. 5 (New York, 1941), 472–87.

74. *Contradictiones* 2.5.9, *Opera* 6:565.

75. "Dum viderem parari mensam Caesari, detergebant sedem, mensam, et pedum, pluteum sustentaculum, mappa: existimant enim venenum aliquod adeo esse potens, ut vel sub calceis vel ephippiis occidat: quod probe confirmatur, pestiferi experimento: ipsum enim ferro, vestibus, canibus, lapidibus, lignisque contactu haerens persaepe necat. Hanc tamen tantam subtilitatem perfidia nostrorum temporum invenit, quod antiqui ignorabant" (ibid., p. 566). The occasion was presumably Charles V's visit to Milan in 1541 (on his return journey from the Diet of Regensburg), when Cardano, as rector of the College of Physicians, held the emperor's canopy during his entry into the city; see VP 30, *Opera* 1:19, and Karl Brandi, *The Emperor Charles V* (London, 1939), pp. 453–55.

76. "Et scias, Princeps illustrissime, ex decem qui venenum bibunt vix unus, nisi repetatur, moritur" (*Contradictiones* 2.5.9, *Opera* 6:565).

77. Cardano, *De venenorum differentiis, viribus et adversus ea remediorum praesidiis ac praesertim De pestis generibus omnibus praeservatione et cura libri III*, printed with his *In septem Aphorismorum Hippocratis particulas commentaria* (Basel, 1564; IA *132. 093), otherwise *De venenis libri tres*, *Opera* 7:275–355.

78. "Sed agedum veritas illa sit: quomodo oculis patri assimiletur, naso matri, non explicat? et rursus, cur avo materno, ut ego qui Iacobo Mi[c]herio materno avo moribus, ingenio et corpore sum persimilis? . . . Sicut igitur in anima est vis imaginandi et ratio e memoria, sensus, ita in corpore sunt multae formae, non solum natura sed loco distinctae. Velut cor meum assimilatur in natura patri meo et avo paterno Antonio Cardano et ita proavo Facio alteri et atavo Aldo cum intercesserint ab illius ortu ad hanc usque diem anni CCXX fuerunt enim omnes vivacissimi, non tamen ut audivi forma similes" (*Contradictiones* 2.6.18, *Opera* 6:652–53).

79. See chap. 8, n. 54; chap. 2, n. 2, and discussion in chap. 9.

80. Some examples of Cardano's treatment of Aristotelian ideas in his natural philosophical works are discussed in Jean-Claude Margolin, "Cardan, interprète d'Aristote," in *Platon et Aristote à la Renaissance. XVIe Colloque International de Tours* (Paris, 1976), 307–33; see also Bianchi, "Scholastische Motive."

81. For some medieval examples, see Nancy G. Siraisi, *Taddeo Alderotti and His Pupils* (Princeton, 1981), pp. 186–201.

82. " . . . sicque mediam inter philosophos et medicos viam amplexus est, quae et meo iudicio etiam verior existit" (*Contradictiones* 2.1.4, *Opera* 6:445).

83. Ibid. 2.6.18, *Opera* 6:646–47; "non igitur male dixit Galenus aut Philosophus aut Hippocrates, sed solum imperfecte" (ibid., p. 652).

84. Ibid., p. 646; ; see Vesalius, *Fabrica* (1543) 5.17, pp. 541–43. *Contradictiones* 2.1.4, *Opera* 6:443; see Vesalius, *Fabrica* (1543) 3.6, pp. 275[375]–276[376]; *Contradictiones* 2.1.4, *Opera* 6:445.

85. *De subtilitate* 2, *Opera* 3:372–74. On Cardano's element theory, see Ingegno, pp. 223–32. I do not here address the question of resemblances between Cardano's element theory and some Paracelsian ideas. Cardano's ideas about the

elements were roundly denounced in the elder Scaliger's famous attack on *De subtilitate*. I have consulted Julius Caesar Scaliger, *Exotericarum exercitationes libri XV de subtilitate ad Hieronymum Cardanum* (Frankfurt, 1592), in which the attack on Cardano's views on the status of fire as an element occurs on pp. 45–53; the first edition was Paris, 1557. Regarding the wide attention attracted by the dispute between Cardano and Scaliger, see Maclean, "The Interpretation of Natural Signs," at p. 231.

86. "Hippocrates quoque in libro de carnibus connumerat terram, aquam, et aerem, aether quod dicit esse immortale, et cuncta cognoscens" (*Contradictiones* 10.26, *Opera* 6:910); "Sed certe sub coelo Lunae nullus est ignis: nam quum [Lyon, 1559: cum] coelum purissima res sit, non decuit sub omnis qualitatis experte re, ardentissimam collocasse. Natura enim semper extrema mediis iungit. Inter carnem enim et os, membranam: inter os et ligamenta, cartilagines: inter os et cerebrum, quod carne cerebrum esset mollius, duplicem membranum, ac duriorem ossi propinquiorem collocavit" (*De subtilitate*, bk. 2, *Opera* 3:372). For the Hippocratic passage, see *Hippocratis Cois medicorum omnium longe principis, opera quae ad nos extant omnia. Per Ianum Cornarium medicum physicum latina lingua conscripta* . . . (Basel, 1546), p. 55, Littré 8:584.

87. "humores in animalibus quatuor sunt: sed quid hoc ad elementa? quid si tantum tria cum Thrusiano expositore artis medicae Galeni esse dicam? Sed tamen sensus ostendit esse quatuor" (*De subtilitate*, bk. 2, *Opera* 3:373). According to Turisanus (Torrigiano de' Torrigiani, fl. early fourteenth century), "Dicemus ergo videri nobis eterogeneitatem illius commixti quod est in venis ex tribus constare manifestis substantiis tantum, scilicet terrestri aquea et spirituali: quarum una proportionatur melancolie: reliqua flegmati, 3a colere ex quibus secundum proportione commixtis resultat sanguinis temperamentum: propter quod aliquando dicimus sanguinem colericum: aliquando melancolicum: aliquando flegmaticum a dominio unius eorum in commixto: non dicimus autem sanguinem sicut a dominatio alicuius quarte substantie preter dictas: sed dicimus eum temperatum a temperantia mixtionis illarum trium secundum decentem proportionem ad opus naturae: et hoc est quod simpliciter dicitur sanguis sine hac additione colericus vel flegmaticus vel melancolicus" (*Turisani monaci plusquam commentum in microtegni Galieni. Cum questione eiusdem de Ypostasi* [Venice, 1512], fol. 54v). On Turisanus, see Siraisi, *Taddeo Alderotti*, pp. 64–66.

88. "Item calor animalium secundum Philosophum est calor non igneus, sed coelestis. . . . Manifestum est autem quod Galenus aliter censet, nam libro de Usu respirationis, vult calorem nostrum igneum, sumpta similitudine, quod non secus ac in fornace ignis prohibita transpiratione extinguatur. Est igitur hic alia inter Galenum et Aristotelem discordia. . . . Verum neque illud concedere cogimur, quod si calor animalis etiam sit igneus, ob id debeat, cum sub forma mixti est, agere in subiectam materiam" (*Contradictiones* 1.1.11, *Opera* 6:308). The decision to muffle his views on the elements in *Contradictiones* was a conscious one; in *De subtilitate* he remarked, "Admirabitur forsan aliquis, quod in contradicentium libris aliter senserim. Sed ubi opiniones antiquorum sequi propositum fuit, hic vero docere veritatem" (*De subtilitate* 2, *Opera* 3:390). The remark is quoted in Maclean, "The Interpretation of Natural Signs," p. 237. A

much fuller and clearer statement of his position on the elements is found in *Contradictiones* 10.26, *Opera* 6:911 (not printed in his lifetime).

89. Ibid. 2.1.1, *Opera* 6:439, with the entire discussion on pp. 437–40. As noted above, when it suited another argument, he was ready to postulate separate forms for different organs of the body.

90. "Formam vero temperamenti dicimus adesse, sed non disiunctam esse ab anima, in belluis: quia vel est ipsa, vel ab ipsa sustentatur. Item dico de homine apud Galenum, et Alexandrum Aphrodiseum. Nobis autem constitutentibus animum humanum immortalem, longa nimis esset disputatio, si vellemus hoc declarare: dictum est etiam partim hoc in libro De animi immortalitate" (ibid. 2.1.1, *Opera* 6:440). On Galen's materialism as regards the soul and its Christian critics, see Owsei Temkin, *Galenism* (Ithaca, 1973), pp. 82–92.

91. "Sed adest dubitatio, nam si forma mixti est forma elementi praedominantis, igitur nullum simplex medicamentum habet facultates contrarias: nam non datur forma sine operatione: cum tamen Galenus dicat, quod Balanus Myrepsica [a suppository with myrrh], seu glans unguentaria, calidam habet terreamque substantium simul, astringentemque vim . . . nisi esset quod et in his partes sunt actu invicem distinctae, quoniam viventis fuerunt herbae: et tunc potentia quidem tales, actu vero formam animae plantae consequebantur [1548: . At] postquam eradicatae, ac mortuae fuerint, unaquaeque in proprium relabitur temperamentum" (*Contradictiones* 2.1.1, *Opera* 6:440).

92. Ibid. 5.44, *Opera* 6:745.

93. Ibid. 1.2.8, *Opera* 6:320–334. For the controversy over derivation and revulsion, see Andreas Vesalius, *The Bloodletting Letter of 1539*, trans. J. B. de C. M. Saunders and C. D. O'Malley (New York, n.d.), introduction, pp. 7–19. Although Cardano referred to bk. 3 of the *Fabrica* in the course of this discussion (*Opera* 6:330; ed. 1545, fol. 45v), I have not found any citation of Vesalius's *Epistola, docens venam axillarem dextri cubiti in dolore laterali secandam* (Basel, 1539) (the so-called bloodletting letter). Essentially, the argument was over whether the object of bleeding should be to direct the blood (and other humors) toward an affected part or to draw them away from it. It involved claims to revive authentic Hippocratic and Galenic procedures, attacks on and defenses of medieval tradition, and extensive differences of opinion about the interpretation of ancient sources.

94. *Contradictiones* 2.2.7, *Opera* 6:467–86; 2.1.4, pp. 442–46, and 4.16–23, pp. 695–704. For discussion of the content of these sections, see chaps. 5 and 7.

95. "Deus an singula quaeque cognoscat" (*Contradictiones* 3.6, *Opera* 6:657–59). For discussion, see chap. 7. The *quaestio* itself was a traditional one and had been discussed by Thomas Aquinas, *Summa Theologiae*, Prima pars, qu. 14, A.11, "Utrum Deus cognoscat singularia."

96. *Contradictiones* 3.6–7, *Opera* 6:657–61; 6. 10, pp. 764–67. The plea for a Maecenas (Cardano's own term) is to be found in *Contradictiones*, epistle *ad lectorem* at end of bk. 2 (Lyon, 1548), p. 464.

97. *De immortalitate animorum* (Lyon, 1545; IA *132. 049); *Opera* 2:456–536.

98. *Theonoston*, bks. 3 and 5, *Opera* 2:403–33 and 448–54. Cardano was at

work on this treatise, which was not published during his lifetime, in 1555 and 1561 (LP 1562, *Opera* 1:112, 118).

99. See Eckhard Kessler, "The Intellective Soul," in *The Cambridge History of Renaissance Philosophy*, ed. Charles B. Schmitt et al. (Cambridge, 1988), pp. 485–507.

100. Cardano, *De immortalitate animorum*, *Opera* 2:529–30. Cardano's views on the soul and the related question of the intellect are discussed in Margolin, "Cardan, interprète d'Aristote," pp. 316–22, and Ingegno, pp. 61–78.

101. "si corpus esset instrumentum animae, aliquae operationes poterunt esse validiores quam pro natura corporis, et ita non erit necessarium temperaturam esse bonam si functio sit bona, quoniam ut videmus in tonsoribus, tonsor unus melius tondet alio cum eadem novacula, et scriptor unus melius scribit alio cum eadem penna, atramento, et papyro, et discrimen hoc est notabile: Et est mirum de Galeno. Et plurimum etiam iuvaret in multis morbis curare animam" (*Contradictiones* 6.10, *Opera* 6:765). For the repudiation of Galen's identification of the soul with the temperament of the body, ibid., p. 767.

102. "At cum ille [Galenus] non omnino affirmet esse mortalem, Hippocrates, et Hasen immortalem est dicant, constat etiam medicorum opinionem ad immortalitatem accedere" (ibid., p. 767).

103. "Hippocrates videtur animam nostram censuisse immortalem cum in libro *De carnibus* haec scripsit. 'Et videtur sane mihi id quod calidum vocamus, immortale esse, et cuncta intelligere, et videre, et audire, et scire omnia tum praesentia, tum futura. Huius igitur plurima pars, quum turbata essent omnia, in supernam circumferentiam secessit. Et videntur mihi ipsum veteres Aethera nominasse. Altera pars inferna, apellatur Terra, frigidum quid et siccum, et multis motionibus obnoxium, et in hac sane multum calidi inest. Tertia pars aeris, medium locum occupavit, calidum quid ac humidum existens. Quarta vero pars terrae proximum locum coepit, humidissimum quid ac crassissimum.' Cum ergo censeat hominem ex his quatuor constare et animam esse calidum illud, haud dubie animam immortalem esse voluit. Idem in primo *De diaeta* haec habet quae etiam alias a me, sed ad aliud propositum recitata sunt. 'Et quidem nullum omnino corpus perit, neque sit quod prius non erat; verum permista et discreta permutantur. Homines autem putant hoc quidem ex orco in lucem auctum generari, illud vero ex luce in orcum imminutum perire ac corrumpi'" (ibid., p. 764). The Hippocratic passages are quoted from the translation of *De diaeta sive victus ratione* (= *Regimen*) by Cornarius; see Hippocrates, *Opera*, trans. Cornarius (Basel, 1546), pp. 55, 125. See also Littré 8:54 and *Regimen* 1.4, *Hippocrates* (Loeb) 4:233. Attention is drawn to the significance of *Regimen* 1.4–6 for Cardano in Ingegno, pp. 226–27. Cardano also cited remarks about the weeping and laughter of infants in *On the Seven Month Child* as evidence for Hippocrates' belief in the immortality of the human soul; see *Contradictiones* 3.7 and 5.10, *Opera* 6:660 and 764, and Hippocrates, *De septimestri partu*, *Opera*, trans. Cornarius (Basel, 1546), p. 64 (Littré 7:450).

104. "Generatio an detur? Et an resurrectio mortuorum" (*Contradictiones* 3.7, *Opera* 6:659–61).

105. "Ne tamen videamur Hippocrati, aut immortalitati animi, vel resurrectioni addicti, respondebimus his quibus ab Aristotele responderi potest" (ibid.,

p. 661). See Ingegno, pp. 226–29, pointing out the further discussion of some of these ideas in Cardano's *Hyperchen, Opera* 1:284–92.

106. "... contra tua de elementis paradoxa argumentarer (quod sane, ut mihi quidam eruditi retulerunt, prius inventum fuit Ioannis Francisci Mirandulensis)" (Camuzio, *Disputationes*, fol. 72r). Pico's chapter on physiology is found in Gianfrancesco Pico, *Examen vanitatis doctrinae gentium et veritatis Christianae disciplinae* (Mirandola, 1520), 1.16, fols. 27v–32r; on this chapter, see Nancy G. Siraisi, "Medicine, Physiology, and Anatomy," pp. 214–29.

107. "ille [Cardanus] ipse velut heresiarcha quidam insignis in arte medica, novam propemodum sectam condiderit, a Galeno quampluribus in locis diversae [*sic*] penitus, Hippocraticum se medicum adfirmans. . . . siquidem in haec Insubria nostra quamplures videas non solum auditores, verumetiam iamdiu promotos ad lauream, quos minime pudeat Cardanum conta Galeni placita veluti Pythiam Apollinem in medium producere" (Camuzio, *Disputationes*, *iiiv).

108. For discussion of some of these features of Cardano's natural philosophy, see, in addition to Ingegno, Margolin, "Cardan, interprète d'Aristote," idem, "Analogie et causalité chez Jérôme Cardan," in *Sciences de la Renaissance. VIIIe Congrès International de Tours* (Paris, 1973), pp. 67–81, and Maclean, "The Interpretation of Natural Signs."

CHAPTER 4
TIME, BODY, FOOD: THE PARAMETERS OF HEALTH

1. He lectured at Bologna on *Aliment* and *Regimen in Acute Diseases* in 1568 and 1569. See chap. 6.

2. *Opus novum cunctis de sanitate tuenda ac vita producenda studiosis apprime necessarium: in quatuor libros digestum. A Rodulpho Sylvestrio Bononiensi Medico, recens in lucem editum* (Rome, 1580; IA *132. 118). It was reissued Basel, 1582 (IA *132. 120), and corresponds to ST, *Opera* 6:8–294.

3. Cardano, *De usu ciborum liber, Opera* 7:1–64; *Liber secundus Theonoston seu De vita producenda, atque incolumitate corporis conservanda, Opera* 2:372–402. These treatises were not published in Cardano's lifetime. Book 2 of *Theonoston*, also known as *De optimo vitae genere*, survives as an independent item in two Vatican manuscripts (Vat. lat. 5849 and Fondo Boncompagni J 51); it was published under the title *Theonoston, seu de vita producenda atque incolumitate corporis conservanda dialogus* (Rome, 1617). I have not seen these manuscripts or editions, and cite the edition from Ingegno, p. 26.

4. The main Hippocratic treatises specifically devoted to diet are *Regimen* (known in its Renaissance Latin versions as *De diaeta* or *De victus ratione*), *Aliment*, and *Regimen in Acute Diseases*, but the subject is, of course, central to Hippocratic medicine and recurs throughout the corpus. Galen treated the subject as part of general regimen in *De sanitate tuenda*, Kühn 6:1–452, and with respect to individual foodstuffs in *De alimentorum facultatibus*, Kühn 6:453–748. In addition, there was a Renaissance forgery of Galen's lost commentary on *Aliment*; see n. 110 to chap. 6. Ancient and medieval developments are summarized in Pedro Gil Sotres, "Le regole della salute," in *Storia del pensiero medico occidentale*, vol. 1, *Antichità e Medioevo*, ed. Mirko D. Grmek

(Rome and Bari, 1993), pp. 399–438. The traditional set of nonnaturals consisted of air and water, food and drink, repletion and excretion, motion and rest, sleep and waking, and the emotions.

5. Only a few relevant studies can be indicated here, notably Nada Patrone, *Il cibo del ricco ed il cibo del povero*, and Massimo Montanari, *The Culture of Food* (Oxford, 1994; originally published as *La fame e l'abbondanza: Storia dell'alimentazione in Europa* [Rome and Bari, 1993]), chaps. 2–4. Regarding dearth in fifteenth-century Florence, see John Henderson, *Piety and Charity in Late Medieval Florence* (Oxford, 1994), pp. 278, 283, 361, 404, 373, 401–2, 404. Also suggestive is Piero Camporesi, *Bread of Dreams: Food and Fantasy in Early Modern Europe* (Cambridge, 1989), esp. chap. 2. Mostly on the basis of Italian evidence, Braudel estimated that one-fifth of the sixteenth-century population of the Mediterranean world lived in extreme poverty (Fernand Braudel, *The Mediterranean and the Mediterranean World in the Age of Philip II* [New York, 1972], 1:453–61); however, Nada Patrone (pp. 18–19) stresses the impossibility of arriving at accurate quantitative results from the available evidence. On upper-class diet in England in the late fifteenth and early sixteenth centuries, see Barbara Harvey, *Living and Dying in England 1100–1540: The Monastic Experience* (Oxford, 1993), pp. 34–71 (with the conclusion that most monks of Westminster must have been obese); Andrew W. Appleby, "Diet in Sixteenth-Century England: Sources, Problems, Possibilities," in *Health, Medicine and Mortality in the Sixteenth Century*, ed. Charles Webster (Cambridge, 1979), pp. 97–116, pointing to a sixteenth-century divergence between the diets of rich and poor. Although, as Cardano and many others noted, northern Europe was a land of butter and beer in contrast to the southern olive oil and wine, the dietary discrepancy between rich and poor, and the prevalence of meat and alcohol in the diet of the former and grains in the diet of the latter, was presumably much the same in both cases.

6. A survey and analysis of the content of numerous diet books written in both southern and northern Europe between 1450 and 1650 is contained in Kenneth B. Albala, "Dietary Regime in the Renaissance," Ph. D. diss., Columbia University, 1993. I am grateful to Dr. Albala for lending me a copy of his dissertation. On the social characteristics attributed to different foods, see Allen J. Grieco, "The Social Politics of Pre-Linnean Botanical Classification," *I Tatti Studies: Essays in the Renaissance* 4 (1991): 131–49; Montanari, *The Culture of Food*, and many of the sources assembled in Massimo Montanari, ed., *Nuovo convivio: Storia e cultura dei piaceri della tavola nell'età moderna* (Rome and Bari, 1991).

7. Michele Savonarola, *Libreto de tute le cosse che se manzano*, ed. Jane Nystedt (Stockholm, 1982); see also the review by Jole Agrimi in *Aevum* 2 (1984): 358–65. The work entitled in Latin *Tacuinum sanitatis* was translated in the thirteenth century from an Arabic treatise by Ibn Botlan (fl. mid–eleventh century); for the late-fourteenth-century illuminated manuscripts, see Luisa Cogliati Arano, ed., *The Medieval Health Handbook: Tacuinum sanitatis* (New York, 1976).

8. I have consulted *Platyne de honesta voluptate et valetudine* ... (Venice, 1475) at the New York Public Library.

9. On the ancient sources for, and development of humanist interest in, regimen for intellectuals, see Kümmel, "Der Homo litteratus und die Kunst, gesund su leben," pp. 67–85. Regarding Renaissance interest in regimen in old age, see Luke E. Demaitre, "The Care of Health in Old Age: The Development of Gerocomy in the Renaissance," in *Aging and the Life Cycle in the Renaissance: The Interaction between Representations and Experience*, ed. Adele Seefe and Edward Ansello (University of Delaware Press, forthcoming), pointing to the increased influence of bk. 5 of Galen's *De sanitate tuenda* from the late fifteenth century (I wish to thank Dr. Demaitre for graciously allowing me to read this article before publication), and Georges Minois, *History of Old Age from Antiquity to the Renaissance* (Cambridge, 1989), pp. 288–99.

10. Marsilio Ficino, *Three Books on Life*, ed. and trans. Carol V. Kaske and John R. Clark (Binghamton, N.Y., 1989). The first edition of *De vita libri tres* was published in Florence, 1489.

11. Gabriele Zerbi, *Gerontocomia, On the Care of the Aged*, and Maximianus, *Elegies on Old Age and Love*, trans. L. R. Lind, Memoirs of the American Philosophical Society, vol. 182 (Philadelphia, 1988).

12. Gregory Lubkin, *A Renaissance Court: Milan under Galeazzo Maria Sforza* (Berkeley and Los Angeles, 1994), p. 111, citing a list of books placed or re-placed in the ducal library in 1469, and therefore presumably either in recent use or new acquisitions.

13. For example, Marisa Milani notes that Savonarola's *Libreto de tute le cosse che se manzano* was reprinted Venice, 1554, and that Ficino's *De vita* appeared in Italian translation, Venice, 1548, as did Galen's *De sanitate tuenda*, Venice, 1549 (Alvise Cornaro, *Scritti sulla vita sobria, elogio e lettere*, ed. Marisa Milani [Venice, 1983], introduction, p. 10).

14. Jean Céard, "La diététique dans la médecine de la Renaissance," in *Pratiques et discours alimentaires à la Renaissance*, ed. Jean-Claude Margolin and Robert Sauzet (Paris, 1982), pp. 21–36. The first chapter of Cardano's *De sanitate tuenda* is entitled "Cur disciplina tuendae sanitatis fuerit neglecta" (*Opera* 6:15).

15. *De malo usu*, MM 1.7–8, *Opera* 7:205–6.

16. "Quod exhibent album cibum aegris, deinde observant res nullius momenti" (MM 1 [= *De malo usu*] 83, *Opera* 7:234–35); Terence Scully, "The Sickdish in Early French Recipe Collections," in *Health, Disease, and Healing in Medieval Culture*, ed. Sheila Campbell, Bert Hall, and David Klausner (New York, 1992), pp. 132–40.

17. The Hippocratic author asserted that one must know the stars "to watch for change and excess in food, drink, and wind and the whole universe, from which diseases exist among men" (*Regimen* 1, chap. 2 [Loeb] 4: 228–29).

18. "Vaticinatio et medicina fere similes sunt" (marginal heading in Hippocrates, *De victus ratione, Diaetave liber* [*Regimen*], trans. Marco Fabio Calvo, in Hippocrates, *Opera* [Basel, 1526], p. 143). "Ego vero artes hominis manifestas, affectionibus, et in manifestis, et obscuris, similes esse declarabo. Vaticinatio tale quid est. Ex manifestis quidem cognoscere obscura . . ." (Hippocrates, *De diaeta sive victus ratione*, trans. Janus Cornarius, in Hippocrates, *Opera* [Basel, 1546], fol. 102v).

19. "Cum autem aqua minus potest quam ignis, si syncera sit horum mistio, corpore hi valent, prudentes sunt, statim hic animus ingruentia sentit, nec saepe mutatur qui cum sit optimae naturae melior tamen sit, si rite victitet" (Hippocrates, *De victus ratione*, trans. Fabio Calvo, p. 147). "Talis autem anima ito percepit allabentia, et non saepe ab una re in aliam transit. Natura quidem igitur talis animae bona est. Melior autem reddetur. . . . Si vero amplius aquae vis ab igne superetur, tali homini necesse est tanto acutiorem animam esse, quanto citius movetur et ad sensus allabi. . . . Conducit etiam talibus a sapientia, ut minime carnosi sint" (*De diaeta sive victus ratione*, trans. Cornarius, fols. 107v–8r). See also *Regimen* 1.35, in *Hippocrates*, ed. and trans. W.H.S. Jones (Loeb), 4:284–91, from which the phrases translated into English are quoted.

20. In the Basel, 1526, edition of the translation of Hippocrates' *Opera* by Fabio Calvo, *De victus ratione, Diaetave liber* is not divided into books but includes the entire contents of bks. 1–4; a small subheading in the text, "De insomniis," marks the beginning of that part of the work. There is no separate entry for *De insomniis* in the table of contents. In the Cornarius translation of the *Opera* (consulted in the edition of Basel, 1546), *De diaeta sive victus ratione* is divided into three books; *De insomniis* follows immediately as a separate work; it is also listed separately in the table of contents. Modern editors accept *De insomniis* as part of *Regimen* (see W.H.S. Jones, introduction, *Hippocrates* (Loeb), pp. xxxviii–xxxix.

21. "Mors enim quatuor modis homini advenit, vel puro casu [i.e., as a result of trauma]. . . . Alius est modus, cum naturaliter pure pereunt: id fit (ut dixi) humido iam toto in amurcam mutato: atque proferri hic docetur, atque in longum produci. Tertius est, in quo etiam plus valet ars nostra, et est cum per continuam mutationem cibi, iam debilitatibus viribus, deterius, efficitur nutrimentum, atque humidum, atque hic modus interitus naturalis non est, sed naturali simillimus. Quartus vero mixtus, qui ex morbo contingit, hocque modo plerique moriuntur: est enim communis maxime omnibus ferme hominibus, constatque natura et casu" (ST 1.8, *Opera* 6:36). For the history of the concept of radical moisture and the contribution of Avicenna, see Thomas S. Hall, "Life, Death and the Radical Moisture," *Clio medica* 6 (1971): 3–23. Galen described the process of aging in *De marcore* (*De marasmo*) 2–5, Kühn 7:669–87, and devoted *De sanitate tuenda*, bk. 5, chaps. 4–10, Kühn 6:330–62, to regimen for the elderly. The main Hippocratic and Galenic loci are collected, and Galen's teaching on the physiology of aging and its modification by medieval Arabic and Latin authors is described and analyzed, in Luke Demaitre, "The Care and Extension of Old Age in Medieval Medicine," in *Aging and the Aged in Medieval Europe*, ed. Michael M. Sheehan (Toronto, 1990), pp. 3–22, with remarks alluded to at p. 9.

22. ST 2.1, *Opera* 6:107–8.

23. ST 4.9, "De victu eorum qui dentibus carent," *Opera* 6:256.

24. Ibid., 1.28, *Opera* 6:74. In the same passage, he stressed the Hippocratic source of his idea. "Accipe quae dicat Hippocrates Epidemiorum sexto. 'Cibus paucus non delassari, non sitire.' Aliter vertit alius 'Cibi paucitas lassitudinem non faciens, nec sitim accendens.' . . . Dubitant autem in hoc quod dixi, optime se habere, reclamabuntque isti, qui se Galenici, nimium iactant, dicentes idem esse et sanum esse perfecte et optime se habere. At mihi plurimum differre vi-

dentur: nam ut ex sententia Hippocratis liquet, delassari non convenit, et cibo pauco uti: at noster Galenus, tam graves iniungit exercitationes, ut et delassari necesse sit quotidie et multo cibo repleri non solum quod immodicus ille labor famem magnam excitet, sed quod etiam si non des, laedetur graviter homo" (ibid., pp. 73–74). Neither version of the Hippocratic quotation resembles the rendering in either the Calvi or the Cornarius translation of *Epidemics* 6 (Hippocrates, *Opera* [Basel, 1526], p. 301, and Hippocrates, *Opera* [Basel, 1546],p. 457).

25. "Quaedam etenim reperiuntur corpora humidum radicale admodum pingue ac purum habentia, quod prae pinguedine et quantitate facile resistit re-solutionibus, et calorem innatum tuetur ac conservat, et talia longissimam ducunt vitam, si convenienti tamen utantur victus regimine, nec sibi ipsis exitium afferant: ut plurimum enim immoderatis laboribus se exponunt, quibus exiccatur humidum substantificum et nimia venere utuntur, et otio, et crapula superexce-denti, et ebrietate, quibus suffocatur calor innatus, et vita quae longissima esse deberet, brevissima sit" (ST 1.8, *Opera* 6:34).

26. "Ex quo cum vehementiore spiritus concitatione, excrementa melius ex-purgantur, itaque obscurum non est Galenum cum sua sapientia non civis, aut studiosi, sed militis, aut athletae, vitam instituisse, cum qua nemo sana mente, neque integris sensibus nec diu vivere possit: nam (ut dixi) tales exercitationes cerebrum saepe collidunt ut ante senectam surdi, aut coeci plerunque fiant, amentes quasi omnes, et immemores" (ibid., 1.27, *Opera* 6:74). The passage of Galen referred to is *De tuenda sanitate* 2.2 and 8, Kühn 6:83–91, 133–37.

27. "qui ad magnam senectutem perveniunt homines sunt frigido et humido corde" (ST 1.18, *Opera* 6:56).

"macilenti, ac etiam pallidi, et minime vividi, quod calor in his admodum parvus sit, ad longissimam senectam perveniunt, quales in coenobiis [1580: Xenobiis], sacras aliquot virgines videre adhuc licet, et multo plures paucis ante annis, quae annum centesimum superaverunt" (ibid., p. 58).

28. Ibid. 1.27, *Opera* 6:73.

29. "Itaque hunc errorem adeo gravem admittit Galenus, quoniam non ani-madvertit exercitium proportione ea aetate minuendum esse" (ibid. 4.9, *Opera* 6:257). The Hippocratic *Regimen* 1.2 contains a striking statement about the need to monitor kinds and amounts of physical activity carefully placed against the marginal heading "Quid possit exercitatio aspicito." In the Calvi translation this runs: "Contraria nanque inter sese sunt, cibaria et labores, tamen utraque sanitati conferunt. Labores enim suapte natura, superflua demunt: cibaria autem et pocula vacua complent. Quare laborum naturalium, et non naturalium vim dignoscito . . ." (Hippocrates, *Opera* [Basel, 1526], p. 141 [*Hippocrates* (Loeb) 4:229]). See also n. 19, above.

30. "Exercitatio igitur maxime in senibus, et praecipue valida, ac celer, vitam abbreviat manifeste, tametsi valetudini conferat conservandae" (ST 1.18, *Opera* 6:55).

31. "Sed iam de agitationis commodis agendum est nec non damnis. Diximus eam esse triplicem, magnam, et haec duplex, inaequalis sed non incommoda, ut in mari vehi, haec igitur movet omnes humores, et totum corpus vomitu evacuat, non solum propter agitationem, sed ob maris odorem, quia nauseam excitat, quibus igitur facilis vomitus est, utilissima, et iuventutem instaurat, a multisque morbis liberat" (ibid., 1.20, *Opera* 6:63).

32. See Zerbi, *Gerontocomia*, pp. 110–12.

33. Cardano, *Consilia*, nos. 53 and 54, *Opera* 9:230–37. The *consilium* for Morone (b. 1509) appears to have resulted from Cardano's personal attendance on the cardinal in a city other than Rome: "Verum in hoc erimus praesentes, sed de his hactenus: posset enim Romam ire" (*Consilum*, no. 53, ibid. p. 230); possibly it was written on the occasion sometime between 1564 and 1570 when Cardano traveled from Bologna to Modena to treat Morone (n. 69 to chap. 2). If so, the comment about sadness and fear may conceivably be an indirect allusion to the efforts of Pius V (1566–72) to reopen accusations of heresy against members of former "spiritual" circles; see Firpo, *Inquisizione romana e Controriforma*, pp. 16–17. On lathe turning as a pastime, see Joseph Connors, "*Ars tornandi*: Baroque Architecture and the Lathe," *Journal of the Warburg and Courtauld Institutes* 53 (1990): 217–36; for another example, see also Robert Klein and Henri Zerner, eds., *Italian Art 1500–1600: Sources and Documents* (Englewood Cliffs, N.J., 1966), pp. 154–55.

34. On the medieval and Renaissance literature of prolongevity, see Gerald J. Gruman, *A History of Ideas about the Prolongation of Life: The Evolution of Prolongevity Hypotheses to 1800. Transactions of the American Philosophical Society*, n.s., 56, pt. 9 (Philadelphia, 1966); Agostino Paravicini Bagliani, "Ruggero Bacone, Bonifacio VIII e la teoria della 'prolongatio vitae,'" in his *Medicina e scienze della natura alla corte dei papi nel Duecento* (Spoleto, 1991), pp. 327–62; Michela Pereira, "Un tesoro inestimabile: Elixir e 'prolongatio vitae' nell'alchimia del '300," *Micrologus* 1 (1993): 161–87.

35. "a Ficino prodigiosum illud, ac pene magicum vivendi genus, quod ferme in omni sua doctrina secutus est, quodque merito contemni poterat a me, nisi illum nonaginta septem, matrem autem illius centum septem et decem annis vixisse accepissem" (ST 1.9, *Opera* 6:38).

36. Ficino was born October 19, 1433, and died October 1, 1499; see Paul Oskar Kristeller, *Marsilio Ficino and His Work after Five Hundred Years*, Quaderni di Rinascimento, vol. 7 ([Florence], 1987), pp. 157 and 166.

37. ST 1.7, *Opera* 6:35; the proem, *Opera* 5:12–14, contains several references to Tommaso Rangone, *Iulio Tertio Sanctissimo. Thomae Philologi Ravenna De vita homini ultra CXX annos protrahenda*. The first edition of this work appeared in Venice, 1550, according to Milani (Cornaro, ed. Milani, p. 11); I have consulted that of Venice, 1553.

38. "Definiamus ergo primum eam nunc esse vitam longam appellandam, quae in Italia non aliis gentibus adeo firma sit: at si neque error, neque casus obstaret, prope centesimum deducere hominem posset circa LXXX adhuc integris sensibus, viribus autem eiusmodi, quae homini gravi exercendo essent necessariae, velut deambulationi, itinere, ad forum brevi orationi, atque similibus" (ST 4.4, *Opera* 6:248). Ibid. 4.3, pp. 243–48, "De vita longitudine, et an optimum sit statim custodia uti, exempla, et modi," collects much anecdotal material about longevity; compare Gruman, *History of Ideas about the Prolongation of Life*, pp. 21–27, 63–65.

39. "mihi enim hoc fuit privilegium a natura datam, ut in iudicanda [1580: diudicanda] aetate, nunquam plus biennio aberraverim, atque eo rarissime" (ST 1.18, *Opera* 6:57).

40. Ibid.

41. I have consulted Alvise Cornaro, *Scritti sulla vita sobria, elogio e lettere,* ed. Marisa Milani (Venice, 1983); the work was first published in 1558 and enlarged by the author with various supplements between 1559 and 1565. It was repeatedly reissued throughout the seventeenth and eighteenth centuries.

42. Cornaro, ed. Milani, pp. 21–22.

43. Ibid., p. 63.

44. ST 1.1, *Opera* 6:15.

45. " . . . utrique [1580: utrunque] in Academia habitatio, et conversatio, illi tamen ut Veneto patritio decora, mihi ut professori honesta" (ibid., 1.9, *Opera* 6:38). The remark seems to refer to place in and manner of life in general, rather than to membership in specific academies. On the multiple meanings of the word *academia* in the Renaissance, see James Hankins, "The Myth of the Platonic Academy of Florence," *Renaissance Quarterly* 44 (1991): 429–75, at pp. 433–36. Cardano was, however, at one time a member of the Accademia degli Affidati of Pavia; see VP 30, *Opera* 1:20.

46. " . . . sententia Cornarii ter sapientis, quem sequi proposui. Ab hoc ergo finem huius instituti, exemplumque vitae, et experimentum operis ipsius desumere non gravabor, aut dedignabor, quamvis ille literas humaniores, aut medicinam non profiteretur" (ST 1.9, *Opera* 6:37).

47. *Theonoston* 2, *Opera* 2:379 and 397. There is also a reference to *Theonoston* in ST 1.28, *Opera* 6:73. The two works, completed in final form around the same time, were evidently intended to go together.

48. Cardano, *Theonoston* 2, *Opera* 2:377.

49. "Sed duo sunt, de quibus dubitamus. Magna enim, primum est voluptas conviviorum, quas omnes gentes celebrant, et a memoria hominum semper in honore habita; nec quicquam tam commune omni genti, omni aetati, pauperibus atque divitibus, regibus quoque ipsis, Iudaeis, Christianis, Idolorum, et Mahumethi cultoribus, viris, pueris, senibus, mulieribus, latronibus, ac probis hominibus. Conviviis vero sobrietas e regione adversatur. . . . Secunda quod ex ea contabescere ventriculus videatur" (ibid., p. 376).

50. "Qui lente mandit bibendo pytissat serius aliquanto incipit, finit ante alios, multa loquitur in medio coenae, huic vix tantum suppetet temporis, ut quod consuevit edere, atque bibere possit. . . . Neque enim accedimus ad convivia ut epulones, aut lurcones, sed ut confabulemur, congaudeamusque. Et quaedam sunt edulia postquam res ipsa pondere definitur suavia admodum, nec valetudini adversa, ex quibus si, vel ut rem ederis, pondus non aequabis duarum unciarum, qualis est lactis spuma ubique nota, sed Mediolani in praecipu usu, maxime in mensis Principum, atque conviviis" (ibid., p. 378). I am unable to identify "foam of milk [*lactis spuma*]" any further. Some form of ricotta or whipped cream seems more likely than the steamed milk froth that springs to the late-twentieth-century mind.

51. Ibid, p. 381.

52. Ibid., pp. 379–81.

53. Ibid., pp. 383–85.

54. For a modern assessment of the effects of drastic calorie reduction in laboratory animals (using carefully planned, nutrient-rich diets), see Richard Weindruch, "Caloric Restriction and Aging," *Scientific American* 274 (1996): 46–52.

55. "Enimvero tametsi multa de hac disciplina clarissimi viri scripserint, Hip-

pocrates sive Polybus et Diocles, totque alii, de quibus alias actum est, multos tamen habent contradicentes . . ." (ST 1.1, *Opera* 6:15) (these are the opening words of the work).

56. "Senes sunt frigidiores et sicciores. . . . Est ergo humidus cibus, utpote vitellus ovi melior, sed tanto facilior concoctu, et minore quantitate praeferendus, sic enim mutationis labor auferetur, et praesertim consuetus, et somni hora, idque optimum cum tum ad humidum, ideoque ad calidum corpus senile retrahat. Quaecunque enim ad humidum retrahunt, eadem si humidum sit pingue, seu coctum, calefaciunt simul: ut olea, carnes, lac, et similia. Qua propter nihil nocentius humido non pingui, sed aqueo, cuiusmodi fructuum non oleosorum, seu horaero[r]um, herbarum, germinum, furculorum, atque radicum omnium, talia enim omnia senibus inimica" (ibid. 4.6, *Opera* 6:253).

57. "Verum docebimus infra, vitam longaevam, neque carnibus, neque ovis, neque vino constare, dico vitam illam admodum longam, de qua proprie vir hic [Tommaso Rangone, see n. 37, above] sermonem habet, sed in fructibus terrae, ut pane, amygdalis, pineis, castaneis, aqua cum saccharo" (ibid., proemium, p. 13). It is perhaps worth mentioning that a partial translation of Porphyry, *De abstinentia animalium* had been made by Marsilio Ficino, and that Porphyry's views are alluded to in Ficino's *De vita* 2.6, ed. Kaske and Clarke, p. 180.

58. ST, proemium, *Opera* 6:12; *Theonoston* 2, *Opera* 2:382, 393. VP contains similar contradictions about diet; it recommends that old men not eat fish at the end of a chapter largely devoted to describing the elderly author's pleasure in doing so (VP 8, *Opera* 1:6–7; on this chapter, see further below).

59. See, for example, *Theonoston* 2, *Opera* 2:379, 400.

60. On the idea of wild food, roots, and vegetables as especially appropriate diet for hermits, see Allen J. Grieco, "Les plantes, les régimes végétariens et la mélancholie à la fin du Moyen Age et au début de la Renaissance italien," in *Le monde végétal (XIIe–XVIIe siècles): Savoirs et usages sociaux*, ed. Allen J. Grieco et al. (Saint-Denis, 1993), pp. 11–29.

61. *Theonoston* 2, *Opera* 2:372; compare VP 1–2, *Opera* 1:1–2; "Ad naturam autem ars plurimum confert; qui vocem habent vitiatam nulla musica canori evadunt; attamen et qui bonam habent vocem, non fiunt sine arte musici" (*Theonoston* 2, *Opera* 2:382). For the argument that Machiavelli was engaged in *Il principe* in constructing a prudential rhetoric that was intended as "an immanent critique of humanist imitation and the humanist pedagogy of examples" (p. 19), see Victoria Kahn, *Machiavellian Rhetoric: From the Counter-Reformation to Milton* (Princeton, 1994), pp. 18–33.

62. See Elizabeth Sears, *The Ages of Man: Medieval Interpretations of the Life Cycle* (Princeton, 1986) pp. 38–53, and J. A. Burrow, *The Ages of Man: A Study in Medieval Writing and Thought* (Oxford, 1986), pp. 1–94.

63. "Omnes leges tum regna et civitates ac familiae non solum fines habent, sed certos quos, nequaquam praeterire licet, verum in statis temporum circuitibus quemadmodum et animalium vita terminantur" (Cardano, *De arcanis aeternitatis tractatus* 11, *Opera* 10:17). For the scheme of fourteens, see ibid., p. 20–21. Cardano's ideas on the astrologically determined fall of states were used, and vigorously criticized, by Jean Bodin in several of his works. See, for example, *Methodus ad facilem historiarum cognitionem*, chap. 6, in Jean Bodin, *Oeu-*

vres philosophiques, ed. Pierre Mesnard (Paris, 1951), pp. 199–201. I am grateful to Anthony Grafton for drawing my attention to Bodin in this connection.

64. "Sic ex ambientis eadem constitutione varios in variis corporibus effectus contingere atque etiam casus" (comm. *Tetrabiblos* 1.2.11, *Opera* 5:102).

65. "Veluti Mediolanum est magis occidentale et Boreale, quam Florentia: Ideo Mediolanenses sunt fortiores, et pulchriora habent corpora, et delicatiores, et laborum patientiores: At contra Florentini sunt magis compti, et ornati, et lingua liberiores, et minus cibo indulgent, et magis amatores scientiarum et disciplinarum mathematicarum" (ibid. 2.3.12., *Opera* 5:178–79). Regarding Cardano's commentary on *Airs Waters Places* and the influence of Ptolemaic and Hippocratic environmentalism, see further chap. 6, below.

66. See, for example, Giovanni Pico della Mirandola, *Disputationes adversus astrologiam divinatricem*, bk. 4, chap. 3, "Quomodo rerum fortuitarum causa sit Deus, quomodo angeli, quomodo nos, quomodo fortuna," ed. Eugenio Garin (Florence, 1946), 1:428–42.

67. ST 1.18, *Opera* 6:56–57.

68. VP 1, 2, and 5, *Opera* 1:1–2, 4–5.

69. ST 2.1, *Opera* 6:108.

70. Alvise Cornaro, *Compendio breve della vita sobria*, in Cornaro, ed. Milani, p. 109.

71. "Platina, qui libellum de honesta voluptate inscripsit, potius ad usum culinarum et voluptatem hel[l]uonum qui popinis tantum indulgent, atque gulae, ventrique sunt dediti, quam ut salubrem arte [*sic*] traderet: et totum studium posuit in arte parandorum ferculorum, varieque in mensarum lautiorum concinnatorum, et bellariorum usu, maximo cum detrimento humanae salutis: siquidem voluptatem tamen secutus est, non autem utilitatem. Est equidem ars haec perniciosa, nisi ut diximus quibusdam coerceatur legibus, quae nobis inserviant ut sanitati consulamus" (Cardano, *De usu ciborum liber* 18, *Opera* 7:43).

72. Yves Pélicier, "Les nourritures à la Renaissance: Essai de typologie," in *Pratiques et discours alimentaires à la Renaissance*, ed. Jean-Claude Margolin and Robert Sauzet (Paris, 1982), pp. 15–20.

73. Galen, *De alimentorum facultatibus*, Kühn 6:453–748, is a work in three books dealing with individual foodstuffs (bk. 1: grains and legumes; bk. 2: fruits, nuts, leafy vegetables, herbs, and roots; bk. 3: foods from animals). A translation by William of Moerbeke was contained in the earliest printed editions of Galen's *Opera*; in the sixteenth century, two new translations into Latin between them appeared in nine separate editions and one of them was included in the Renaissance editions of Galen's *Opera*; in the same period the work was also translated into French and Italian; see Richard J. Durling, "A Chronological Census of Renaissance Editions and Translations of Galen," *Journal of the Warburg and Courtauld Institutes* 24 (1961): 283, no. 13.

74. ST, *Opera* 6: grains and legumes, 2.3–16, pp. 112–21; leafy vegetables, herbs, gourds, melons, and cucumbers, 2.17–39, pp. 121–34; roots, tubers, and fungi, 2.40–49, pp. 134–43; fruit, 2.50–69, pp. 143–57; meat, 3.1–9, pp. 158–66; shellfish and turtles, 3.10, pp. 166–68; milk and milk products, 3.11–13, pp. 168–72; birds and eggs, 3.14–23, pp. 172–79; "fish" (including cetaceans and salted fish), 3.24–73, pp. 180–214.

75. *De subtilitate,* bk. 10, *Opera* 3:537–42; RV 7.37, "Piscium differentia ac genera," *Opera* 3:112–39; 7.38, "Piscium cura, et proprietates," ibid., pp. 739–44.

76. *Contradicentium medicorum liber primus [-secundus]* (Lyon: Sebastianus Gryphus, 1548); *De subtilitate libri XXI* (Lyon: Gulielmus Rouillius, 1550, 1551). See Ian Maclean, "Cardano and His Publishers," Kessler, pp. 317–18.

77. Guillaume Rondelet, *Libri de piscibus marinis* (Lyon: Matthias Bonhomme, 1554). As Rondelet explained in the preface, the work had been in preparation for years and various people saw his drawings and manuscript before publication(sigs. A2v, A5v).

78. Pierre Belon, *L'histoire naturelle des estranges poissons marins* . . . (Paris, 1551). The Latin version was published in Paris, 1552.

79. RV 13.65, *Opera* 3:261.

80. "Haec vero generaliter dicta sint, si quis autem singula prosequi desiderat, non solum in libris antiquorum se exerceat, ut Aristotelis, Athenaei, et Plinii, tum nostrae aetatis Rondeletii, ac Bellonii: verum etiam in ipsa rerum inspectione, cunctaque ad haec quae scripsimus conetur referre" (RV 7.38, *Opera* 3:138).

81. Ibid. 7.37, p. 113; VP 48, *Opera* 1:47. On Rondelet's critique of Cardano's confusion over the *echineis—torpedo—remora* (in *De subtilitate* 10, *Opera* 3:539), see Brian P. Copenhaver, "A Tale of Two Fishes: Magical Objects in Natural History from Antiquity through the Scientific Revolution," *Journal of the History of Ideas* 52 (1991): 389.

82. ". . . Bellonius . . . ostendat se non solum pisces vidisse, sed piscium singulorum viscera, quae ignorasse Rondelletium haud obscurum est" (*Theonoston* 2, *Opera* 2:386).

83. For example, Rondelet, Belon, Pliny all appear on one page, RV 7.37, *Opera* 3:117. For the allusions to Cardano's own experiences cited, see ibid. 7.37, pp. 117, 121, 122, 128.

84. Conrad Gesner, *Historiae animalium liber IIII, qui est de Piscium et Aquatilium animantium natura* (Zurich, 1558), prefatory list of acknowledgments; see Alfredo Serrai, *Conrad Gesner,* ed. Maria Cocchetti (Rome, 1990), p. 316.

85. Compare RV 3.37, *Opera* 3:134–35, and ST, *Opera* 6:211–12.

86. Gianfranco Folena, "Per la storia della ittionimia volgare: Tra cucina e scienza naturale," *Bollettino dell'Atlante Linguistico Mediterraneo* 5–6 (1963–64): 61–137.

87. "Grande fatica e quasi non possibile seria a nominare tuti i pessi che se manzano" (Savonarola, *Libreto,* p. 116).

> Or s'io volessi de' pesci contare,
> e tante forme diverse narralle,
> sarebbe come in Puglia annumerare
> le mosche, le zenzare e le farfalle.

(Luigi Pulci, *Morgante* 25.332.1–4, quoted in Folena, "Per la storia della ittionimia volgare," p. 63.

88. See RV 7.37, *Opera* 3:124, 135, 138, 139.

89. Paolo Giovio, *De piscibus*, in his *Opera*, vol. 9, ed. Ernesto Travi and Mariagrazia Penco (Rome, 1984), pp. 11–64. The first edition was in 1524. On Giovio, see now the excellent biography by T. C. Price Zimmerman, *Paolo Giovio: The Historian and the Crisis of Sixteenth-Century Italy* (Princeton, 1995). Ippolito Salviani, *Aquatilium animantium historia liber primus* (Rome, 1554 [1558]). Rondelet accused Salviani of plagiarism; for his outraged denial, see fols. 231r–232r of the *Aquatilium animantium liber*. Regarding Aldrovandi's interest in these works, his visit to a Roman fish market, and his personal contacts with Salviani, see Findlen, *Possessing Nature*, pp. 175–76. Cardano was among the many who visited Aldrovandi's museum at Bologna (ibid., p. 140).

90. Salviani's tables occupy fols. 1–56 of the *Aquatilium animantium liber*. The parts of them relating to vernacular nomenclature are edited in Folena, "Per la storia della ittionimia volgare," pp. 103–37. In a number of instances, Cardano gives the same Roman name for various species as does Salviani, although this is not, of course, necessarily evidence of dependence.

91. See Folena, "Per la storia della ittionimia volgare," pp. 77–78.

92. UC 2.2, *Opera* 2:47. The work was begun in 1557 and first published in 1561.

93. ST 3.88, "De cervisia et aliis potibus artificialibus, atque eorum nocumentis" (*Opera* 6:229–30).

94. "Et licet primo gustui ingrata appareat cervisia, usu tamen suavior redditur" (Cardano, *De usu ciborum* 25, *Opera* 7:53). The account of beer making in this passage is even more detailed than that cited in the previous note.

95. UC 2.2, *Opera* 2:47 (first published Basel, 1561; IA *132. 082). Thus although Cardano's illness took place before Cornaro's book was published (1558), the book in which he recorded it appeared subsequently. On the illness that preceded the change of regime, see further chaps. 8 and 10, below.

96. On the complexion and characteristics of snails and turtle, see for example, Leonardo Legio, *Practice ordinarie ibidem interpretis fabrica regiminis sanitatis* (Milan, 1522), fol. 17r–v (work dedicated to the duke of Milan). A recipe for snail soup is, however, included in *Opera di M. Bartolomeo Scappi cuoco secreto di Papa Pio Quinto* (Florence, 1570), bk. 6, chap. 166.

97. ST 4.10, "De propria victus institutione, dum sexagesimum sextum annum agebam" (*Opera* 6:258–59).

98. Ibid., p. 259.

99. "cum irata esset mihi ancilla, nec auderem committere salutem meam illi, quippe ut coqueret panem et madefactum aqua non existamabam utilem, nimis enim crudus erat, et inflasset: ob id ergo consilium coepi, ut panem infunderem in aquam more solito inde cum hora adveniret (neque ob legendi munus, et curarum negotium coquendi panem coram me tempus suppetebat) expressum more communi infundebam iuri carnium ferventi, quod paratum erat pro omnibus, ut nulli periculo me exponerem . . ." (ibid.). With reference to the modifications he introduced in 1570, he added, "non arrideret, ancilla enim inepta erat" (ibid.).

100. VP 8, *Opera* 1:6–7; see also chap. 52, p. 52.

101. "Questa vita [sobria] consiste se non in queste due cose: quantità e qualità. La prima, che è la qualità consiste solo in non mangiare cibi né bevere

vini contrarii allo suo stomaco. . . . Le quali quantità e qualità debbon pur esser conosciute da l'huomo come è pervenuto alla età delli XXXX anni o L o LX; e quello che tiene tali dui ordini vive vita ordinata e sobria, la quale ha tanta virtù e forza che gli humori di quel corpo si fanno perfettissimi, concordi, et adunati" (Cornaro, *Compendio*, in Cornaro, ed. Milani, p. 108).

CHAPTER 5
THE USES OF ANATOMY

1. "Ex laudabilibus etiam, minime, cognoscendis plantis ob memoriae defectum: neque agriculturae, quod exercere oporteat magis quam scire: ab anatomia autem multa me deterruere. Nec etiam pangendis carminibus, nisi necessariis et valde parum. . . . In proprio agro destituor chirurgiae usu" (VP 39, *Opera* 1:31).

2. The horoscope of Vesalius is no. 93 in Cardano, *Liber de exemplis centum geniturarum* (= the fifth book in his *Libelli quinque* [Nuremberg, 1547; IA *132. 054], fol. 178r), *Opera* 5:500. See also Giuseppe Ongaro, "Girolamo Cardano e Andrea Vesalio," *Rivista di storia della medicina* 13 (1969): 51–61, which includes a review of the earlier literature; O'Malley, *Andreas Vesalius*, pp. 28 (noting that the horoscope provides the sole evidence for Vesalius's birth date), 95, 234, 467; Eckman, *Jerome Cardan*, p. 52. Cardano acknowledged the horoscopes given him by Rheticus as follows: "Forte fortuna Georgius Ioachimus in Italiam ex Germania venit, vir humanus et in mathematicis haud mediocriter eruditus. Sed in primis, primo more officiosus, ac syncerus, hic clariorum virorum genituras, quas secum habebat, mihi obtulit ultro. Vessalii, Ioannis Monteregii, Cornelii Agrippae, Politiani, Iacobi Mycilli, Osiandri, quarum aliquot addidi huic operi ad centenarium explendum, dubias enim omnes reieci." *De exemplis centum geniturarum*, no. 67 (horoscope of Heinrich Cornelius Agrippa), *Opera* 5:491. The passage was first noted in McNair, "Poliziano's Horoscope," p. 270, cited from the edition of Nuremberg, 1547. On Cardano's relation with Rheticus, see McNair, "Poliziano's Horoscope," and Grafton, "From Apotheosis to Analysis."

3. On the nature of medical prognosis in Galen and parallels with astrological practice of his day, see Tamsyn S. Barton, *Power and Knowledge: Astrology, Physiognomics, and Medicine under the Roman Empire* (Ann Arbor, Mich., 1994), chap. 3; see ibid., pp. 140–43, for an example, and discussion, of retroactive analysis by Galen.

4. VP 39, "Eruditio, vel repraesentatio" (*Opera* 1:31). Listed as "disciplinae malae, aut perniciosae, aut vanae" are chiromancy, the art of compounding poisons, physiognomy, and magic using incantations for summoning daemons or souls of the dead. Cardano did not necessarily use incantations to summon his daemon or the ghost of his father, but he certainly believed both visited him; physiognomy is the subject of Cardano, *Metoposcopia* (Paris, 1558; IA *102. 076; I have not seen this edition).

5. I make no attempt to indicate the copious bibliography on Renaissance anatomy and its ancient and late medieval antecedents. A helpful recent study of Renaissance anatomy in cultural context is Andrea Carlino, *La fabbrica del corpo: Libri e dissezione nel Rinascimento* (Turin, 1994). On the relation of anatomy

and natural philosophy, see Roger French, *William Harvey's Natural Philosophy* (Cambridge, 1994), pp. 3–17.

6. Helpful recent studies addressing these developments include Reeds, *Botany in Medieval and Renaissance Universities*; Findlen, *Possessing Nature*; Giuseppe Olmi, *L'inventario del mondo: Catalogazione della natura e luoghi del sapere nella prima età moderna* (Bologna, 1992); N. Jardine, "Epistemology of the Sciences," in *Cambridge History of Renaissance Philosophy*, ed. Schmitt et al., pp. 685–711; William B. Ashworth, "Natural History and the Emblematic World View," in *Reappraisals of the Scientific Revolution*, ed. David C. Lindberg and Robert Westman (Cambridge, 1990), pp. 304–32. There is, of course, evidence of interest in assembling descriptions of plants and animals in the Middle Ages (notably, for example, in the paraphrase of the Aristotelian books on animals by Albertus Magnus), but the status of such "empirical" knowledge remained relatively low.

7. Since the classic studies of Erwin Panofsky the connections between developments in anatomy and Renaissance art have been examined from a number of standpoints. The literature is too diverse to be listed here, but among more recent studies mention may be made of John B. Schultz, *Art and Anatomy in Renaissance Italy* (Ann Arbor, 1985).

8. On negative and positive traditions of moralizing about anatomy, see William Schupbach, *The Paradox of Rembrandt's "Anatomy of Dr. Tulp,"* *Medical History*, supplement no. 2 (London, 1982), pp. 41–49.

9. Giovanna Ferrari, "Public Anatomy Lessons and the Carnival: The Anatomy Theatre of Bologna," *Past and Present* 117 (1987): 51–106, esp. pp. 58, 74–106.

10. Bylebyl, "School of Padua"; Carlino, *La fabbrica del corpo*; Ferrari, "Public Anatomy Lessons"; Giovanni Martinotti, "L'insegnamento dell'anatomia in Bologna prima del secolo XIX," *Studi e memorie per la storia dell'Università di Bologna* 2 (1911): 3–146; Peter Murray Jones, "Thomas Lorkyn's Dissections," *Transactions of the Cambridge Bibliographical Society* 9 (1988): 209–30.

11. "ac prorsus emortuam humani corporis partium scientiam, ipse tot praestantium virorum exemplo provocatus, huic pro mea virili, ac iis quibus possem rationibus opem ferendam duxi. . . . hoc naturalis philosophiae membrum ita ab inferis revocandum putavi" (Vesalius, *Fabrica* [1543], preface, *3r).

12. Vivian Nutton, "Wittenberg Anatomy," in *Medicine and the Reformation*, ed. Ole Peter Grell and Andrew Cunningham (London, 1993), pp. 11–32; Sachiko Kusukawa, *The Transformation of Natural Philosophy: The Case of Philip Melanchthon* (Cambridge, 1995), pp. 114–23.

13. Ferrari, "Public Anatomy Lessons," p. 68; Bylebyl, "School of Padua," pp. 361–62.

14. Vesalius, *Fabrica* (1543) 3.7, p. 280[380]. For discussion, see Nancy G. Siraisi, "Vesalius on Human Diversity," *Journal of the Warburg and Courtauld Institutes* 57 (1994): 60–88, and Glen Harcourt, "Andreas Vesalius and the Anatomy of Antique Sculpture," *Representations*, no. 17 (1987): 28–61.

15. Ladislao Münster, "La medicina legale in Bologna dai suoi albori fino alla fine del secolo XIV," *Bollettino dell'Accademia Medica Pistoiese Filippo Pacini* 26 (1955): 257–71; Park, "The Criminal and the Saintly Body."

16. *Il primo processo per San Filippo Neri,* ed. G. Incisa Della Rochetta et al., 4 vols. (Vatican City, 1957–63), vol. 1, no. 40, p. 153; no. 63, pp. 235–36; no. 75, pp. 265–66; vol. 2, no. 160, p. 44; no. 224, pp. 220–22; nos. 225–226, pp. 222–227; no. 241, pp. 259–67; vol. 3, nos. XLI–XLII, pp. 437–45; L. Belloni, "L'aneurisma di S. Filippo Neri nella relazione di Antonio Porto," *Rendiconti dell'Istituto Lombardo di Scienze e Lettere. Classe di scienze* 83 (1950): 665–80; Gianbattista Carcano Leone, *Exenterationis cadaveris illustrissimi Cardinalis Borrhomaei Mediolani Archiepiscopi . . . verissima, atque elegantissima enarratio* (Milan, 1584). See also Giulia Calvi, *Histories of a Plague Year: The Social and the Imaginary in Baroque Florence* (Berkeley, 1989).

17. Richard Palmer, "Medicine at the Papal Court in the Sixteenth Century," in *Medicine at the Courts of Europe,* ed. Vivian Nutton (London, 1990), pp. 49–78, at p. 67.

18. For example, the late-fifteenth-century autopsy reports recorded in Benivieni, chaps. 33–37, pp. 563–57, are much shorter and less anatomically precise than the late-sixteenth-century reports cited in n. 16, above.

19. Siraisi, "Giovanni Argenterio," pp. 177–78. Regarding syncretism and the absorption of influences in sixteenth-century Aristotelianism, see Charles B. Schmitt, *Aristotle and the Renaissance* (Cambridge, Mass., 1983), especially pp. 89–109.

20. Giovanni Costeo, *Disquisitionum physiologicarum . . . in primam primi Canonis Avicennae sectionem libri sex . . .* (Bologna, 1589), pp. 398–451; for discussion, see Siraisi, *Avicenna,* pp. 328–32.

21. Girolamo (fra' Scipione) Mercurio, *La commare o riccoglitrice,* excerpts from the edition of Venice 1601 [1606] edited in Maria Luisa Altieri Biagi et al., *Medicina per le donne nel Cinquecento: Testi di Giovanni Marinello e di Girolamo Mercurio* (Turin, 1992), pp. 86–87. The first edition appeared in 1596 (ibid., p. 41). In the introduction, Altieri Biagi stresses that the intended audience of this book did not consist of midwives themselves (most of whom would have been illiterate) but rather the fathers of families who were their employers (ibid., p. 13).

22. "Nunc vero satis sit monuisse, debere medicos singulis annis corpora hominum dissecare, qui ex morbo in xenobiis [*sic*] mortem oppetunt. Nec in illis cum difficulter hoc fiat, absolutam totius quaerere dissectionem, sed membri proprie quod morbi affectum creditur, in laterali morbo pectoris: in coli dolore intestinorum: in phthoe tabeque pulmonum: duo enim potius sunt quam unus. Nam et hoc addendum in narratione ipsa fuerat, in febribus cordis ac iecoris, in attonito morbo cerebrum cum corde, in asclite renes, omentum, iecur, peritoneon. Namque alia sunt ut principia, alia autem ex morbo oblaeduntur. In arcuato [Venice, 1545: arquato] fel et sima seu cava iecoris: in mala concoctione ventriculus [Venice, 1545: vermiculus): at in doloribus satis manifesta est ratio, dicente Hippocrate, quod ubi dolor, ibi est morbus." ("Quod raro et oscitanter adminstrationem exercent anatomicam," MM sectio 1 [= *De malo usu*], 89, *Opera* 7:238.)

23. VP 4, *Opera* 1:4; VP 25, *Opera* 1:16. Salvatore Spinelli, *La Ca' Granda, 1456–1956* (Milan, 1956), p. 97. The younger Cardano and his wife were housed in the Ospedale Maggiore while he taught in this school because he held

a salaried position in a subsidiary institution of the hospital—not because they were paupers in the workhouse, as is stated in some of the secondary literature.

24. Spinelli, *La Ca' Granda*, pp. 97–109, 116–29, 161–64; *La Ca' Granda: Cinque secoli di storia e d'arte dell'Ospedale Maggiore di Milano* (Milan, 1981), pp. 100–102.

25. Charles D. O'Malley and J. B. de C. M. Saunders, *Leonardo da Vinci on the Human Body: The Anatomical, Physiological, and Embryological Drawings of Leonardo da Vinci* (New York, 1952, 1982), p. 10.

26. Bylebyl, "School of Padua," pp. 346–49; idem, "Teaching *Methodus medendi* in the Renaissance," in *Galen's Method of Healing*, ed. Fridolf Kudlien and Richard J. Durling (Leiden, 1991), pp. 157–89, at pp. 184–89.

27. VP 4, *Opera* 1:4; VP 32, *Opera* 1:23. Cardano never met Vesalius in person—"Brasavolum, ut qui Ferrariensis esset, et Ferrariae moraretur, nunquam vidi: ut neque Vesalium, quamquam intimum mihi amicum" (LP 1562, *Opera* 1:138). Regarding the horoscope, see n. 2, above.

28. ". . . nam pictorem omnia necesse est scire, quia omnia imitatur. Et [Lyon, 1557: Est] philosophus pictor, architectus, et dissectionis artifex. Argumento est praeclara illa totius humani corporis imitatio, iam pluribus ante annis inchoata a Leonardo Vincio Florentino, et pene absoluta: sed deerat operi tantus artifex, ac rerum naturae indagator, quantus est Vesalius" (*De subtilitate* 17, *Opera* 3:609). Leonardo bequeathed his notebooks to his disciple Francesco Melzi (d. 1570), who kept them at his villa at Vaprio near Milan and showed them to a few visitors; see O'Malley and Saunders, *Leonardo da Vinci on the Human Body*, p. 33. Guglielmo Bilancioni, "Leonardo e Cardano," *Rivista di storia delle scienze mediche e naturali* 12 (1930): 302–29, alludes to another mention of Leonardo in *De subtilitate*, as well as to the possibility that Leonardo was acquainted with Fazio Cardano. Leonardo himself regarded both *imitatio* of nature and *inventio* (in the sense of finding out nature) as essential to painting; see Martin Kemp, "From 'Mimesis' to 'Fantasia': The Quattrocento Vocabulary of Creation, Inspiration, and Genius in the Visual Arts," *Viator* 8 (1977): 347–99, at pp. 376–77.

29. *De subtilitate* 17, *Opera* 3:609–12.

30. In *De subtilitate* bks. 11–14 are on mankind, with the titles, respectively, *De hominis necessitate et forma, De hominis natura et temperamentum, De sensibus, sensibusque et voluptate, De anima et intellectu, Opera* 3:549–86. In *De rerum varietate*, bk. 8, *De homine* contains chaps. 40–46 on, respectively, *Hominum natura, Sensus, Mens, Hominis mirabilia, Cura morborum superstitiosa, Communes calamitates, Humanarum rerum substantia, Opera* 3:146–77.

31. *De subtilitate* 11, *Opera* 3:555–56. On the history of Renaissance enthusiasm for theories of human proportion (most ultimately derived from Vitruvius), see Erwin Panofsky, "The History of the Theory of Human Proportions as a Reflection of the History of Styles," in his *Meaning in the Visual Arts* (Garden City, N.Y., 1955), pp. 55–107, and F. Zöllner, *Vitruvs Proportionsfigur: Quellenkritische Studien zur Kunstliteratur im 15. und 16. Jahrhundert* (Worms, 1987). For Vesalius's interest in proportion theory and the figure of the *homo ad circulum*, see *Fabrica* (1543) 5.3, p. 389[489] (much abbreviated in *Fabrica* [1555] p. 595). See also Pigeaud, "Formes et normes dans le *De fabrica* de

Vésale," idem, "Homo quadratus: Variations sur la beauté et la santé dans la médecine antique," *Gesnerus* 42 (1985): 337–52, and idem, "Les problèmes de la création chez Galien."

32. "Similiter est ferme, sed quasi divinius, quod medicina meditatur per has constitutiones temporum, salubritatem corporum, et morborum genera praedicere . . ." (*De subtilitate* 16, *Opera* 3:605). The passage continues on the next page; it follows a discussion of meteorological portents and phenomena and at the end merges into a discussion of divination.

33. Ferrari, "Public Anatomy Lessons," pp. 66–69; Eugenio Dall'Osso, "Aranzio, Giulio Cesare," *Dictionary of Scientific Biography* 1 (New York, 1970): 204; C. D. O'Malley, "Varolio, Costanzo," ibid., 13 (New York, 1976): 587–88; Dorothy M. Schullian, "Coiter, Volcher," ibid., 3 (New York, 1971), 342–43; Robert Herrlinger, *Volcher Coiter* (Nuremberg, 1952), pp. 18–25.

34. The date is established by the presence of Fracanzano, who taught at Bologna only for the years 1562–64; Umberto Dallari, ed., *I rotuli dei lettori legisti e artisti dello Studio bolognese dal 1384 al 1799* (Bologna, 1889), 2:156, 159.

35. For example, Galen, *De temperamentis* (*De complexionibus*) 2.6, Kühn 1:631–32; Mondino de' Liuzzi, *Anothomia*, ed. Piero P. Giorgi and Gian Franco Pasini (Bologna, 1992), p. 208. However, the editors endeavor to save Mondino by interpreting his statement "Alter ramus magnus descendit ad intestinum duodenum, ut vidisti superius, et iste bifurcatur quia ab ipso ramus parvus ramificatur, qui vadit ad fundum stomachi . . ." as referring to the main pancreatic duct.

36. Galen, *On the Usefulness of the Parts of the Body* 5.1, trans. May, 1:249.

37. VP 12, *Opera* 1:10. Ferrari, "Public Anatomy Lessons," pp. 64, 70, notes instances of the noisy and disorderly character of anatomies, and the concern of the authorities to regulate them.

38. At any rate in 1540, the lectures by Matteo Corti given jointly with Vesalius's dissection at Bologna took place in the cloister and church of San Salvatore, whereas the dissection itself was held in a room at the cloister and church of San Francesco nearby. Professors and students moved from one location to the other in a disorderly mob, according to Baldasar Heseler; Baldasar Heseler, *Andreas Vesalius' First Public Anatomy at Bologna 1540: An Eyewitness Report*, ed. Ruben Eriksson (Uppsala, 1959), p. 85, p. [344], and plate 5. After the construction of the Archiginnasio (1562–63), Aranzio carried out public anatomies in a temporary wooden anatomy theater erected inside the building each year.

39. Ibid., p. 158.

40. Alessandro Benedetti, *Historia corporis humani sive Anatomice*, (Venice, 1502), fol. 20v, translated in L. R. Lind, *Studies in Pre-Vesalian Anatomy: Biography, Translations, Documents* (Philadelphia, 1975), p. 95; I have consulted Carpi in the edition of 1535: Jacopo Berengario da Carpi, *Isagoge breves perlucide ac uberime [sic] in Anatomiam* (Venice, 1535), fol. 14r, translated in *A Short Introduction to Anatomy (Isagoge Breves)*, trans. L. R. Lind (Chicago, 1959), p. 62.

41. Niccolò Massa, *Anatomiae liber introductorius* (Venice, 1559 [colophon, 1536]), chap. 14, fol. 25v, translated in Lind, *Studies in Pre-Vesalian Anatomy*, p. 193; Vesalius, *Fabrica* (1543) 5.8, pp. 509–11.

42. Falloppia, *Observationes anatomicae*, fols. 177r–179r.

43. The only edition is Cardano, *Anathomiae Mundini cum expositione*, *Opera* 10:129–67.

44. Martinotti, "L'insegnamento dell'anatomia in Bologna," pp. 63–65; Dallari, *I rotuli* 2:93; Bylebyl, "School of Padua," pp. 356–57; on the extent to which contemporary debates were introduced into some commentaries on traditional medical texts, see Siraisi, *Avicenna*, pp. 221–352.

45. Durling, *Catalogue*, nos. 1058–60, lists editions of Corti's commentary on Mondino, published in Pavia, 1550, and Lyon, 1551; a third edition appeared in Venice, 1580. For Cardano's personal relations with and estimate of Corti, his former teacher, see chap. 2, above.

46. " . . . circa quam etiam hallucinantur Curtius" (comm. Mondino, *Opera* 10:143); "Verum non est credendum quod Curtius, qui fuit vir tanti ingenii et eruditionis, haec non intellexerit, quae vel initiatus medicinae vel philosophiae per se intelligeret" (ibid.); "Curtius multa dicit de triplici cute, quae omnino sunt inania" (ibid., p. 149); "Mundinus autem deteriores habuit translationes Galeni quam Princeps" (ibid., p. 155). Other examples could be cited.

47. "Nos ergo cum dirigamus totam hanc tractationem ad utilitatem medici . . . " (ibid., *Opera* 10:151).

48. Ibid., pp. 131, 150. Andreas Vesalius, *Anatomicarum Gabrielis Falloppii observationum examen* . . . (Venice, 1564).

49. *Contradictiones* 4.16, "Venarum fibrae, an opus peculiare habeant"; 17, "Ventriculi tunica interior an trahat"; 18, "Musculi an moveantur a fibris"; 19, "Musculi abdominis an octo"; 20, "Musculi recti abdominis, an ab osse pubis oriantur"; 21, "An musculi recti sint superiores obliquis?"; 22, "Musculi substantia an caro, vel fibrae et tendo"; "Musculus quilibet an in tendonem finiatur? Ligamenta an sentiant et valde. Musculo cuique an oppositus musculus factus est?"; *Opera* 6:695–704. References to Falloppia on pp. 695, 696, 700–701, and an allusion to Vesalius as alive and almost fifty years old on p. 703 (Cardano had learned Vesalius's birthdate at the time he cast his horoscope) establish that this group of *quaestiones* was written between 1561, when Falloppia's *Observationes anatomicae* were published, and 1563.

50. "Utrum vero anathomia debeat dici scientia, ars, neutrum, sed sola cognitio sensus, dico quod ut habetur *secundo Posteriorum* ex experimentis pluribus fit experientia, ex experientia fit ars, et ideo dico quod primum est ars, quia est recta ratio agendorum. Declaro modo quod sit scientia quoniam cum demonstrantur posteriora ex prioribus fit scientia, sed in anathomia hoc contingit et Aristoteles tradit scientiam *in libris de animalibus* et non potest haberi scientia nisi ex his quae sint per intellectum vel sapientiam vel per sensum, cognitio autem connexorum seu orationum necessario est non per sensum, licet medio sensus, cum ergo additur causa, et fit generalis transit in scientiam, ergo anathomia sine cognitione huius partis est ars, et cum ex cognitione est scientia" (Cardano, *In primam primi Hasen [= Avicenna, Canon 1.1] commentarii* 1.29, *Opera* 9:487). These lectures were delivered both at Pavia in 1561 and at Bologna in 1563 (ibid., pp. 455, 458).

51. "Exemplum adhibeo de oculo, oculum etiam patet sensu rursus et partes illius, sed non quod sint partes oculi hoc enim ad rationem pertinet, post quod oculus videat non sensu ipso deprehenditur. Sed videre sensu deprehendimus,

oculo ergo oculum video, communi sensu deprehendo me videre; ratione igitur adhibita cum cognoscam clauso oculo me non videre, aperto videre, ex his construo rationem igitur homo videt per oculum si igitur addantur his rationes ut pote quod oculus est lucidus et quod, species relucet in eo tamquam in speculo et illa species est ibi ergo deprehenditur spiritu quia est instrumentum animae ergo anima videt per oculum si enim supponamus quod anima potest comprehendere, et istud est altioris scientiae, itaque aut omnino nihil scimus aut haec est vera scientia, concludo ergo quod anathomia est vera scientia sicut sunt reliquae quicquid enim dixeris de hoc, dicam ego, de aliis etiam obiiciam partibus philosophiae naturalis; anathomia ergo scientia est et praeclara" (ibid., p. 487).

52. "Non eadem est ratio in artibus quae in scientiis praefationis, neque numerus idem eorum quae ante exercitationem atque traditionem novisse oportet. Quippe artes praeter certam tradendi viam aut inveniendi, exercendi quoque modum docere debent" (comm. Mondino, proem, *Opera* 10:129).

53. "Porro haec ars ad hanc usque diem minime recte tradita est, non solum quod omnis ars et praesertim difficillima, qualis ista est, quotidie suscipiat incrementam, sed quoniam qui eam tradiderunt artis dialecticae penuria laborarunt, quam neque nos ad annum usque quinquagesimum octavum attigimus. Itaque cum una tantum dialecticae regula, Ptolomaeus [*sic*] tria pulcherrima opera construxerit, magnam scilicet compositionem, astrorum praenotiones, et divinam Musicam, secum quisque reputet, quantum ex quadraginta quatuor regulis (tot enim invenimus, ipsa enim ars seipsam docet, quemadmodum et inter maechanicas fabrilis sibi maleum et incudem fabricat) proficere potuerimus" (ibid.). Regarding the composition of Cardano's *Dialectica*, *Opera* 1:293–308, see LP 1562, *Opera* 1:113. On sixteenth-century concepts and accounts of discovery, invention, and enlargement or accumulation of knowledge, see Paolo Rossi, *Philosophy, Technology and the Arts in the Early Modern Era* (New York, 1970), pp. 66–99.

54. "Quarta est consensus vinculumque partium quae pro instrumentis habentur: velut ventriculi cum iecore, quae cum pulcherrima esset ac medicinae utilissima, quaeque rem prae oculis ipsis poneret, hanc tamen omnes anatomici quantum diligentes praetermisere, ob difficultatem credo" (ibid.).

55. Ibid., pp. 129, 137.

56. "adeo ut viderim aliquos (male curatos tamen) quorum dolor renali ex lapide (lithiasin Graeci vocant) duravit ferme per tres menses. quorum unum ex familia lanceorum nomine Simonem curavi in paulo plus quam sex horis ex scientia anathomica" (ibid., p. 165).

57. "Itaque si hominem dissecuerimus corporum sanandorum causa, anatomia medicae artis pars est: si ut naturae diligentiam contemplemur, et satrapae sapientiam et Dei maiestatem, nostr[or]umque omnium curam, naturalis philosophia est et divina ac theologia prorsus; sin ludibrii causa, amentia, sin odii, crudelitas: ergo dissectionis opus, quod trium maximarum disciplinarum partem non vulgarem occupet, minime inter mediocria reponendum est" (ibid., p. 130).

58. Ibid., pp. 134–36. On his use of the term *foliata*, see further below; Andrew Cunningham, "Fabricius and the 'Aristotle Project' in Anatomical Teaching and Research at Padua, " in *The Medical Renaissance of the Sixteenth Century*, ed. Andrew Wear, Roger French, and I. M. Lonie (Cambridge, 1985),

pp. 195–222; Findlen, *Possessing Nature*, pp. 208–20; Schullian, "Coiter, Volcher."

59. "Nec placet ut novo mortis genere ac magis terribili occidantur ob spectaculum, neque enim tanti est discrimen suffocati ab eo qui laqueo suspensus est ut crudeliter homines occidamus, verum suffocare aquis lentus [*sic*] est mortis genus" (comm. Mondino, *Opera* 10:136).

60. "Nec placet quod qui ostendit, loquatur de morbis ac symptomatibus, sed hoc pertinet ad professorem medicinae. Curatio vero quae pendet ex anathomia debet docere ab ipso professore [*sic*] verbo: modus autem operandi ab eo qui dissecat" (ibid.).

61. Ibid., pp. 130–31. On Mondino, see Siraisi, *Taddeo Alderotti*, pp. 66–71; Piero P. Giorgi, introduction to Mondino de' Liuzzi, *Anothomia*, pp. 1–91. One of Mondino's scholastic commentaries has been edited, namely, *Mondini de Leuciis Expositio super capitulum de generatione embrionis Canonis Avicennae cum quibusdam quaestionibus*, ed. Romana Martorelli Vico (Rome, 1993).

62. Following a passage denouncing princes for their failure to patronize good medicine, Cardano added, "non potest Caesar vituperari inter caeteros, qui Vesalium apud se habeat, hominem antiquam redolentem ingenuitatem" (*Contradictiones* 1.2.8, *Opera* 6:323). Some of Cardano's remarks about Vesalius, including those in the commentary on Mondino, are discussed in Ongaro, "Girolamo Cardano e Andrea Vesalio."

63. " . . . viro clarissimo et amico nostro . . ." (VP 4, *Opera* 1:4). On Rheticus and Cardano's horoscope for Vesalius, see n. 2 to this chapter. Cardano is also said to have written a (lost) biography of Vesalius in the form of an independent work; see Ongaro, "Girolamo Cardano e Andrea Vesalio," pp. 55–56.

64. In fact, Vesalius left a daughter.

65. "Nec hoc dixerim ut Vesalii gloriae aliquid detraham, quem non divinum (absit enim hoc) appellabo, huiusmodi faciunt hi, qui viventi perperam adulabantur hoc nomine, rebus autem ipsis insidiabantur et contradicebant: verum hominem ego appellabo humana conditione altiorem, et inventis admirabilem, qui eam partem tantum omisit ut lucro et ambitioni satisfaceret, qua in re omnes alios praeclaros viros secutus est, quod ei male cessit. Gloriae enim inter mortales plus satis habuit, non solum quam speraverit, sed etiam quam concupierit, medicus Caesaris, medicus Philippi regis omnium regum quorum memoria extat potentissimi, servato illi sua arte a morte evidenti Carolo unico eius filio, ita ut e faucibus orci vere rectus dici posset. Verum ipse invidiae stimulis vexatus, praeposteram navigationem aggressus, mortuus est paulo maior quinquagesimo anno, sine sobole, addicatus a studio litterarum, gloriam suam fraudavit, opes dispersit, magnum cumulum verisimile est peccatorum se contulisse, hi fructus anlarum [*sic*: aularum] regiarum et immoderatae cupiditatis, tam labilis boni" (comm. Mondino, *Opera* 10:153).

66. Jean Matal (Metellus), letter to George Cassandre, April 15, 1565, printed in J.-P. Nicéron, *Mémoires pour servir à l'histoire des hommes illustrés dans la république des lettres* (Paris, 1731), 10:153–54. A letter by Matal to Arnold Birckmann on the same topic, published in *Illustrium et clarorum virorum epistolae selectiores, superiore saeculo scriptae vel a Belgis, vel ad Belgas* (Leiden, 1617), ep. 72, pp. 370–85, is translated in O'Malley, *Andreas Vesalius*, pp. 310–11. Jean

Matal (1510–97) spent much time in Italy in the 1540s and 1550s, when he was joined with Antonio Agustín in investigating texts of Roman law; subsequently, Matal spent much of the latter part of his life in Cologne. See Jean-Louis Ferrary, ed., *Correspondance de Lelio Torelli avec Antonio Agustín et Jean Matal (1542–1553)* (Como, 1992) (which does not, of course, contain the letters about the death of Vesalius), and Ron Truman, "Jean Matal and His Relations with Antonio Agustín, Jerónimo Osório da Fonseca and Pedro Ximenes," in *Antonio Agustín between Renaissance and Counter-Reform*, ed. M. H. Crawford, Warburg Institute Surveys and Texts 24 (London, 1993), pp. 247–63.

67. See, for example, VP 32, *Opera* 1:23–24.

68. In Cardano's dialogue *Carcer* the speakers are Lucilius and Hieronymus.

L. Sed tu eras dives tum.

H. Neque eram, neque sum, cum nec habeam in redditibus centum coronatos, sextam partem annuae impense.

L. Hui non plus.

H. Non.

L. Existimabam, ut alii etiam multi credunt, te divitem.

H. Sed falso.

L. Verum putant te habere pecunias?

H. Habeo ex patrimonio vendito: sed ubi agellum emero, vix redditus impense quatuor mensium sufficient, id est tertia partis anni.

L. Non plus?

H. Non.

L. Habes tamen domum?

H. Nil aliud.

L. Valde pauper es.

H. Magis quam vellem.

L. Gaudeo quod videam te hilari animo paupertatem ferentem. (Biblioteca Apostolica Vaticana, MS Chigi E. V. 171, Hieronymi Cardani dialogus cui nomen Carcer, fol. 18r)

Lucilius was identified by Leone Allaci as Lucillo Maggi, a professor of medicine at Pavia, imprisoned by the Inquisition in 1563, but a Stoic allusion (to Seneca's correspondent Lucilius) may well be present simultaneously. Regarding this dialogue, see Eugenio Di Rienzo, "Cardaniana: Su alcuni manoscritti inediti di Cardano conservati alla Biblioteca Vaticana," *Rivista di storia e letteratura religiosa* 25 (1989): 102–10. I am grateful to Alfonso Ingegno for drawing my attention to this article.

69. A. Bertolotti, "I testamenti di Girolamo Cardano, medico, filosofo e matematico nel secolo XVI," *Archivio storico lombardo* 9 (1882): 615–60.

70. Comm. Mondino, proem, *Opera* 10:133.

71. Ibid., pp. 151, 132.

72. Ibid. On the durable connections between public dissection and punishment of criminals, see Carlino, *La fabbrica del corpo*, passim.

73. "Prima est oratio quae debet esse continua, ordinata, dilucida, diffusaque, ut res ipsa oculis subiiciatur, quae partes aliquo modo magis desiderantur in Vessalio [*sic*] quam Galeno, idque obtigit quod Galenus florenti eloquentia Asiatica

praeditus esset, quae nulla in parte opportunior est, quam in huiusmodi tracta-
tione. At contra Vessalius aridus, brevis, succinctus, asper, mente intenta potius
quam proloquio leni, minime huic negotio accommodatus nisi alter Vessalius
eum legat ac interpretetur: praetereaquam brevi tempore et maxime iuvenis
mirum dictu scilicet trigesimo tertio anno aetatis suae, quo ego tempore nondum paginam scripseram quam non flammis mandaverim, aut mandari cupiam"
(comm. Mondino, *Opera* 10:133). Vesalius was actually twenty-nine when the
Fabrica was published.

74. Ibid.

75. See Vesalius, *Fabrica* (1543), two pages of plates at end of bk. 3, following p. 312[412]; Andreas Vesalius, *De humani corporis fabrica librorum Epitome* (Basel, 1543; copy with cutout and pasted figures, New York Academy of
Medicine); J. B. de C. M. Saunders and Charles D. O'Malley, *The Illustrations
from the Works of Andreas Vesalius of Brussels* (Cleveland, 1950; New York,
1973), pp. 220–26. On anatomical fugitive sheets, see Leroy Crummer, "Early
Anatomical Fugitive Sheets," *Annals of Medical History* 5 (1923): 189–209, and
Andrea Carlino, "'Knowe thyself': Anatomical Figures in Early Modern Europe," *Res 27, Anthropology and Aesthetics* (Spring 1995): 52–69.

76. "Demum ad tertium genus repraesentationis transeundum divisis foliatis
in ichnographicas descriptiones quas ex Vessalio velut satis absolutas desumere
licebit" (comm. Mondino, *Opera* 10:133). The suggestion would not have
pleased Vesalius, who vigorously denounced unauthorized combinations of his
plates with other texts.

77. Charles Estienne, *De dissectione partium corporis humani libri tres* (Paris,
1545).

78. "Defecit [Vesalius] quoque quod ichnographiam tantum partium humani
corporis licet cum umbris scripserit, cum necessarium fuisset foliatum, vel saltem
ichnographiam cum oratione luculenta, quae ascensum, decensum, accessum, re-
cessum, flexionem, crassitiem, magnitudinem, colorem, substantiam, regionem,
propinquitatem ad notissima loca, formam, et ad totius membri partium compa-
rationem describere. Defecit et ea in parte quam diximus negligenter ab omnibus
tractatam, quaeque plurimum necessaria est, et maxime pulchra, scilicet in partium quae instrumenti vicem gerunt progressu, situ, forma, comparatione.
Verum cum his omnibus tanto quod ad anatomiam pertinent ordine, perfec-
tione, veritate, repraesentationeque Galenum antecellit, quanto Galenus omnes
reliquos qui nunc extant. Post illum descripsit Carolus Stephanus anatomiam
quandam ex Vessalio sumptam, cuius tamen ne meminet quidem satis facilem, et
multo satis imperfectiorem: hoc unum tantum addens quod ichnographiam mediam ac ad foliatum accedentem opposuit. Namque lineis eductis, quae supra sint
quaeque infra iaceant, indicat, minuens etiam inventionis laborem, qui apud Ves-
salium certe non levis est, sed facile est inventis addere. Referunt et quosdam
esse nunc claros viros, qui nonnulla invenerint Vessalio incognita ab eo perperam
tradita, de quibus locis suis agemus. Vidimus et ichnographiam Leonardi Florentini pictoris manu descriptam, pulchram sane et tam celebri artifice dignam,
sed prorsus inutilem: quod eius esset qui nec numerum intestinorum nosceret.
Erat enim purus pictor non medicus nec philosophus" (comm. Mondino, *Opera*
10:131).

79. "Quod vero praeter libros maximam afferre posset utilitatem . . . esset constructio sceleti, non illius vulgaris ex ossibus humanis sed totius corporis, sic ut nihil prorsus desideraretur. Itaque ex dura materia conficere ipsum oporteret, ne tantus labor totque annorum, tantaque impensa brevi periret, sed et ductili ut minima quaeque effingi possent et flecti et dirigi quaqua versum. Quamobrem neque lapide, neque ligno, nec ebore, nec cera nec terra fingi debet, sed metallo. . . . ex aere purgato atque molli partim albo partim naturali, rubroque, tum aliis infecto coloribus prout in libro de secretis docuimus per chymicum conficiatur. Sed et ratio structurae ibi declarata est, ea enim constat sic ut quemadmodum in dissectione partes a partibus auferri possint, singulae a singulis et ut repositae continuitatis ratio atque species servetur viginti annorum hoc opus esset, spectataeque doctrinae medico indigeret, atque plastico artifice singularis industriae atque subtilitatis: dignum certe opus principe aliquo praestanti, cum tot pecunias in scurras nullo usu, alii in adulatores, alii in lenones cum infamia effundant, quidam in bella intempestiva, in quibus praeter hominem caedes et incendia aedificiorum nobilium nihil spectatur commodi aut lucri, alii in moles maximas, alii in aedes magnificas, alii in machinas, quae coeli motum repraesentant, nulla tamen utilitatis ratione aut certi finis scientia immensos thesauros profundunt. Hac vero fabrica quid generosius, quid praeclarius, quid pulchrius, quod [sic] utilius, quam posse semetipsum videre, qualiter se interius habeant omnia viscera sensus, penetraliaque naturae; idque posse etiam ostendere philosophiae ac veritatis studiosis, quandoquidem nullum sit illustrius spectaculum, aut admirabilius sub luna structura humani corporis, idque etiam medicis ut sine horrore ullo aut tetri odoris periculo spectare possint, quotidie, quae non tam sunt utilia ac salubria, quam etiam necessaria saluti aegrotantium, quorum magna pars perit ex ignoratione medicorum, circa ea, quae ad compositionem, situm, consensum, magnitudinemque membrorum interiorum attinent. Tum vero in chirurgis tanta necessitas est huius scientiae . . ." (ibid., pp. 133–34).

80. Judging by the reference to size of the internal organs in the passage just quoted.

81. Thomas N. Haviland and Lawrence C. Parish, "A Brief Account of the Use of Wax Models in the Study of Medicine," *Journal of the History of Medicine and Allied Sciences* 25 (1970): 52–75.

82. Herrlinger, *Volcher Coiter*, pp. 104–15; Schullian, "Coiter, Volcher." The model does not survive. On Nicholas Neufchatel, the artist, and his activity in Nuremberg, see Ulrich Thieme and Felix Becker, *Allgemeines Lexikon der bildenden Künstler*, ed. Hans Vollmer, vol. 25 (Leipzig, 1931), p. 407. Two copies of the portrait, without the anatomical model, were also painted in the sixteenth century.

83. "Firmissima artis medicae fundamenta iactavimus, dum descripta humani corporis consectione, omnes eius particulas singillatim ob oculos proposuimus. . . Itaque ut ad historiae fidem geographia, sic ad rem medicam corporis humani descriptio pernoscenda" (Fernel, *Universa medicina*; *Physiologia* 1.16, "Consectionis ratio" (pp. 41–45), concluding "Peroratio"; ibid., *Pathologia* 5.10, "Pulmonum morbi, symptomata, causae et signa" (pp. 269–72). On the latter chapter see Esmond R. Long, "Jean Fernel's Conception of Tuberculosis," in *Science, Medicine and History*, ed. E. Ashworth Underwood, 2 vols. (Oxford, 1953),

1:401–7; clinical observations similar to Fernel's had been made previously but not their correlation with specific lesions of the lungs.

84. "Indicio duo sunt quae publice Bononiae pollicebar. . . . Aliud (ut tamen liberum esset conditionem mihi recipere vel non) ut si moriturus esset ager, locum morbi ostenderem, et si mortuo illo aberrassem, teneri poena centupli acceptarum pecuniarum: Itaque cum plurimi aperte primum sperantes me arguere posse, quod aberrassem, corpora dissecuissent, ut Senatoris Ursi, Doctoris Peregrini, Georgii Ghisileri [*sic*]: In quo illud visum est admirabile praedixisse me morbum fore in iecore, cum urinae essent optimae? incolumem vero ventriculum qui perpetuo doleret: post clam multos alios, nunquam errare me invenerunt, nec conditionem recipere ausi, nec ut reciperetur consuluerunt" (VP 40, *Opera* 1:33); similarly VP 42, *Opera* 1:36, where the fee is specified as ten crowns, but the odds reduced to ten to one. For Cardano's other challenge, see chap. 2, above.

85. Comm. *Prognost.*, bk. 3 (of commentary), *prognosticon* 59, *Opera* 8:705–6. The first edition is Cardano, *In Hippocratis Coi prognostica opus divinum. . . . Atque etiam in Galeni prognosticorum expositionem, commentarii absolutissimi* (Basel, 1568; IA *132. 102). The work was completed in December 1566 (*Opera* 8:584) and is based on lectures given at Bologna in the 1565–66 academic year (*In Hippocratis Coi prognostica* [Basel, 1568], cols. 7–8).

86. "Ita cum nunc invecta sit anatomia corporum humanorum ignota Galeno, atque Hippocratis aetate sic amissa, quae tum nota erat ars curandi empycos, pectus secando aegrorum nunc est. Ergo cum sint tria genera signorum. Pathognomicon quod in pretio non est, quoniam de his non est quae sensu vulgaribus possint ostendi: velut si quis dicat, 'hic homo laborat obstructione, aut ardente febre,' dicunt plebei homines, et imperiti, 'qui scit? ita dicit, quia coargui de hoc non potest. Deus novit: forsan ita est, forsan non' " (comm. *Prognost.* 3.59, *Opera* 8:705).

87. "Alterum est prognosticum celebre quidem, et in quo ars medici illustratur, sed parum tamen ad authoritatem medici utilis est ob duas causas. Una quidem, quod huiusmodi divinatio medicinae a pluribus esse non creditur. . . . Altera causa potentior est: quoniam haec praedictio ad salutem infirmi tametsi utilis sit, non tamen quantum satis esset, quod utilis adeo sit, imo ne *gry* quidem, ut Graeci dicere solent, conferre videtur" (ibid.).

88. "Unde emersit tertium genus signorum nobilissimum, in quo ego fortunatissimus fui atque primus qui id aetate mea et forsan primus omnium etiam ante nos qui id introduxerim, aususque fuerim in medium praeponere atque tentare: scilicet ut dicerem quo morbo et in qua parte corporis quove in membro laboraret aeger, quod si quispiam aliorum medicorum curationi nostrae obniteretur, ut ostenderem ubi ille periisset, dissecto cadavere, me vera docuisse, culpa alterius illum mortuum esse, quod cum saepe et saepe ut dixi fecisse, eo redacta est, ut summa felicitate, cum omnes qui sanare possent, sanarentur, et maxima cum autoritate curarem in posterum aegros, contradicente nemine. Hoc genus signorum percelebre est, cui ego evidentium nomen imposui" (ibid., pp. 705–6).

89. Heinrich Von Staden, "Anatomy as Rhetoric: Galen on Dissection and Persuasion," *Journal of the History of Medicine and Allied Sciences* 50 (1995):

47–66; more generally, on the influence of classical *exempla* on scientific activity in the Renaissance, see Findlen, *Possessing Nature*, pp. 193–354.

90. "Aetate autem hac adeo ea mire fortunatus fui, ut non solum id facile obtinerem, sed necessarii vel ultro offerent, vel etiam rogarent. Nec vilis personae, ob tonsoris proemium, sed nobilium omnium fuere cadavera. Quin etiam principum, ut scitis, mos est, ut servare corpus possint, secare illa, et eximere viscera et cerebrum" (comm. *Prognost.* 3.59, *Opera* 8:706).

91. N. 38, above.

92. ". . . postquam adeo clare omnia inspexerunt, etiam contra Galeni praecepta et ut dicebant, medicinae axiomata, velut in patricio fratre Hectoris Ghislerii (quem honoris causa nomino) quem ego levitate intestinorum laborantem, et ventriculi symptomate, cum optimis urinis morientem, bis, aut ter iam inspectum, pronunciassem, ventriculum habere illaesum, iecur autem exustum, atque putrefactum totum, ac nigrum, cum etiam modica siti laboraret, atque ita inventum est, dissecto cadavere in aede B. Francisci astantibus medicis Antonio Gandulfo, Camillo Montagnana, et Caesare Arantio praeclaro anatomico admirantes" (comm. *Prognost.* 3.59, *Opera* 8:706). For the autopsy of this individual, see also n. 84, above.

93. "Ita constat, quod hoc genere signorum si quis profecerit, dicta illius in arte pro oraculis accipienda esse, etiam ab aemulis: neque enim aliorum ad evidentium genus est nulla comparatio" (ibid.).

94. Ibid. 2.2–3, *Opera* 8:649–50. The passage specifies "haec scribo VII scilicet Idus septembris anni MDLXVI," and states of Pellegrini "mortuus est enim ieri." See further chap. 8.

95. "Rogatum igitur ut dissecarem, accessi cum Germano anatomico egregio, et qui artem profitebatur, Folcherio, et dissecuimus: nec in musculo partis dextrae, nec in iecore, nec in ullo viscerum inferiorum inventus est scirrhus, nec aliquid duri, solum iecur languidioris coloris, et dilutioris, scilicet [ad] albedinem tendentis, conspeximus, verum ipsum non solis vinculis transversis, ut in caeteris hominibus, annexum erat septotransverso, sed eidem ferme totum per alia vincula connexum erat, ut tota illa pars eidem iungeretur: similiter et ventriculus ipse connexus erat per ligamenta, praeter naturam, ipsi septo rursus pulmo totus ima parte eodem modo per vincula iunctus erat eidem septotransverso undique, et circumcirca membranae costas succingenti ante, retro, et a lateribus, quod etiam dicebat ipse Folcherius observasse in aliis multis, qui praesertim ex phtisi [*sic*] obierant, erat praeterea pulmo maximus, ut pene totum pectus occuparet et pericardio annexum: plenus autem totus scirrhis, ac vesicis aqua plenis" (ibid.).

96. Cardano, comm. 1 *Epid.* 1, *Opera* 10:205; comm. 1 *Epid.* 2, ibid., p. 261 (referring to a different occasion). Cardano's lectures on the *Epidemics* were given in the academic year 1563–64 (see further chap. 6) and were probably written as he went along.

97. Harvey Cushing, *A Bio-Bibliography of Andreas Vesalius* (New York, 1943), pp. 124–25, describing the English edition of Thomas Geminus, *Compendiosa totius Anatomie delineatio* (London, 1553). For this edition, the indexes to the Vesalian plates were translated by Nicholas Udall. For the text of Vesalius's *Epitome* (used in the Latin edition of 1545) Geminus and Udall sub-

stituted a text similar to that used by Thomas Vicary in his *Anatomie of the Bodie of Man* (1548), rearranged to follow the order of Mondino. This text was drawn from a fourteenth-century English translation of Henri de Mondeville's work.

CHAPTER 6
THE NEW HIPPOCRATES

1. *De subtilitate libri XXI* (Lyon, 1550), bk. 16, pp. 524–27. Cardano allowed that literary figures (Homer, Virgil) were also gifted, but not with subtlety. In this passage, he seems to have been thinking of subtlety both as a personal quality and as one that involved mathematical or other technical knowledge.

2. "Neque est unum genus subtilitatis in quo auctores celebrantur, sed plura. Aristotelis ab ingenio, cuius aemuli Theophrastus et Scotus. Ab ingenio, ac imaginatione, ut Calculatoris. A sensu cum imaginatione, ut Euclidis. A iudicio: ut Algebra. A sensu atque experientia, ut Vitruvii. . . . Atque hi omnes ingenio praestiterunt, sed qui humanas vires supergressi propioresque divinitati cuipiam [*sic*] fuisse videntur, tres sunt: Ptolemaeus Alexandrinus, Hippocrates Cous, et Plotinus" (*De subtilitate libri XXI* [Basel, 1560], bk. 16, p. 1013 [with the entire list and discussion, pp. 1010–15]; *Opera* 3:607–8). Hippocrates and Plotinus do not appear at all in the first version of the list. The list still appears in its original form in *De subtilitate libri XXI* (Lyon, 1559), pp. 569–70. Margolin, "Cardan, interprète d'Aristote," pp. 308–10, discusses the list of twelve and its revision without commenting on the second set of three introduced in the revised version. The three separate editions of *De subtilitate*, each issued in a number of printings, are distinguished in *The First Book of Jerome Cardan's De Subtilitate*, ed. and trans. Myrtle Marguerite Cass (Williamsport, Pa., 1934), pp. 16–18.

3. "Nam sublimia illa atque divina queque nemo preter Plotinum attigit, ortumque mortalium rerum omnium et finem septem libris *de Aeternitatis arcanis* amplexi sumus" (RV [Basel, 1557], dedicatory epistle, fol. bb v); this passage and that cited in the previous note are quoted and the role of Plotinus in Cardano's philosophy of nature is discussed in Eckhard Kessler, "*Alles ist Eines wie der Mensch und das Pferd*. Zu Cardanos Naturbegriff," Kessler, pp. 91–114. Brian Copenhaver, "Renaissance Magic and Neoplatonic Philosophy: 'Ennead' 4. 3–5 in Ficino's 'De vita coelitus comparanda,'" in *Marsilio Ficino e il ritorno di Platone: Studi e documenti*, ed. Gian Carlo Garfagnini (Florence, 1986), 2:451–69, calls attention to the influence of Plotinus on Renaissance magic. The only modern study specifically devoted to Cardano's Hippocratism known to me is Pigeaud, "L'Hippocratisme de Cardan."

4. "Nam cum universum opus prognosticum sit totum, ad futurorum expectationem ac divinationem spectat. . . . Res divina est prorsus divinatio, quae a divinitate originem nominis sumpsit. Eo nomine oracula omnia illustrata tum Sibillaes [*sic*] tum vero Astrologi, Medici, Physiognomi, Metoposcopi, Aruspices, Augures, Chiromantici, Brixomantes, Nautae, agricolae, bellique duces: tum singuli quique e prophetarum genere ac vatum atque alii multi in clarissimos viros evasere, et pro diis habiti sunt" (Cardano, comm. *Epid.*, proem, *Opera* 10:194). Barton, *Power and Knowledge*, provides a thought-provoking account

of parallels among interpretative practices in late ancient physiognomy and astrology and Galen's medical prognosis.

5. See chaps. 3 and 4.

6. There is very little astronomical material of any kind in the Hippocratic
corpus, but what there is is concentrated in the treatises named; see Otta Wenskus, *Astronomische Zeitangaben von Homer bis Theophrast*, Hermes: Zeitschrift
für klassische Philologie, Einzelschriften 55 (Stuttgart, 1990), pp. 93–123.

7. Medieval Latin manuscripts of works attributed to Hippocrates are listed
in Pearl Kibre, *Hippocrates latinus* (New York, 1985).

8. For example, there were a number of signs of interest in Hippocrates in
Florentine humanist and medical circles in the 1490s. A recently copied manuscript of the corpus in Greek (now Biblioteca Laurenziana cod. 74. 1) belonged
to Lorenzo de' Medici; see André Rivier, *Recherches sur la tradition manuscrite
du traité hippocratique "De morbo sacro"* (Berne, 1962), pp. 122–25. About
1490, Poliziano undertook a (lost) retranslation of Galen's commentary on the
Aphorisms (which includes the text); Lorenzo Lorenzani, a professor of medicine
at Pisa and a member of Poliziano's circle, published a translation of the same
work in 1494 (it was also translated by the doyen of medical humanists, Niccolò
Leoniceno of Ferrara, ca. 1490). Lorenzani and Manente Leontini, physician to
Lorenzo de' Medici, duke of Urbino, were both interested in further Hippo-
cratic translation projects. For these and related developments, see Augusto
Campana, "Manente Leontini Fiorentino, medico e traduttore di medici greci,"
La Rinascita 4 (1961): 499–15, and A. Perosa, "Codici di Galeno postillati da
Poliziano," in *Umanesimo e Rinascimento: Studi offerti a Paul Oskar Kristeller*,
ed. Vittore Branca et al. (Florence, 1980), pp. 80–87.

9. *Hippocratis Octoginta volumina . . . per M. Fabium Calvum Latinitate donata . . .* (Rome, 1525); . . . *Omnia opera Hippocratis* (Venice, 1526) (on these
editions, see G. Maloney and R. Savoie, *Cinq cent ans de bibliographie hippocratique, 1483–1982* [St.-Jean-Chrysostome, Québec, 1982], nos. 92 and 102). On
Calvo, his translation, and its publication, see Giovanni Mercati, "Su Francesco
Calvo da Menaggio primo stampatore e Marco Fabio Calvo da Ravenna primo
traduttore latino del corpo ippocratico," *Notizie varie di antica letteratura medica e di bibliografia, Studi e testi* 31 (Rome, 1917): 47–71; *Oeuvres complètes
d'Hippocrate*, ed. E. Littré (Paris, 1861), 10:LXI; Giovanni Mercati, "Altre notizie di M. Fabio Calvo," *Bessarione* 25 (1919): 159–63; Johann Ilberg, "Zur
Ueberlieferung des hippokratischen Corpus," *Rheinisches Museum für Philologie*
21 (1887): 436–61, at pp. 444–46.

10. . . . . *Hippocratis Coi . . . libri omnes ad vetustos codices summo studio col-
lati et restaurati* (Basel, 1538; Maloney and Savoie, *Cinq cent ans*, no. 167) and
*Hippocratis Coi, medicorum omnium longe principis, opera quae apud nos extant
omnia. Per Janum Cornarium . . . Latina lingua conscripta* (Basel, 1546; Maloney and Savoie, *Cinq cent ans*, no. 231). Cornarius's translation was also published in Venice and Paris in 1546 (Maloney and Savoie, *Cinq cent ans*, nos.
228–30, 232). For a listing of Hippocratic publications (editions, translations,
commentaries, and compendia, including reissues) in the fifty years following the
appearance of the Aldine edition, see Maloney and Savoie, *Cinq cent ans*, pp. 38–
73.

11. Anthony Grafton, *Joseph Scaliger: A Study in the History of Classical Scholarship*, vol. 1, *Textual Criticism and Exegesis* (Oxford, 1983), pp. 180–82. On Renaissance Hippocratism, see Vivian Nutton, "Hippocrates in the Renaissance," in *Die hippokratischen Epidemien: Theorie-Praxis-Tradition*, ed. Gerhard Baader and Rolf Winau, *Sudhoffs Archiv*, Beiheft 27 (Stuttgart, 1989), 420–39; also Wesley D. Smith, *The Hippocratic Tradition* (Ithaca and London, 1979), pp. 13–19; Iain M. Lonie, "The Paris Hippocratics," in *The Medical Renaissance of the Sixteenth Century*, ed. A. Wear, R. K. French, and I. M. Lonie (Cambridge, 1985), pp. 155–74; Thomas and Ulrich Rütten, "Melanchthons Rede 'De Hippocrate,'" in *Melanchthon und die Naturwissenchaften seiner Zeit* (Sigmaringen, 1996).

12. Nutton, "Hippocrates in the Renaissance, pp. 422–25. Galen's influence on subsequent understanding of the Hippocratic corpus extended from his own day until long after the Renaissance; see Smith, *Hippocratic Tradition*, pp. 61–176.

13. Nutton, "Hippocrates in the Renaissance," pp. 435–38.

14. "librum primum inchoavi vagantium morborum. . . . Magnitudo ut epidemiorum Hippocratis" (LP 1544, *Opera* 1:56); "Anno autem MDXXVI cum in Saccense oppidum me contulissem . . . conscripsi Epidemiorum libros, satis exiles, et ut Hippocratis narrationi conferrentur prorsus indignos" (LP 1562, *Opera* 1:97).

15. Calvo's translation of all seven books of the *Epidemics* was preceded by that of Manente Leontini, made between 1513 and 1521 and dedicated to Pope Leo X, which, however, remained unpublished and survives in a single manuscript. Six other complete or partial Latin translations followed before the end of the century. See Innocenzo Mazzini, "Manente Leontini, Übersetzer der hippokratischen Epidemien (cod. Laurent. 73, 12): Bemerkungen zu seiner Übersetzung von Epidemien Buch 6," in *Die hippokratischen Epidemien: Theorie—Praxis—Tradition*, ed. Gerhard Baader and Rolf Winau, *Sudhoffs Archiv*, Beiheft 27 (Stuttgart, 1989), pp. 312–320, at pp. 312–15.

16. It seems unlikely that he could have been inspired to make his collection of descriptions of local diseases by the medieval "*Epidemics*," that is, a work incorporating parts of the disjointed bk. 6, which survives in a number of manuscripts and was printed in early editions of the medical handbook known as the *articella* (for example, *Articella nuperrime impressa* [Lyon, 1515], fols. lxi r–lxvii r). The most recent editors of *Epidemics*, bk. 6, believe that the medieval Latin manuscripts probably all contain either a commentary on *Epidemics* 6 by Johannes Alexandrinus, translated from Greek possibly by Bartolomeo of Messina (fl. 1258–66), or a compilation of the lemmata from the commentary in that translation; see Hippocrates, *Epidemie libro sesto*, ed. and trans. Daniela Manetti and Amneris Roselli (Florence, 1982), pp. LXII–LXIII, LXX. The twenty manuscripts in question are listed in Kibre, *Hippocrates latinus*, pp. 138–39, although with the probably incorrect attribution of a translation from Arabic to Simone of Genoa and the assertion that a commentary on *Epidemics* 6 by Galen circulated in the Middle Ages.

17. Regarding the place of the *Aphorisms*, *Prognostic*, and *Regimen in Acute Diseases* in the Latin compilation of teaching texts formed in the twelfth and

thirteenth centuries and subsequently known as the *articella*, and the Latin tradition of commentary, see Paul Oskar Kristeller, "Bartolomeo, Musandino,
Mauro di Salerno e altri antichi commentatori dell' 'Articella,' con un elenco di
testi e di manoscritti," reprinted with an expanded list of manuscripts in his *Studi
sulla scuola medica salernitana* (Naples, 1986), pp. 97–151, which makes some
corrections to the relevant entries in Kibre, *Hippocrates latinus.* On the modified
collection used in the fifteenth-century Italian universities, see Tiziana Pesenti,
"Le 'articelle' di Daniele di Marsilio Santosofia (d. 1410), professore di medicina," *Studi petrarcheschi* 7 (1990): 50–92.

18. At any rate the final published version of his commentary appears to be
mainly based on Leoniceno's translation; see further below.

19. "[In 1544] academia [of Pavia] in urbem nostram translata est: abeun-
tibus etiam professoribus ob inopiam rei pecuniariae, locum eius accepi, qui
Papie iam anno MDXXXVI pro me fuerat subrogatus, medicinamque professus
Mediolani, inde Papiae usque ad MDLI, nisi quod MDXLVI intermisi: scripsi
igitur his annis commentaria in duas primas sectiones Aphorismorum, foliis
CCLXXV, quorum initium est, 'Intermissum diu ac pene interruptum legendi
munus.' Haec autem cum Epidemiorum interpretatione in quatuordecim libros
digeram, nec solum hos, sed omnes germanos Hippocratis libros haec expositio
complectitur, non tamen verba sed solum sententias aphoristicas. . . . Quatuor
enim artes totas quatuor voluminibus complexus sum . . ." (LP 1557, *Opera*
1:69–70). The incipit does not match that of his published commentary on the
Aphorisms.

20. "Erunt autem, ut reor, si ex ungue leonem, ad chartas mille ducentas,
textus vero ipse trecentum: ut opus necesse sit in duo volumina, seu tomos di-
videre" (LP 1562, *Opera* 1:107).

21. See Silvia Rizzo, *Il lessico filologico degli umanisti* (Rome, 1984), pp. 28–
31.

22. "Ipsa tamen opera [sc. on arithmetic, astrology, music, and Hippocratic
medicine], quae dixi, quatuor praestantissima sunt meo iudicio omnium quae a
me conscripta sunt, tametsi non ignorem multos alios libros e nostris maiori in
pretio apud multitudinem habendos, velut libri de Subtilitate, de Varietate
rerum, de Arcanis aeternitatis et de Fato" (LP 1557, *Opera* 1:70).

23. "At commentaria haec in universam Hippocratis doctrinam praeter id
quod totam artem amplectuntur, historia delectant, et utilitatem secum coni-
unctam habent, scribunturque eruditis, nobilibus, divitibus; ipsa ars in venera-
tione, ipsa autoris fama inclyta, cuius nomen colitur apud omnes, ad quos
memoria eius pervenit" (LP 1562, *Opera* 1:107; and similarly in LP 1557,
Opera 1:70).

24. LP 1557, *Opera* 1:64.

25. VP 44, *Opera* 1:40.

26. He wrote three other short medical commentaries, all apparently unfinished: on Mondino's *Anatomia*, discussed in the previous chapter; on Galen's
Ars medica (lost; LP 1562, *Opera* 1:107; Bertolotti, "I testamenti," p. 651), and
on Avicenna, *Canon* 1.1 (*Opera* 9:453–567; Siraisi, *Avicenna*, pp. 256–62). Lectures on the last two would have been a routine obligation for a professor of
medical *theoria*, though Cardano's treatment of Avicenna was not routine. The

colophon, in a different and perhaps somewhat later hand than the text, of a commentary on Avicenna, *De febribus* (i.e., *Canon* 4.1) in Rome, Biblioteca Nazionale Centrale, MS S. Francesca a Ripa 33, fols. 1r–177v, reads, "explicit tractatus de febribus ca. p. Hieronimi Cardani mediolanensis in accademia Bononiense publice profitentis 1556," but I think this must be a misattribution. Cardano was not teaching at Bologna in 1556; *Canon* 4.1 was normally a text in medical *practica*, whereas his chair at both Pavia and Bologna was in *theoria*; and although I have not attempted a detailed study of this commentary, it appears to be a conventional production with no traces of his style or interests.

27. Regarding Cardano's appointment and activities at the University of Bologna, see Costa, "Gerolamo Cardano allo Studio di Bologna"; Simili, "Gerolamo Cardano, lettore e medico a Bologna," pp. 384–507; Dallari, *I rotuli* 2:155–77. The only one of his Hippocratic commentaries that is not based on lectures given at Bologna is *Examen XX aegrorum Hippocratis* (from *Epidemics* 1 and 3), *Opera* 9:36–46, which was written in 1574 (*Opera* 9:36) or 1575 according to *Libellus cui titulus est Examen XXII aegrorum Hippocratis, quem edidit Cardanus annum agens lxxiv* (Rome, 1575). I have not seen this very rare edition, which is not included in IA, and cite it from Ingegno, p. 25.

28. The commentary on the *Aphorisms* was reduced to writing in its final form in 1563, since the dedication to Pius IV is dated in the fourth year of his pontificate (*Opera* 8:215).

29. Biblioteca Apostolica Vaticana, MS vat. lat. 5848, fol. 1r, heading: "Hieronymi Cardani Mediolanensis civisque Bononiensis Professoris supra ordinarii Medicinae in expositione primorum Librorum Epidemiorum praefatio anni MCDlxiii" (the seventy-one numbered *lectiones* continue to fol. 106v). This work corresponds to *Commentarii tres in primum Epidemiorum Hippocratis librum. Commentarii duo in secundum Hippocratis [Epidemiorum] librum, Opera* 10:168–387. The division into three commentaries on *Epidemics* 1 and two on *Epidemics* 2 is found in both the manuscript and the printed edition; the division into *lectiones*, present in the manuscript, has been stripped out of the printed edition. Both manuscript and edition are incomplete and break off at the same point. The preface (fols. 1r–v and *Opera* 10:193–94) is addressed to the clergy, senate, professoriat, and students, evidently of Bologna; it refers to Cardano's exile from his homeland and his teaching of the *Aphorisms* in the previous year.

30. "Hieronymi Cardani . . . medici medicinam supra ordinariam Bononiae profitentis, in Prognosticorum Hippocratis librum, libri quatuor, Bononiae, Anno MDLXV enarrati" (Cardano, *In Hippocratis Coi prognostica* [Basel, 1568], cols. 7–8); the work was still being reduced to writing in September 1566 (comm. *Prognost.* 2.2 and 3, *Opera* 8:649).

31. "Concluditque illud dirum esse portentum, ver sine temperie, aestate sine calore, quae ambo, ut dixi, hoc anno MDLXVIII experti sumus" (comm. AAL 7.6, *Opera* 8:163); but, p. 162, "hoc anno MDLXVII." Both dates are similarly found in the edition of 1570.

32. *Hieronymi Cardani . . . in librum Hippocratis de alimento commentaria praelecta dum profiteretur supraordinariam medicinae, Bononiae anno MDLXVIII* (Rome, 1574).

33. Biblioteca Nazionale Centrale, MS S. Francesca a Ripa 11, fol. 1r, heading: "Hieronimi Cardani Mediolensis medici civisque Bononiensis professoris supraordinariam publice profitentis in libro de victu in acutis commentaria anno 1569." The manuscript (125 folios) contains 102 numbered lectures divided into four "books" of *De victu in acutis,* and part of a second copy, as follows: fols. 1r–98v, lectures 1–85 on bks. 1–3; fols. 100r–111r, lectures 1–19 on bk. 4 (some lectures from this sequence appear to be missing); fols. 111v–115v blank; fols. 116r–25, second, partial, copy of lectures 6, 7, 13, 14, 16–19 from the first set. Thus Cardano delivered a full set of lectures on this text, although only a fraction of his commentary, breaking off at a point corresponding to the middle of lecture 13 and fragmentary up to that point, is included under the title *Commentaria in libros Hippocratis de victu in acutis* in *Opera* 10:168–92.

34. *In septem Aphorismorum Hippocratis particulas commentaria* (Basel, 1564; IA *132. 093; *Opera* 8:213–580); *In Hippocratis Coi prognostica, opus divinum.* . . . *Atque etiam in Galeni prognosticorum expositionem, commentarii absolutissimi. Item in libros Hippocratis de septimestri et octomestri partu, et simul in eorum Galeni commentaria, Cardani commentarii* (Basel, 1568; IA *132. 102— in fact, no commentary on *De octimestri partu* is included; *Opera* 8:581–806, 9:1–35); *Commentarii in Hippocratis de aere, aquis, et locis opus* (Basel, 1570; IA *132. 107; *Opera* 8:1–212); *In librum Hippocratis de alimento commentaria* (Rome, 1574; IA *132. 109; *Opera* 7:356–515).

35. I have consulted Jacques Dubois (Sylvius), *Ordo et ordinis ratio in legendis Hippocratis et Galeni libris* (Paris, 1548). In it works are divided under the headings physiology, hygiene, pathology, etiology, semiotics, and therapy. I am grateful to Vivian Nutton for drawing my attention to this work.

36. Cardano, comm. *Epid., Opera* 10:197–98, 195.

37. Comm. AAL, preface, *Opera* 8:2. On the list of Hippocratic books in the tenth-century Byzantine encyclopedia known as the *Suda,* see Jody Rubin Pinault, *Hippocratic Lives and Legends* (Leiden, 1992), pp. 20–21.

38. The opposite was strongly maintained by, for example, Giovanni Manardi. See Daniela Mugnai Carrara, "Epistemological Problems in Giovanni Mainardi's Commentary on Galen's *Ars parva,*" forthcoming.

39. "Etenim Hippocrates cum utriusque philosophiae tam naturalis quam moralis tum [1564: tamen] medicinae principaliter fuerit studiosus, omnes suos libros tres ad fines conscripsit: aut ut medicum in moribus instrueret, aut in principiis philosophiae naturalis, aut in artis ipsius medicae operibus. . . . In naturali philosophia quinque proposuit sive fines, primum, ut de omnium rerum initiis disputaret, idque in primo de Diaeta ostendens, quod et nos declaravimus . . . quod aperte in libro de Carnibus docet . . ." (Cardano, comm. *Aph.* 7, proem, *Opera* 8:532). The passages quoted from *De diaeta* (*Regimen*) and *Fleshes* are the same ones that he used in other contexts in direct support of his views on immortality and the elements; see chap. 3, n. 103.

40. "Post principia mortalium rerum ex quibus hae componerentur docuit, atque ea quatuor, in libro de Humana natura, elementa siquidem seu calidum, frigidum, humidum atque siccum, seu quatuor humores, qui in hominibus pluribusque aliis animalibus vicem quatuor elementorum obtinent. . . . Ab his tota philosophia Peripatetica defluxit, adeo ut quicquid habemus traditum ab

Aristotele de huiusmodi sensilibus principiis, id totum ipsi Hippocrati debeamus" (ibid.).

41. Ibid., pp. 532–33.

42. VP 18, *Opera* 1:14.

43. On the figure of Hippocrates in the Renaissance, see Nutton, "Hippocrates in the Renaissance," pp. 422–24. In addition to Hippocratic texts, humanist scholarship brought to light an epitome of a *Life* of Hippocrates attributed to Soranus (included in Calvi's Latin edition of the corpus), the list of Hippocrates' works in the *Suda*, and the Hippocratic pseudepigrapha, a collection of letters and documents giving a novelistic account of various episodes in the life of Hippocrates. For early-fifteenth-century humanist translations into Latin of letters ascribed to Hippocrates and his correspondents, see Kibre, *Hippocrates latinus*, pp. 158–62. The letters were also translated by Fabio Calvi and included in his printed Latin *Opera* of Hippocrates; see *Hippocratis Coi medicorum longe principis, opera ... nunc tandem per M. Fabium Rhavennatem, Guilielmum Copum Basiliensem, Nicolaum Leonicenum, et Andream Brentium, viros doctissimos Latinitate donata* (Basel, 1526), pp. 479–80. Scholarship on late ancient and Byzantine biographical and bibliographical accounts of Hippocrates and their interrelationship is summarized and evaluated in Pinault, *Hippocratic Lives and Legends*, pp. 1–34; for the pseudepigrapha, see Hippocrates, *Pseudepigraphic Writings*. For the portrait of Hippocrates in this material, see Owsei Temkin, *Hippocrates in a World of Pagans and Christians* (Baltimore, 1991), pp. 51–75. Thomas Rütten, *Demokrit lachender Philosoph und sanguinischer Melancholiker: Eine pseudohippokratische Geschichte* (Leiden, 1992), presents some interesting examples of Renaissance uses of the Hippocratic pseudepigrapha. For a summary of the post-Renaissance history of Hippocratic scholarship and ideas about Hippocrates, see Smith, *Hippocratic Tradition*, pp. 13–44.

44. I. M. Lonie, "Cos versus Cnidus and the Historians: Part 1," *History of Science* 16 (1978): 49; however, Nutton, "Hippocrates in the Renaissance," p. 423, notes that Mercuriale was still largely following Galen's judgment. See Girolamo Mercuriale, *De morbis puerorum. Item de venenis et morbis venenosis. Quibus adiuncta est Censura Hippocratis* (Basel, 1584; Maloney and Savoie, *Cinq cent ans*, no. 525). The *Censura* is separately paginated at the end of the volume.

45. *Galeni in libros Hippocratis et aliorum commentarii*, ed. G. B. Rasario (= *Galeni omnia quae extant*, vol. 7) (Venice, 1562), p. 2. The commentary is a forgery, presumably by Rasario, containing elements from genuine works of Galen. See further below, and works cited in n. 110.

46. ACP, *Opera* 7:192–94.

47. Cardano's appointment as a professor of medical theory at Bologna was described as *ordinarius* in the morning hours (and therefore necessarily involving lectures on a book in the standard curriculum) only for 1562–63; see Dallari, *I rotuli* 2:155–77. Subsequently, it seems likely that he was free to select his texts.

48. See n. 17, above.

49. See Siraisi, *Avicenna*, pp. 99–103.

50. Cardano, comm. SP, *Opera* 9:2. Fernando Mena's commentary on the same text was published at Antwerp in the same year, 1568 (Maloney and Savoie, *Cinq cent ans*, no. 424).

51. "... Antonius Fracanzianus Vincentinus, qui paucis ante annis medicinam hoc eodem loco clare profitebatur recto iudicio censuit in his Commentariis, quae in manibus omnium habentur ..." (Cardano, comm. *Aliment.*, *Opera* 7:358). Antonio Fracanzano, *In librum Hippocratis De alimento commentarius* (Venice, 1566). As noted, Cardano's lectures were given in 1568–69. As far as I have ascertained, only one other commentary on *Aliment* was published before this date, namely, Francisco Valles, *In aphorismos, et libellum De alimento Hippocratis* (Alcalá, 1561; Maloney and Savoie, *Cinq cent ans*, no. 383).

52. Cardano, comm. *Aliment.*, *Opera* 7:359–60.

53. Leonhart Fuchs, *Hippocratis medicorum omnium longe principis Epidemiorum Liber Sextus.... Addita est luculenta universi eius libri expositio, ... Leonardo Fuchsio authore* (The Hague, 1532); Gianbattista Da Monte, *In tertium primi Epidemiorum sectionem explanationes* (Venice, 1554). In addition, a commentary on *Epidemics* 2 was published by Pedro Jaime Esteve (Valencia, 1551; Maloney and Savoie, *Cinq cent ans*, no. 274).

54. Cardano, comm. *Epid.*, proem and preface, *Opera* 10:193–97. For citations of bks. 5 and 7, see nn. 97–98, below.

55. On the relation of the *Epidemics* to Cardano's own medical narratives, see further chap. 9, below.

56. "Tertia intentio fuit ut constitueret fundamenta artis ex experimento" (comm. *Epid.*, proem, *Opera* 10:196); "Nam cum universum opus prognosticum sit totum, ad futurorum expectationem ac divinationem spectat, quae pars etiam divina est. Etenim cum praeterita sint memoria pollentium, praesentia prudentium, atque solertium, futura sunt divinorum: atque ille probe divinus etiam videtur qui futura praevidet" (ibid., p. 194); "Epidemii, in quibus solum narratur essentia rei, nil agendum docetur, unde theorici sunt" (ibid., p. 197).

57. "Secunda utilitas est qua ego utebar in iuventute, experiendo me, et erat ut legerem quicquid acciderat aegro absque exitu, et dijudicarem, an obiret, an non, et quando: et si in paucis homo hos [*sic*] assequitur, quid sperabit in exercendo gloriae, et si in multis melior est, et si in omnibus, et plene, tunc norit se iam esse perfectum" (ibid., p. 195).

58. Regarding ancient, medieval, and Renaissance environmental theories, see Clarence J. Glacken, *Traces on the Rhodian Shore: Nature and Culture in Western Thought from Ancient Times to the End of the Eighteenth Century* (Berkeley, 1967), pp. 80–115, 254–87, 429–60. Bodin expounded his theories of climatic and astrological influence on the character of societies in both the *Methodus ad facilem historiarum cognitionem* (1566), chap. 5, and the *Six livres de la République* (1576) 5.1. For discussion, see Marian J. Tooley, "Bodin and the Medieval Theory of Climate," *Speculum* 28 (1953): 64–83, and Glacken, *Traces*, pp. 434–47.

59. "lectio huius libri tum praecipue tamen medicis, philosophis, geographis atque astrologis utilissima sit" (comm. AAL, bk. 1, preface, *Opera* 8:2).

60. "Quod si quis in eodem genere iam tibi amicus scripserit, seu argumento novo, seu exponendo aliena opera, ut nuper mihi contigit in Adriano Alemano,

Lutetiano medico, qui commentaria quatuor in librum de Aere et aquis Hippocratis scripsit, et quamvis non e facie vel ulla alia causa notus mihi sit, cum tamen multa adducat ex nostris commentariis in secundum de Iudiciis astrorum librum Ptolemaei, non sine magna nostri laude (hoc enim maximum est quod cuiquam tribui possit, ut integrae pagellae vel periodi ad verbum transcribantur, illius non suppresso nomine) nos vero cum antea multo quam liber in manus nostras pervenerit, decrevissemus commentaria in totum Hippocratis volumen conficere . . ." (LP 1562, *Opera* 1:139). L'Alemant (1527–59) was a professor of medicine at Paris. *Hippocratis medicorum omnium principis, de aere, aquis, et locis, Liber olim mancus nunc integer . . . Ab Adriano Alemano apud Parisios medico commentariis quatuor illustratus* (Paris, 1557), in marginal headings on fols. 29r and 32r, indicates Cardano as the source of lengthy passages on astrology. L'Alemant's commentary includes the Greek text of the Hippocratic work, which Cardano's does not.

61. "Nonnihil etiam ad lucidiorem sensum adiutus opera utraque, et interpretationis, et explanationis Adriani Alemani Sorcenois, qui et librum illius de Flatibus exposuit, medici non vulgaris, ac Lutetiae professoris, cui [*sic*] extant vulgata in hunc librum Commentaria, quae etiam apud unumquemque vestrum cupio esse, consulendo facilitati si cui nostra graviora aut difficiliora nuper initiatis videbuntur" (comm. AAL 1.1, preface, *Opera* 8:1). Remarks critical of or correcting L'Alemant are scattered throughout the commentary.

62. Ibid. 1.2, *Opera* 8:4.

63. Ibid. 6.80 (divisions are into books and *lectiones*), *Opera* 8:151; 6.79, 8:149; 1.119, 8:16; 7.90, 8:172; 4.68, 8:126.

64. "Sunt et aliae multae generosae et praedivites urbes, inter quas Xandu, Taidu, Ezina, Lop, Saion [1570: Sachion], sed omnium praeter Cambalu celeberrimae. Quinsa, id est, sunt, et Cianglu et Ciangli, Tudinsu, Tapinzu . . . [the list continues]. Pianfu, Pazanfu . . . similiter est aliud paradoxum quod cum sic vivant et ferarum ritu, se tamen ingeniosissimos affirmant: solosque qui duobus oculis cernant mortales alios praecipueque Latinos commemorant uno. Id etiam ostendunt cum tres artes calleant Chymiam, Lymiam, Hymiam, Chymia est quam nos vocamus Alchymiam ad metallorum, et gemmarum transmutationem, quam illi longe melius norunt quam nos, tametsi enim argentum aut aurum efficere nequeant, mutant tamen nonnullas gemmas, ut discerni a veris nequeant, metalla vero difficillime. Lymia est ars amatoria, cuius vix vestigium est apud nos, extat tamen et apud Turcas credo in usu esse. Scymia [1570: Symia] est praestigiatrix qua plurimum illi valent, nec solum ut deludant oculos atque fallant, sed eo profecerunt ut ad magiam accedat, cogentes ventos, imbres, grandines avertentes" (ibid. 7.90, *Opera* 8:172).

65. For example, ibid. 2.22, *Opera* 8:36 and 2.62, 8:114. On the role of the *Problemata* in sixteenth-century encyclopedic natural philosophy, see Ann Blair, "The *Problemata* as a Natural Philosophical Genre" (forthcoming).

66. Comm. AAL 4.55, *Opera* 8:103.

67. Ibid. 1.12, *Opera* 8:21.

68. "Honestissima voluptas est ocium peregrinationis, adeo ut pro negotio censeri possit, velut et pro negotio ocium haberi, tantum in eo est iucunditatis: movetur corpus, quiescit animus" (ibid. 1.2, *Opera* 8:3).

69. Ibid. 4.65, *Opera* 8:117; 1.2, 8:4–5.

70. Text: "Qui vero macra, aquis carentia, et nuda loca tenent, et quae temporum mutationibus non sunt permista, horum formas necesse est esse asperas et vegetas, flavas magis quam nigras: mores etiam eorum rigidi sunt, pertinaces et contumaces." Comm.: "Est descriptio huius regionis, certe oppido nostro, unde oriundi sumus, valde accommodata, distat enim Cardanum oppidum . . . , prope Gal[l]aratum ad mille passus, ab urbe Medolani XXIV M. P." (ibid. 8.104, *Opera* 8:203).

71. Pigeaud, "L'Hippocratisme de Cardan," passim.

72. "Verum unde mala eveniunt, cum sit Deus bonus?" (comm. AAL 7.94, *Opera* 8:181); ibid. 8.99, *Opera* 8:192.

73. "Sola Christiana optimos efficit, si vel in simplices vel vere sapientes homines incident. Sed si in sophistas fiunt dolosi, subdoli, vafri" (ibid.).

74. The concept of environmental influence on such characteristics as courage and generosity and their opposites was explicitly accepted by Cardano, no matter what qualifications he may have introduced about the soul; see ibid. 8.108, *Opera* 8:212.

75. "Coniugationes autem sunt pene infinitae, ut ita dicam. . . . et fient bis mille nonagentae triginta sex. Intelligit ergo per mutationem victus in speciali, si Anglus cogatur multum se exercere et parum comedere . . . et generaliter, si regio assueta abundantiae tritici et vini et carnium, ut Insubrum, cogatur esurire, comedere herbas" (ibid. 1.11, *Opera* 8:19). The larger number comes from *Examen* prefatory epistle, *Opera* 9:36.

76. "Triplex est genus cognitionis de rebus mortalibus apud mortales. . . . At vero quae non ordinibus constat, partim quidem, et quo ad nos, et quo ad nostram scientiam effugit nomen ipsum scientiae, et coniecturalis vocatur, qualis quae in unoquoque est eorum, tamen scientia est apud meliores nobis quae extenditur ad singulas gentes non solum, sed etiam homines singulos, et singulas operationes, et casus fortuitos, sed ista sunt comprehensa rationibus infinitis, velut si quis comprehendat in cubito quod divisus bifariam aequabitur sibiipsi, et trifariam dimidio, et quae in proportionibus dicta sunt a nobis, et horum infinitorum ea scientia est apud incorporea, ex qua fatum et causae naturalium et singulorum et tempora et modi et eventus, de quibus nobis nec coniectura est nedum scientia. Ergo de hac neque loquitur Hippocrates, sed de priore, de qua apud nos, per ordines, coniectura est" (comm. AAL 8.108, *Opera* 8:211).

77. "Ultima classis [of the works of Hippocrates] est selectorum dictorum, septem digesta sectionibus, ut dixi; ex omni congerie operum Hippocratis selecta praeter primum. Quo fit ut cum Aphorismum aliquem alibi exscriptum invenerimus, illinc vera sit expetenda interpretatio; si vero nullibi inveniatur, periisse librum illum in quo scriptus erat credendum sit" (comm. *Aph.*, proem, bk. 7, *Opera* 8:533).

78. "Qui negant hos aphorismos esse continuos venia digni non sunt" (ibid. 1.14, *Opera* 8:242).

79. "nullus liber apud Aristotelem vel Galenum tanto ordine conscriptus sit" (ibid. 1.11, *Opera* 8:230).

80. Ibid., proem, bk. 7, *Opera* 8:533; proem, bk. 4, *Opera* 8:346–47.

81. "Nam octo annis in hoc almo Ferrariensi gymnasio dialecticae gyros interpretati sumus. Deinde philosophiam naturalem novem annis. Nunc vero eandem naturalem philosophiam sub alio nomine interpretari auspicabimur, nempe medicae rei theoriam naturalis philosophiae partem summi viri censuerunt" (Antonio Musa Brasavola, *In octo libros Aphorismorum Hippocratis et Galeni commentaria et annotationes* [Basel, 1546], p. 1).

82. "Quaestiones illae de principiis primis nec absolutae, nec satis firmae, nescio cui bono sint, aut auxilio ad medicinam perdiscendam, utiliores enim essent disputationes Ricardi Suiset Angli, quod de rebus magis sint quam elenchi illi circa ea quae qualia sint nondum constat" (Cardano, comm. *Aph.*, proem, bk. 4, *Opera* 8:347).

83. "Unde causa errorum in medicina est, quoniam qui contemplantur non medentur, velut Galenus, Paulus, et Princeps, . . . et hodie omnes medicinae professores: ideo loco regularum et dogmatum scribunt somnia. Et qui medentur non contemplantur, nec sunt exercitati in philosophia, nec dialecti[c]a nec animadvertunt in tanta multitudine aegrorum adeo occupati communia pluribus similia, ac dissimilia. . . . Et ideo ex recentioribus non inveni meliorem L. Iachimi, qui fuit, ut ego, professor post longam artis iam exercitationem, amator virtutis, et vixit satis senex" (Cardano, comm. *Prognost.* 2.60 [bk. 3 of commentary], *Opera* 8:708). Cardano used a version of the *Prognostic* that divided the text into three books, and within each book into numbered short maxims on the model of the *Aphorisms*. He divided his commentary into four books: bk. 1, commentary on *Prognostic*, bk. 1; bk. 2, commentary on *Prognostic* 2.1–42; bk. 3, commentary on *Prognostic* 2.43–74; bk. 4, commentary on *Prognostic*, bk. 3.

84. *Hieronymi Cardani in Hippocratis Coi Prognostica, opus divinum, superans humani ingenii captum, quo nihil unquam, omnium sapientum virorum testimonio, perfectius scriptum est, utilissimum non duntaxat ad praedictionem in morbis sed et curationem. Atque etiam in Galeni prognosticorum expositionem commentarii absolutissimi. Item in libros Hippocratis de Septimestri et Octomestri partu, et simul in eorum Galeni Commentaria, Cardani Commentarii. . . . Fuerunt hi viri Hippocrates et Cardanus, praeter summum doctrinam, longo felicique usu et experientia in operibus artis admirandi, cum haec scripserunt, uterque ultra LX annorum aetatem.* Cf. "Itaque jure merito haec commentaria omnibus nostris operibus praestant. Siquidem maturo iam annis consilio conscripti sunt" (LP 1557, *Opera* 1:70). Also, "Fuit ergo intentum Hippocratis in hoc volumine multiplex. . . . Secunda [*sic*] fuit, ut recordaretur in senio eorum quae in iuventa observaverat" (comm. *Epid.*, *Opera* 10:195).

85. "Postquam ergo hoc facile est perdiscere autem medicinae artem ut ab Hippocrate atque nobis tradita est" (comm. *Aph.*, proem, bk. 4, *Opera* 8:347).

86. "Cumque ex his qui non ferro neque vi pereunt duae quintae partes obeant ex erroribus medicorum" (comm. *Aliment.* lecture 38 on text 40 [48], *Opera* 7:440).

87. Cardano, comm. *Prognost.* 3.7 (bk. 4 of commentary), *Opera* 8:747–48.

88. See Peter Brain, *Galen on Bloodletting: A Study of the Origins, Development and Validity of His Opinions, with a Translation of Three Works* (Cambridge, 1986), pp. 112–21, where it is noted that, despite Galen's claims that

Hippocrates highly valued bleeding, there are only about seventy references to bloodletting in the entire Hippocratic corpus and (as Cardano noted) many more to purgatives.

89. "Dico ergo quod cum Hippocrates sua aetate magis reformidaret sectionem venae, quam purgationem: ergo multo minus illam fecisset in his temporibus, quam medicamentum purgans exhibuisset . . . neque in febribus, neque in magnis fracturis mittebat sanguinem, sed potius exhibebat elleborum et inedia summa utebatur quam vellet sanguinem mittere. At in interioribus inflammationibus sanguinem mittebat ob maximam necessitatem. . . . In senectute tamen Hippocratis [*sic*] magis adhaesit sectione venae, quia videbat aegros nolle pati exquisitam illam inaediam. Unde etiam in periculo phlegmonis mittebat sanguinem. Et ex hoc patet concordia Hippocratis, Galeni, et etiam Erasistrati: omnes enim bene dicebant et bene faciebant, sed diversa ratione" (comm. AAL 2.62, *Opera* 8:115).

90. "Neque vero rectum est, quod est ut se habet docere velle omissa authoris sententia, ut facit Iulius Scaliger dum Theophrastum exponit: neque ita sequi authorem, ut rei ipsius historiam omittas. . . . Primum igitur mente Hippocratis explicare decet, quae mens ei, qui sensus: Deinde quomodo res se habeat universa declarare: demum unum alii coaptare: ut rem ipsam per Hippocratem intelligamus, et Hippocrati rem ipsam accommodemus" (ibid. 5.66, *Opera* 8:121).

91. I have consulted *Hippocratis Coi medicorum omnium sine controversia principis Aphorismorum sectiones septem recens e Graeco in Latinum sermonem conversae, et luculentissimis, iisdemque breviss. commentariis illustratae et expositae . . . per Leonhartum Fuchsium* (Paris, 1545). For Brasavola's commentary, which, like Cardano's, is based on Leoniceno's translation of the *Aphorisms*, see n. 81, above.

92. His use of Leoniceno's translation of the *Aphorisms* has already been noted. For *Prognostic* he used the translation of Lorenzo Lorenzani, and for *Airs Waters Places* and *Aliment* that of Cornarius (Maloney and Savoie, *Cinq cent ans*, nos. 422, 432, 451). Comparison of the lemmata in Cardano's expositions of *On the Seven Month Child* and *Epidemics* 1 and 2 (*Opera* 9:1–35 and 10:168–387) with Hippocrates, *Opera*, trans. Cornarius (Basel, 1546), pp. 61–64 and 397–415 (Cardano's commentary on *Epidemics* 2 being incomplete), shows that he also used the Cornarius translation for those works. I have not identified the translation used as the basis for his commentary on *Regimen in Acute Diseases*. Possibly the commentary on *Prognostic*, as well as that on the *Aphorisms* (see n. 18, above), was begun before the publication of Cornarius's translation. Comparison of a few lemmata in Cardano's commentary on the *Aphorisms* with Leoniceno's translation revealed occasional minor variations, but I have made no systematic investigation. The supposition of deliberate emendation is, however, supported by, e.g., Cardano's accusation that Leoniceno did not correctly understand the Greek text of *Aph.* 4.80 (*Opera* 8:416).

93. *Galeni in primum Hippocratis de morbis vulgaribus librum commentarius primus Hermanno Cruserio Campensi interprete* (Paris, 1534 [title page missing in the New York Academy of Medicine copy]; first edition in 1531).

94. For example: "Quia ut dixi prius poterat hic textus bifariam legi: Galenus

qui gloriae potius quam veritati studuit (quis enim aliter sentiat) tertium sensum, ex utroquo compositum invenit. . . . Sed ut dixi Cornarii lectio omnino absurditate vacat, reliquarum minus mala est Galeni" (comm. 1 *Epid.* 1, *Opera* 10:221). He made similar comparisons between the Aldine text of the *Aphorisms* and Fuchs's edition; see, for example, comm. *Aph.* 7.48, *Opera* 8:569.

95. *Contradictiones* 1.4.10, *Opera* 6:369; the table of contents (Greek and Latin) of the Aldine Greek Hippocrates (Venice, 1526) carries the note "De alimento quem esse Hippocratis negat Galenus." For the contrary view, see Cardano, comm. *Aliment.*, proemium, *Opera* 7:358–60. Galen's acceptance of *Aliment* as an authentic work of Hippocrates, his lost commentary on it, and his frequent references to it are established in the introduction and notes to *De l'Aliment*, in *Hippocrate*, vol. 6, pt. 2, ed. and trans. Robert Joly (Paris, 1972), pp. 131, 136, 141, 142, 143, 145. Joly dates *Aliment* to the second or third century B.C.

96. Comm. *Aph.* 6.36 (by Cardano's enumeration; that is, 6.38), *Opera* 8:504–6 (carcinoma, etc.); comm. *Aliment.*, lecture 24 on text 26, *Opera* 7:412 (pustules and contagious childhood diseases); ibid., lecture 25 on text 26, *Opera* 7:413–16 (lepra).

97. Comm. *Aph.* 4.76–77, *Opera* 8:410. For an example of the use of a whole series of cases from the *Epidemics* 1, 3, and 7, see comm. *Prognost.* 3.16 (bk. 4 of commentary), *Opera* 8:757–58.

98. Comm. *Prognost.*, 1.20–21, *Opera* 8:613–14.

99. "Novi (famulusque is meus fuit) hominem, qui decem octo annis in triremi vinctus fuit apud Afros Hortensium nomine, patria Brixiensem, qui etiam uxorem duxerat, cum oculos clauderet, nullamque sui corporis partem moveret, in nullo a mortuo potuisse dissimilem dici. Ita pallor, macies, extensa cutis, arctae nares, color plumbeus ac ferrugineus cum tumore quodam iuxta oculos illum mortuo similem fingebant. Palam est autem, quod, qui talis erat, sanus non fuit: hunc tamen sanum appellat Hippocrates, qui possit muniis sanorum fungi" (ibid., 1.8–9, *Opera* 8:595).

100. *Aphorisms* 5.47 (5.45 by Cardano's enumeration) in *Hippocrates*, ed. and trans. W.H.S. Jones (Loeb), 4:170, translating the second clause "tents must be employed."

101. *Expositio Ugonis Senensis super Aphorismos Hippocratis* . . . (Venice, 1517). I cite Giacomo's views via Brasavola's commentary on the *Aphorisms*, 5.47, p. 852 in the edition cited in n. 81, where they are not necessarily represented fairly.

102. Ibid.; on p. 853 Brasavola pointed out that Galen used the word in this sense. Fuchs, commentary on the *Aphorisms*, pp. 428–30 in the edition cited in n. 91. Brasavola's understanding of the word appears to be supported by other uses in the Hippocratic corpus (Gilles Maloney, Winnie Frohn, and Paul Potter, eds., *Concordantia in Corpus Hippocraticum* [Hildesheim, Zurich, and New York, 1986], 2:1413) and is that of modern translators of the *Aphorisms* (Littré and W.H.S. Jones).

103. Comm. *Aph.* 5.45, *Opera* 8:453–54. At p. 453: "Ubinam [1564: ubi nam] gentium? Barbaros Germanus Italos vocat?"

104. ". . . genuinus sensus est explicandus. At nemo putet haec alio animo a

me esse dicta, nisi quod consulam ut homines solum amplectantur eos qui vel vertant e lingua in linguam vel sua prodant inventa: dico res, non nugas, vel demonstrent veros auctorum sensus continua serie erutos ac firmo consensu continuae orationis elisos. . . . Emmoton ergo ulceris nomen erat, quod non nisi longo specillo curari poterat" (ibid., p. 454).

105. "Incitavit autem me ad hoc felix quaedam interpretatio primum in *Aphorismos*, cum vidissem Galenum adeo oscitanter [1585; *Opera*: oscitantes] illos exposuisse, ut ne umbram quidem sensuum Hippocratis videatur assecutus" (LP 1562, *Opera* 1:107). The generally anti-Galenic stance in Cardano's Hippocratic commentaries is noted in both Pigeaud, "L'Hippocratisme de Cardan," and Simili, "Gerolamo Cardano, lettore e medico a Bologna." Donato Mutti, a physician of Ragusa, had previously criticized Galen's commentary on the *Aphorisms* in his *In interpretatione Galeni super quatuordecim Aphorismos Hippocratis dialogus* (Basel, 1547), which I have not seen.

106. "Ergo nunc primum audietis Hippocratem nova lingua loquentem ac disserentem, non minus quam existimatis nova esse quae in geometria et arithmetica invenimus" (LP 1562, *Opera* 1:107). See G.E.R. Lloyd, "Galen on Hellenistics and Hippocrateans: Contemporary Battles and Past Authorities," in his *Methods and Problems in Greek Science* (Cambridge, 1991), pp. 398–416, esp. pp. 401–2. I am grateful to Vivian Nutton for drawing my attention to this point and article.

107. Smith, *Hippocratic Tradition*, pp. 122–72.

108. Kibre, *Hippocrates latinus*, lists numerous manuscripts of this type.

109. For translators and early printed editions of Galen's Hippocratic commentaries, see Durling, "Chronological Census," pp. 294–95, nos. 149–60.

110. Galen's commentaries on *Humors* and *Aliment* are lost (Smith, *Hippocratic Tradition*, p. 124); that on *Epidemics* 2 survives in Arabic and was translated from that language for the first time in Galen, *In Hippocratis Epidemiarum libros I et II*, ed. Ernst Wenkebach and Franz Pfaff, *Corpus Medicorum Graecorum* V 10, 1 (Berlin, 1934). Regarding the Renaissance forgeries of these commentaries, see, respectively, Smith, *Hippocratic Tradition*, pp. 172–5; Hippocrates, *De l'Aliment*, p. 136; Ernst Wenkebach, *Praefatio, Corpus Medicorum Graecorum* V 10, 1, p. XXIII. On ancient and Renaissance forgery and text criticism more generally, see Anthony Grafton, *Forgers and Critics: Creativity and Duplicity in Western Scholarship* (Princeton, 1990), and Paul Gerhardt Schmidt, "Kritische Philologie und pseudoantike Literatur," *Die Antike-Rezeption in der Wissenschaften während der Renaissance* (Weinberg, 1983), pp. 117–27.

111. "Plerisque in locis magis necessaria omisit: multis in locis quam sit opus prolixior est. . . . [E]go ab expositione commentariorum Galeni, et ab omnium insectatione abstinebo" (Cardano, comm. *Aph.*, proem, bk. 1, *Opera* 8:216–17).

112. For example: (1) "Si Galenus non videt ullam difficultatem in tanta ambiguitate sensus, laudo hominem excellentissimi ingenii, qui difficillima intelligeret perfecte ac facillime: si vidit laudo consilium, qui prorsus non attigerit. Mihi res omnino tota difficilis videtur" (Cardano, comm. 1 *Epid.* 1, *Opera* 10:234); (2) "Et hic rursus Galenus dubitat, involvit, denique fugit expositionem, quae clarissima est, sed uno verbo mutato" (comm. 2 *Epid.* 1, *Opera* 10:262); (3) "Et haec est lectio genuina, quam Galenus dissimulavit, quia non

intellexit" (comm. 3 *Epid.* 1, *Opera* 10:287). Galen's commentary on *Epidemics* 1 was first translated into Latin in 1531 (Durling, "Chronological Census," no. 152). In his commentaries on *Prognostic* and *Regimen in Acute Diseases* Cardano also expounded Galen's commentaries on those works; in the former the treatment of Galen is often critical but does not seem particularly so in the latter.

113. Cardano, proem to comm. *Epid.*, *Opera* 10:194.

114. Comm. *Epidemics*, bk. 2, *Opera* 10:366–67. Cardano here showed considerable perspicuity. He knew Galen's discussion in the form of a separate short work that circulated under the title of *Quomodo simulantes sint deprehendi*, or some variant thereof. This had been translated into Latin by Niccolo da Reggio in the fourteenth century (manuscripts, which I have not seen, are listed in Lynn Thorndike and Pearl Kibre, *A Catalogue of Incipits of Mediaeval Scientific Writings in Latin*, 2d ed. [Cambridge, Mass., 1963], col. 1143) and was subsequently included among Galen's printed *Opera*. In the twentieth century, discovery of the Arabic translation of Galen's commentary on *Epidemics* 2 revealed *Quomodo simulantes* to be a fragment of that work. The passage in question is translated from the Arabic version of Galen's commentary into German in Galen, *In Hippocratis Epidemiarum libros I et II*, ed. Wenkebach and Pfaff, *Corpus Medicorum Graecorum* V, 10, 1, pp. 206–10; the fragment of Greek text is edited in Karl Deichgräber and Fridolf Kudlien, *Die als sogenannante simulantenschrift griechisch überlieferten Stücke des 2. Kommentare zu den Epidemien II*, in *Galens Kommentare zu den Epidemien des Hippokrates, Corpus Medicorum Graecorum* V, 10, 2, 4 (Berlin, 1960), pp. 107–16. The work is extensively discussed (with French translation) in Danielle Gourevitch, *Le triangle hippocratique dans le monde gréco-romain: Le malade, sa maladie et son médecin* (Rome, 1984), pp. 73–135. It is indeed Galen's commentary on the passage to which Cardano applied it.

115. "nil me optasse magis, quam ut Galeni commentaria in hunc librum invenirentur, cum ex ratione arithmeticae censeantur multo maiora fuisse prognosticorum commentariis, quae habemus, et super tam paucis verbis miram quandam artem expressisse, Galenum verisimile sit" (comm. *Aliment.*, proem, *Opera* 7:360). Cardano noted the loss of Galen's commentary on *Airs Waters Places* (comm. AAL 1. 1, *Opera* 8:1) and rejected as inauthentic a supposed Galenic exposition of *On the Seven Month Child*, which I have not succeeded in identifying (comm. SP, proem, *Opera* 9:1). Galen's authentic commentary on that work survived in Arabic and was first translated from that language in 1935 (Smith, *Hippocratic Tradition*, p. 154). Fragments of his commentary on *Airs Waters Places* survived in Hebrew and were first translated into Latin in the late seventeenth century (ibid., p. 166); the complete commentary survives in Arabic; see Gotthard Strohmaier, "Hellenistische Wissenschaft im neugefundenen Galenkommentar zur hippokratischen Schrift 'Über die Umwelt,' " in *Galen und das hellenistische Erbe*, ed. Jutta Kollesch and Diethard Nickel, *Sudhoffs Archiv*, Beiheft 32 (Stuttgart, 1993), pp. 157–64.

116. "Adeo ut ausus sit dicere primo de Fracturis commentatoris officium non esse demonstrare quae dicuntur ab auctore esse vera, aut illum a calumniatoribus tueri, posse tamen nos id facere. . . . Et alibi: 'Officium boni expositoris non esse demonstrationes dictorum afferre sed solum quae ab illo dicta sunt

verba explicare.' Interrogo te, o Galene, in quo opus est medico ad interpretationem librorum medicinae si solum verba auctoris sunt explicanda? nam si de dictionibus agendum est ac sensibus grammatici hoc opus est" (comm. *Aph.* 6.42 [6.44], *Opera* 8:513).

117. "Galenus coniectura tantum potuit assequi quid voluerit Hippocrates; homo fuit, et multis modis decipi potuit. At Galenum, quid senserit, quandoquidem certi simus id voluisse quod Hippocrates voluit, ubi constiterit quid voluerit Hippocrates, iam plane etiam sciemus quid Galenus voluerit" (ibid. 1.17, *Opera* 8:251).

118. "Hippocratis gloriae, quem adeo videtur extollere, maxime invidit" (comm. *Prognost.* 2.37, *Opera* 8:680).

119. "id cum carnifices medici hoc tempore evertant, demonstrare decet, neque enim pudore contemptae authoritatis Hippocratis hi detinentur. . . . Quamobrem Galenum venia dignum non iudico, in re tanti momenti tam ieiune scribentem" (comm. *Aph.* 1.8, *Opera* 8:227); "Inde in insolubiles nodos contrarietatis incidit . . ." (ibid., 1.15, 8:247); "Deinde praecepta illa nec cum principiis propriis, nec cum Hippocrate, nec cum experimento concordant" (ibid. 1.17, 8:252). Brasavola also noted some discrepancies between Hippocrates and Galen (for example, in his commentary on *Aphorisms* 1.18), but his tone seems less polemical. However, I have not attempted any systematic comparison.

120. "Pauca enim experimenta internorum morborum vidit Galenus et pauciora observavit" (*Examen, Opera* 9:39); "Et rerum quidem difficilium nihil attingit Galenus" (ibid., p. 40); ". . . ob nimiam in illis [sc. libri de grammatica] eruditionem et studium minus se exercuit in seriis et utilioribus" (ibid., p. 44). This brief work contains a number of other similar comments.

121. Luca Gaurico, *Super diebus decretoriis (quos etiam criticos vocitant) axiomata, sive aphorismi grandes utique sententiae brevi oratione compraehensae. Enucleavit item pleraque Hippocratis, et Galeni theoremata, quae medici rerum coelestium expertes vix olfecerunt. Isagogicus astrologiae Tractatus medicis admodum oportunus . . .* (Rome, 1546).

122. "Quae vero nugatur Brasavolus circa astrorum ortum [1564: et] occasum, quanto plura, tanto magis risum movent" (comm. *Aph.* 4.5, *Opera* 8:353).

123. "Dico ergo quod nemo potest dissolvere hanc difficultatem nisi quid [1568: qui] calleat artem Hippocraticam Ptolomei [*sic*]" (comm. *Prognost.* 3.5 [bk. 4 of commentary], *Opera* 8:746).

124. "Haec igitur est summa dierum criticorum, numerus, ordo, explicatio, causa, iuxta veritatem, et Hippocratis sententiam, quam Galenus tot nugis involuit false, confuse, inconstanter, adeo ut qui eam secuti sint finem nullum invenire potuerunt" (ibid. 3.1 [bk. 4 of commentary], *Opera* 8:741). The whole discussion of critical days occupies pp. 741–47.

125. See n. 6, above.

126. "At dicetis: In idem tu vitium incidis, reprehendendo Galenum. Non: nam ego id ago, ne seducti lectores auctoritate viri, quod nunc vitium maxime regnat, veritatem inquirere negligant" (comm. *Aph.* 4.58, *Opera* 8:398).

127. "Ubi omnes Hippocratis libros diligenter intellexeris, etiam iubeo, non consulo solum, ut sex Galeni libros de Locis affectis et decem ac septem de Usu partium, quatuordecim Methodi medendi, quinque primos et tres ultimos de

Simplicibus medicamentis, decem de Compositis secundum locos et septem secundum genera, qui in universum sunt sexagintaduo, evolvas. A reliquis eius libris si abstinueris, non solum id temporis lucri feceris, quod esses impensurus,
sed minus perplexus haerebis in his quae ab Hippocrate clare tradita sunt" (ibid.,
proem, bk. 4, *Opera* 8:348).

128. ACP, *Opera* 7:192.

129. On Argenterio's critique of Galenic teaching on diseases, signs, symptoms, and causes, see Siraisi, "Giovanni Argenterio."

130. Nutton, "Hippocrates in the Renaissance," p. 436.

131. Comm. *Prognost.* 3.59, *Opera* 8:705.

132. Comm. *Aph.* 4.78, *Opera* 8:411–13; 6.31, 8:499–501; comm. *Prognost.*
3.15 (bk. 4 of commentary), *Opera* 8:756–57. The English translations of the
Hippocratic aphorisms are from *Aphorisms*, trans. W.H.S. Jones, 4.78 and 6.32
(*sic*), in *Hippocrates* (Loeb) 4:157, 187, and *Prognostic*, sec. 22, in *Hippocrates*
(Loeb) 2:45–47.

133. Cardano, comm. 1 *Epid.* 2, *Opera* 10:350–51.

134. *Airs Waters Places* 17, in *Hippocrates*, ed. and trans. W.H.S. Jones
(Loeb), 1:117. Regarding the ancient sources of the Amazon myth, see Josine
Blok, *The Early Amazons: Modern and Ancient Perspectives on a Persistent Myth*
(Leiden, 1995).

135. Comm. AAL 7.83, *Opera* 8:155–56. For other remarks about soldiers,
see above, chap. 4.

136. Ibid. 7.83, *Opera* 8:156. H. C. Agrippa, *De nobilitate et praecellentia
foeminei sexus: Edition critique d'après de texte d'Anvers 1529*, ed. R. Antonioli
et al. (Geneva, 1990); on the dissemination of the work, see the editor's introduction to Henricus Cornelius Agrippa, *Declamation on the Nobility and Preem-
inence of the Female Sex*, trans. and ed. Albert Rabil, Jr. (Chicago, 1996),
pp. 27–29, and bibliography there cited (especially with reference to Italy and
related Italian treatises on p. 28). See also Ian Maclean, *The Renaissance Notion
of Woman: A Study in the Fortunes of Scholasticism and Medical Science in European Intellectual Life* (Cambridge, 1980). Some recent studies of the medieval
and Renaissance fortuna of the Amazon myth and of Renaissance attitudes to
Amazons and other women warriors, both in supposed history and in literature,
include Abby Wettan Kleinbaum, *The War against the Amazons* (New York,
1983), pp. 5–137; Alison Taufer, "The Only Good Amazon Is a Converted
Amazon: The Woman Warrior and Christianity in the *Amadis Cycle*," in *Playing
with Gender: A Renaissance Pursuit*, ed. Jean R. Brink, Maryanne C. Horowitz,
and Allison P. Coudert (Urbana, 1991), pp. 35–51; Pamela Joseph Benson, *The
Invention of the Renaissance Woman: The Challenge of Female Independence in the
Literature and Thought of Italy and England* (University Park, Pa., 1992). I have
been unable to identify the episode Cardano had in mind when he referred to
women or a woman fighting "pro patria . . . nostra tempestate Eunei in Sabau-
dia, seu agro Taurino."

137. "Et certe hoc aliud est quam infibulare aut circumcidere puerum, ad
mammas enim venae satis magnae et multae prodeunt, et quanto maiores exti-
terint, sed nervi pauci et tenues et arteriae similiter, eoque magis in puellulis, ut
author est Vesalius (libro 5, cap. 68, et figur. 25) ubi etiam docet multas in adul-

tis esse carnes glandosas, sed in puellis paucas, e regione tamen papillae est glans satis magna, in cuius ambitu sunt multae aliae minores: et nervus maior est ex septimo pari spinalis medullae in intervallo quartae costae: ut certe tanta incisio non sine incommodo fiat, ablatis tot glandibus, venis, nervis, arteriis, amplum spatium etiam occupantibus, quia tamen non sunt membra necessaria vitae nec nervi nec vasa valde ampla et omnia externa, et non adsunt musculi, et locus abundat carne, nec est e regione membri principalis, ideo vacat quasi periculo haec operatio. Modus autem incisionis erat, ut tollerentur carnes omnes glandosae . . . " (AAL 7.83, *Opera* 8:156).

138. " . . . ergo post initium octavi anni erat cum minore periculo, timor autem tollitur occulato facto et praeparatione. Dolor vero ex vinculis ideo debet vinciri stricte mamma constringendo prius per momentum solum ne locus inflammetur: nam dolor augeretur: et post abscindi et exuri ne sanguis erumpat ex vasis, et ut nervi effugiant periculum convulsionis, et omne incrementum partis prorsus tollatur. . . . Dico quod in his qui iam creverunt locus debilitaretur, sed cum illa puellae crescerent et exercerentur, ideo locus trahit plus materiae pro membro, et membrum id est humerus et brachium, et musculi eorum augentur" (ibid., p. 157).

139. Ibid., pp. 154, 156.

140. The surgical description is highly unlikely to have been extrapolated from experience of amputation as a remedy for cancer of the breast in adult women. Cancer of the breast has been known, and recognized as potentially fatal, since antiquity. But prior to the eighteenth century, medical authorities very seldom recommended surgical treatment, regarding it as ineffectual; see, for example, Celsus, *De medicina* 5.28 (Loeb) 2:130. See Pamela Sanders-Goebel, "Crisis and Controversy: Historical Patterns in Breast Cancer Surgery," *Canadian Bulletin of Medical History* 8 (1991): 77–90.

141. *In Aphorismos Hippocratis commentaria luculentissima cum graeco textu* (Pavia, 1653) (see Peter Krivatsky, *A Catalogue of Seventeenth Century Printed Books in the National Library of Medicine* [Bethesda, 1989], no. 2147); *In librum Hippocratis de alimento* (Basel 1582; IA *132.121).

142. "In haec Insubria nostra . . . videas non solum auditores, verum etiam iamdiu promotos ad lauream, quos minime pudeat, Cardanum contra Galeni placita veluti Pythiam Apollinem in medium producere" (Camuzio, *Disputationes* 3.5; see also n. 41 to chap. 3, above, and Jensen, "Cardanus and His Readers," p. 281. In his *Disputationes*, in addition to the rhetorical assault on Cardano, Camuzio devoted seventy-one folios to a point-by-point rebuttal of specific criticisms of Galen made by Cardano in the commentary on the *Aphorisms*.

143. "Ultimum genus paradoxorum est cum quaedam falso recepta sunt ab hominum consensu, velut quod sol sit longe minor terra; qui enim dixerit solem esse maiorem paradoxum dicere videbitur, cum tamen meram dicat veritatem. In huiusmodi ergo genere est quod ab omnibus receptum sit pro constanti, credendum esse magis expositoribus de opinione authoris qui exponitur, quam authori de opinione expositoris; existimant enim plerique, magis credendum Galeno exponenti Hippocratem, et Avicennae de Galeni opinione quam Galeno de Avicennae opinione et Hippocrati de Galeni opinione. Et tamen secus est . . ." (comm. *Aph.* 1.17, *Opera* 8:251).

CHAPTER 7
THE HIDDEN AND THE MARVELOUS

1. See, for example, RV 8.43, *Opera* 3:150–61; VP 37–38, 43, 47, *Opera* 1:27–30, 37–39, 44–45, and n. 97 to chap. 6. Regarding dreams, see further chap. 8.

2. Jensen, "Cardanus and His Readers," pp. 270–73, provides examples. Cardano's contemporaries did not, of course, base their opinions on the material from the *Vita* cited in the previous note (first published in the mid–seventeenth century), but on *De subtilitate* and *De rerum varietate.*

3. Contributions include Jean Céard, "La notion de 'miraculum' dans la pensée de Cardan," in *Acta conventus neo-latini turonensis,* ed. Jean-Claude Margolin (Paris, 1976), 2:924–37; Ingegno, esp. chaps. 1–4; Maclean, "The Interpretation of Natural Signs"; Margolin, "Analogie et causalité chez Jérôme Cardan"; Eugenio Di Rienzo, "La religione di Cardano," Kessler, pp. 49–76; Giancarlo Zanier, "Cardano e la critica delle religioni," *Giornale critico della filosofia italiana* 54 (1979): 89–98.

4. I make no attempt to give a complete bibliography or to summarize the often acrimonious historiographical controversies that have arisen over the sources, nature, and historical significance of Renaissance magic and occultism. Some principal contributions over the last forty years include D. P. Walker, *Spiritual and Demonic Magic from Ficino to Campanella* (London, 1958); Frances Yates, *Giordano Bruno and the Hermetic Tradition* (London, 1964); Eugenio Garin, *Lo zodiaco della vita* (Bari and Rome, 1976); Paolo Rossi, *Immagini della scienza* (Rome, 1977); Brian Vickers, ed., *Occult and Scientific Mentalities in the Renaissance* (Cambridge, 1984); Edward Grant, "Medieval and Renaissance Scholastic Conceptions of the Influence of the Celestial Regions on the Terrestrial," *Journal of Medieval and Renaissance Studies* 17 (1987): 1–23; Brian Copenhaver, "Astrology and Magic," in *The Cambridge History of Renaissance Philosophy,* ed. Charles Schmitt et al. (Cambridge, 1988), 264–300; Paola Zambelli, *L'ambigua natura della magia* (Milan, 1991).

5. One Renaissance medical author who was strongly influenced by Ficino and whose attitude to occultism was almost as ambiguous as Cardano's was Symphorien Champier; see Brian Copenhaver, *Symphorien Champier and the Reception of the Occultist Tradition in Renaissance France* (The Hague, 1978), pp. 175–241. Regarding Pomponazzi's *De incantationibus* and medical examples, see n. 16 to chap. 1.

6. "Complexionatum vero, quod tantum est medicina, manifeste corpus immutat. . . . Activarum autem virtutum quaedam sunt communes omnibus complexionatis, et hae sunt quatuor qualitates primae, quas omnes medicus, ut supra, vocat activas. Aliae vero sunt propriae, et ideo proprietates dicuntur, et a quibusdam virtutes specificae, quia formam specificam consequuntur: Similiter etiam, quia tales virtutes communes sunt omnibus in individuis speciei, propterea operatio ipsarum dicitur a tota specie fieri, et quidam dicunt a tota substantia. . . . multi medicorum vocaverunt proprietatem virtutem occultam. . . . dicitur occulta, quoniam ea quibus res cognoscitur omnino sunt apud humanam rationem ignota: omnis enim res determinate cognoscitur, vel causis immediatis, vel ef-

fectu immediato, quorum utrunque in proprietatibus ignorat humana ratio. . . . effectus autem proprietatis nequit ratione cognosci, cum priora sint in eis occulta, nec etiam colligi potest rationabili experimento, scilicet tantummodo casuali" (Arnald of Villanova, *Speculum introductionum medicinalium*, in his *Opera omnia* [Basel, 1585], cols. 47–48). I am grateful to Chiara Crisciani for this reference.

7. On the interest in contagion and disease transmission, see Vivian Nutton, "The Seeds of Disease: An Explanation of Contagion and Infection from the Greeks to the Renaissance," *Medical History* 27 (1983): 1–34; idem, "The Reception of Fracastoro's Theory of Contagion: The Seed That Fell among Thorns," *Osiris* 6 (1990): 196–234. See also the discussion of the "new" diseases of the sixteenth century in Ann Carmichael, "Diseases of the Renaissance and Early Modern Europe," in *The Cambridge World History of Human Disease*, ed. Kenneth R. Kiple (Cambridge, 1993), p. 283.

8. See Wolf-Dieter Müller-Jahncke, *Astrologisch-magische Theorie und Praxis in der Heilkunde der frühen Neuzeit, Sudhoffs Archiv*, Supplement (Stuttgart, 1985). The scope of Renaissance writing on the marvelous and monstrous is far too vast to be indicated here. Useful studies include Jean Céard, *La nature et les prodiges: L'insolite au XVIe siècle en France* (Paris, 1977); Margaret Hodgen, *Early Anthropology in the Sixteenth and Seventeenth Centuries* (Philadelphia, 1964, 1971); Anthony Grafton, *New Worlds, Ancient Texts* (Cambridge, Mass., 1992), pp. 97–157; Katharine Park and Lorraine J. Daston, "Unnatural Conceptions: The Study of Monsters in Sixteenth- and Seventeenth-Century France and England," *Past and Present* 92 (1981): 20–54. Helpful analysis of sixteenth-century interest in marvels and the preternatural is contained in Daston, "Marvelous Facts," pp. 93–100. For the medieval tradition and an important text, see Bert Hansen, *Nicole Oresme and the Marvels of Nature: A Study of His "De causis mirabilium" with Critical Edition, Translation, and Commentary* (Toronto, 1985); also John B. Friedman, *The Monstrous Races in Medieval Art and Thought* (Cambridge, Mass., 1981). The historical development of the entire tradition of natural marvels has now been examined in Park and Daston, *Wonders and the Order of Nature*. I am most grateful to the last-named authors for allowing me to read their work in manuscript.

9. "Qui multo tempore et multis medetur, varia et multa admiratione digna cognoscit" (Benivieni, p. 523). The remark is from Benivieni's original preface, which is included in the Costa and Weber edition, along with other material omitted from the edition of 1507. The first edition of 1507 is reproduced in facsimile, accompanied by English translation, in Antonio Benivieni, *De abditis nonnullis ac mirandis morborum et sanationum causis*, trans. Charles Singer (Springfield, Ill., 1954).

10. Benivieni, p. 523.

11. The edition of Benivieni's work published in 1507 consists of a selection posthumously edited for publication by a medical colleague, at the request of Antonio's brother Girolamo; see Benivieni, *De abditis*, ed. Singer, pp. 2–6. Benivieni's manuscript was lost in the mid–nineteenth century, but fortunately not before the author's own preface and the cases omitted from the early printed edition had been transcribed; see Benivieni, ed. Costa and Weber, pp. 460–82.

Although the sixteenth-century editor may in a few instances have grouped several similar cases under one head, there is no evidence to suggest that he undertook any major reorganization. For suggested identifications in terms of twentieth-century pathology of some of Benivieni's cases, see Esmond R. Long, "Antonio Benivieni and His Contribution to Pathological Anatomy," pp. xxxv–xli, in Benivieni, *De abditis*, ed. Singer.

12. "preceptor meus . . . Christophorus Landinus" (Antonio Benivieni, *Encomion Cosmi ad Laurentiam Medicem. Riproduzione dell'autografo con proemio e trascrizione*, ed. Renato Piattoli [Florence, 1949], 31). He referred to his studies in philosophy and medicine in the preface of his regimen of health for Lorenzo de' Medici; see Enrico Coturri, "L'inizio di una 'Practica' lasciata incompiuta e ancora inedita di Antonio Benivieni," *Episteme: Rivista critica di storia delle scienze mediche e biologiche* 8 (1974): 3–25, at p. 5.

13. Poliziano addressed a poem in praise of the Benivieni brothers to Antonio (a third brother, Domenico, was a Scotist theologian and poet); see Angelus Politianus, *Opera omnia*, ed. Ida Maier, vol. 2, *Opera ab Isidoro del Lungo edita Florentiae anno MDCCCLXVII* (Turin, 1970), pp. 236–38. Antonio Benivieni's career, education, and associations in Florence are summarized, with comprehensive bibliography, in U. Stefanutti, "Benivieni, Antonio," *Dizionario biografici degli italiani* 8 (Rome, 1966), 543–45.

14. The texts of his other surviving medical works are edited in G. M. Nardi, "Antonio Benivieni ed un suo scritto inedito sulla peste," *Atti e memorie dell'Accademia di Storia d'Arte Sanitaria* 4 (1938): 124–33, 190–97; Coturri, "L'inizio di una 'Practica,'" and Antonio Benivieni, *De regimine sanitatis ad Laurentium medicem*, ed. Lugi Belloni (Milan, 1952). I have not been able to secure access to the last; I rely on the description of it in Coturri, "L'inizio di una 'Practica,'" 10.

15. Benivieni's own list of his books, found in the manuscript of his *ricordi* (Florence, Archivio di Stato, Notarile Antecosmiano 2338 [formerly 1324]), is edited in Bindo De Vecchi, "I libri di un medico umanista fiorentino del sec. XV dai 'Ricordi' di maestro Antonio Benivieni," *La bibliofilia* 34 (1932): 293–301. The medical portion of the library is discussed in Susanna Sclavi, "La biblioteca di Antonio Benivieni," *Physis* 17 (1975): 255–68.

16. De Vecchi, "Libri," no. 164; Benivieni, ed. Costa and Weber, pp. 482–96 and Appendice II: "I brani del De medicina di A. Cornelio Celso assimilati nel De abditis," pp. 720–805. The work of Celsus was little known between the early Middle Ages and the fifteenth century; it was first printed in 1478.

17. De Vecchi, "Libri," no. 151. On Theodore of Gaza's translation, see J. Balme, introduction to Aristotle, *Historia animalium, Books VII–X* (Loeb), 49; Livia Martinoli Santini, "Le traduzioni dal Greco," in *Un pontificato ed una città: Sisto IV (1471–1484). Atti del Convegno, Roma 3–7 Dicembre, 1984*, ed. Massimo Miglio et al. (Rome, 1986), pp. 81–101, esp. pp. 81–83; Lotte Labowsky, "An Unknown Treatise by Theodorus Gaza: Bessarion Studies IV," *Medieval and Renaissance Studies* 6 (1968): 193.

18. De Vecchi, "Libri," nos. 10, 11, 95, 110, 14, 86, 87, 165; he owned two copies of Pietro d'Abano's commentary; on this work, see Nancy G. Siraisi, "The *Expositio problematum Aristotelis* of Peter of Abano," *Isis* 61 (1970): 321–39.

19. De Vecchi, "Libri," nos. 32, 60, 117 (he had two copies of Pliny), 141.

20. Most of this material is to be found in pt. 4, chaps. 2–4, and pt. 5, chap. 8, in *Avicenna latinus. Liber de anima seu sextus de naturalibus IV–V*, ed. S. Van Riet with introduction by G. Verbeke (Louvain, 1968).

21. *Andreae Cattanii Imolensis opus de intellectu et de causis mirabilium effectuum* (n.p., n.d., but thought to be Florence, ca. 1502). See Eugenio Garin, *Medioevo e Rinascimento* (Bari, 1961), pp. 42–45.

22. Armando F. Verde, *Lo studio fiorentino 1473–1503: Ricerche e documenti*, vol. 2, *Docenti-dottorati* (Florence, 1973), pp. 20–21 (Cattani taught during 1499, 1501–2, 1505–6); "[C]um superiore anno libros de anima Aristotelis publice ordinarie interpretaremur. . . . in Mariae novae hospitalibus aegris pro recuperanda sanitate illic manentibus iam diu praesedimus praesidemusque" (Cattani, *Opus de intellectu*, fol. a2r).

23. Cattani, *Opus de intellectu*, Tractatus III, "De causis mirabilium effectuum," fols. e2r–f8r.

24. The passage appears to echo the ideas about statues expressed by Ficino in *De vita* 3.26, although I do not attempt to explore this connection here.

25. The treatise is edited in Nardi, "Antonio Benivieni ed un suo scritto inedito sulla peste," the astral causes of plague being discussed on pp. 126–28.

26. Antonio's brother Girolamo Benivieni was a leading literary figure among Savonarola's followers. On the activities of the Benivieni brothers on behalf of Savonarola, see Lorenzo Polizzotto, *The Elect Nation: The Savonarolan Movement in Florence, 1494–1545* (Oxford, 1994), pp. 68–75, 108–17, 139–67.

27. Benivieni, chaps. 7, 30, 71, and 97, pp. 537, 561, 599, 619.

28. Ibid., chaps. 48, 50–52, and 54, pp. 575, 577–83.

29. Ibid., chaps. 3, 32–37, 73, 79, 81, and 99, pp. 531–33, 561–67, 601, 607, 621–23. Some of these cases perhaps involved cancers.

30. *Aphorisms* 6.18.

31. "Tenuioris intestini morbo, quem Graei ileon vocant, urgeri commune est: sed urgeri, ut sic viam tollat, inauditum" (Benivieni, chap. 76, p. 603). The related passage from Celsus, *De medicina*, is identified in ibid., p. 768.

32. Grieco, "Social Politics."

33. Benivieni, chaps. 13, 59, and 109, pp. 543–45, 585–87, 631, 673. Grieco, "Social Politics," pp. 132–34, points out that physiological and social categories overlapped for both medical writers and authors of *novelle*.

34. Benivieni, chap. 75, p. 603; chap. 54, pp. 581–83; "Quare autorum tandem sententiis nixus, quibus docetur medicus, cum causae morbi abditae sunt his praesidiis uti, quae conferre quidem possint, nocere non possint: coepi primum lenire pectus . . ." (chap. 24, p. 555).

35. "Igitur ii, qui rationalem medicinam profitentur, haec necessaria esse proponunt: abditarum et morbus continentium causarum notitiam. . . . Abditas causas vocant, quibus requiritur, ex quibus principiis nostra corpora sint. . . . Neque enim credunt, posse eum scire, quomodo morbos curare conveniat, qui unde sint ignoret" (Celsus, *De medicina*, bk. 1, proem [Loeb 1:8], quoted in Benivieni, ed. Costa and Weber, p. 484).

36. ". . . sapientis viri consilium esse duximus, nihil omnino de incertis et occultis morbis statuere" (Benivieni, chap. 94, p. 617).

37. "Natura enim multa operatur que miranda medicis videntur, et moriturum ex faucibus Orci sepius revocat" (ibid., p. 665).

38. See n. 35, above.

39. See, for example, Avicenna, *Canon* 1.2.1.1–6.

40. "VIII. Mulier a spiritu malo oppressa. Accidit his temporibus novum et admirandum morbi genus . . ." (Benivieni, chap. 8, pp. 537–39). "De morbo quem vulgo gallicum vocant caput primum. Novum morbi genus, anno salutis nonagesimosexto supra mille quingentos a christiana salute non solum Italiam, sed fere totam Europam irrepsit" (ibid, p. 523).

41. For example, ibid., chap. 72, pp. 599–601, chap. 26, p. 557, chap. 45, pp. 571–73, and 637–39. Also "Ramice vexabatur Michelotius noster. Cumque sacerdoti cuidam, qui hanc artem [sc. medicinam] profiteretur, se se curandum tradidisset. . . . ingens exorta inflammatio. . . . Ex quo paucis dein horis e vita discedens, utile nobis documentum sua morte reliquit, languentium scilicet corpora non sacerdotibus, quibus tantum animarum cura demandata est, sed doctioribus medicis tradi oportere" (ibid., chap. 73, p. 601).

42. Cattani, *Opus de intellectu*, fols. fr–f2r.

43. Benivieni, p. 638.

44. "hoc solo nutu Dei per fidem et orationem sanctissimi illius viri factum fuisse" (ibid., chap. 45, pp. 571–73, with the remark quoted at 573). See also ibid., chap. 9, pp. 539–41. Domenico Buonvicini of Pescia, O.P., was burned at the stake along with Savonarola.

45. "Quod et nos non solum vidimus: sed et propriis (ut aiunt) manibus attrectantes geniculum ipsum" (Benivieni, chap. 9, p. 541); chap. 45, pp. 571–73; pp. 641–43.

46. Benivieni's work was reprinted at least five times in the sixteenth and early seventeenth centuries, always in collections with other works; see Durling, *Catalogue*, nos. 1179–80, 1917, 2015, and 4168.

47. "Prosecutus igitur iter, amice satis cum Pharnelio, et Sylvio, alioque Regis medico quos ibi [sc. Paris] reliqueram . . ." (VP 29, *Opera* 1:18).

48. A bibliography of Fernel's works is included in Charles Sherrington, *The Endeavour of Jean Fernel* (London, 1946; reprint, Folkestone and London, 1974). I have consulted (on microfilm), Jean Fernel, *Universa medicina tribus et viginti libris absoluta. Ab ipso quidem authore ante obitum diligenter recognita, et quatuor libris nunquam ante editis, ad praxim tamen perquam necessariis, aucta* (Lyon, 1581; Durling, *Catalogue*, no. 1469, not in Sherrington). This edition is a reissue of one prepared by Fernel's pupil Guillaume Plancy in 1567. It consists of *Physiologia*, bks. 1–7 (a revision of the work originally published under the title *De naturali parte medicinae* in 1542 and subsequently included in *Medicina* in 1554); *Pathologia*, bks. 1–7 (first published in *Medicina*, 1554); *Therapeutices*, bks. 1–7 (bks. 1–3 were first published in *Medicina*, 1554, and bks. 4–7 added in *Universa medicina*, 1567). The total of twenty-three books is made up by the inclusion of *De abditis rerum causis*, bks. 1–2. Pagination is continous throughout. On Fernel, see also Jacques Roger, *Jean Fernel et les problèmes de la médecine de la Renaissance*, Les Conférences du Palais de la Découverte, ser. D, no. 70 (Paris, 1960), and works cited in the previous note and below.

49. See n. 83 to chap. 5.

50. See Siraisi, "Giovanni Argenterio," p. 161.

51. See James J. Bono, *The Word of God and the Languages of Man: Interpreting Nature in Early Modern Science and Medicine*, vol. 1, *Ficino to Descartes* (Madison, 1995), pp. 92–97. This and the following paragraph owe much to the entire discussion of Fernel, at pp. 85–103.

52. Guillaume Plancy, *Vita Fernelii*, translated by Sherrington, in *Endeavour*, p. 162.

53. Ibid., p. 159. The strong repudiation of divinatory astrology attributed to Fernel in Plancy's *Vita* of Fernel may owe more to Plancy than to Fernel.

54. In addition to Bono, *Word*, Müller-Jahncke, *Astrologisch-magische Theorie*, pp. 113–16; Linda Deer Richardson, "The Generation of Disease: Occult Causes and Disease of the Total Substance," in *The Medical Renaissance of the Sixteenth Century*, ed. Andrew Wear, R. K. French, and I. M. Lonie (Cambridge, 1985), pp. 175–94.

55. See James J. Bono, "Medical Spirits and the Medieval Language of Life," *Traditio* 40 (1984): 91–130; Copenhaver, *Symphorien Champier*, pp. 183–84.

56. Fernel, *De abditis rerum causis* 2.7–8 and 10–13, in *Universa medicina* (1581), pp. 606–13, 617–33; Richardson, "Generation of Disease," pp. 181–84; Bono, *Word*.

57. Fernel, *De abditis rerum causis* 1.9–10, in *Universa medicina* (1581), pp. 575–84.

58. Ibid. 1.11, in *Universa medicina* (1581), pp. 584–88. At p. 588: "Si quos enim spiritus orbe toto volitare et vagare compertum habemus, eosque sensu non attingi, incorporeos esse immortales, et intelligentiae participes: constans id et firmum esse debet, animum quem in nobis sentimus intelligentiae capacem, incorporeum simul et immortalem haberi: et eundem, quum e corpore emigravit, in perpetumm vivere, referrique in spirituum greges."

59. Ibid. 2.16, in *Universa medicina* (1581), pp. 641–44. The case of possession is described on p. 641.

60. "Omnis investigatio ab eo quod sensibus perspicuum est in abstrusas occultatasque causas deducit: quodque ortu et causarum ordine postremum est, investigatione primum occurrit: nempe aut morbus aliquis manifestus, aut certe symptoma. Hoc autem sive laesa functio, sive excrementum, sive dolor fuerit, tum ex situ, tum ex specie nos in aliquam partis affectae suspicionem primum adducet" (Fernel, *Universa medicina* [1581], *Pathologia* 2.9, p. 202).

61. Sherrington, *Endeavour*, pp. 19–22.

62. On the dating of *De naturali parte medicinae*, see ibid., p. 22. *De abditis rerum causis* was published in 1548, but as it is referred to in *De naturali parte medicinae*, it must have been written before 1542. *De abditis* includes a reference to an epidemic of dysentery in 1540 (Fernel, *De abditis rerum causis* 2.13, in *Universa medicina* [1581], p. 630).

63. "Nam duos de Abditis causis adiecimus non ad totius integritatem, sed ad Physiologiae, Pathologiae et Therapeuticae locorum difficiliorum diffusiorem et enucleatiorem per dialogismum explicationem." The remark comes from Plancy's preface to his comprehensive posthumous edition of Fernel's *Universa medicina* (1567), reprinted in the edition of 1581.

64. RV 8.44, *Opera* 3:165–74.

65. "Sunt qui cum alio iuvene bonorum morum duplici fistula, alii unica, commutare sanguinem posse sperent: quod si fiat, commutabuntur et mores" (ibid., p. 172). As this remark suggests, a number of early speculations about ways of improving the blood preceded the well-known pioneering actual transfusions—some of them disastrous—attempted by followers of Harvey in the 1660s; see, among much other literature, Robert G. Frank, Jr., *Harvey and the Oxford Physiologists* (Berkeley, 1980), pp. 169–78.

66. "Praecantationes an in cura aliquid possint" (*Contradictiones* 2.2.7, *Opera* 6:467–86 [Lyon, 1548, pp. 72–113]). The *quaestio* is analyzed from the philosophical standpoint in Ingegno, pp. 56–61.

67. "Haec [sc. Plato's views on daemons] inquam ut ex grandissimo autore sic minus clara: quae tamen ab ipso Pomponazzi maxima ea parte in suo libro de incantationibus sustulimus" (*Contradictiones* 2.2.7, *Opera* 6:468 [Lyon, 1548, pp. 74–75]). Pomponazzi's treatise (n. 16 to chap. 1), written in 1520, was first published in 1556. On its circulation in manuscript, see Zanier, *Ricerche*, pp. 17–25; regarding Pomponazzi's views on occultism and natural magic, see Brian P. Copenhaver, "Did Science Have a Renaissance?" *Isis* 83 (1992): 387–407.

The chapter in *De rerum varietate* (on which Cardano began to work in the mid-1530s [LP 1557, *Opera* 1:65]) was also written before *Contradictiones* 2.2.7: "Cum vero plurima talia sint, ea qua manifesta sunt in tertium librum de rerum varietate retulimus" (*Opera* 6:467 [1548, p. 73]).

68. "Haec sunt quae non solum falsa et impia, sed etiam a Peripateticis aliena magna ex parte, ac etiam ridicula invicemque pugnantia scripsit Pomponatius" (*Contradictiones* 2.2.7, *Opera* 6:478); Ingegno, pp. 60–61; see also Zanier, *Ricerche*, pp. 106–11.

69. "Tria tamen maximam hic afferunt difficultatem. Primum est, quod ut habetur in secundo posterorum [1548: posteriorum], quaestio Quid est et propter quid est, praesupponunt quaestionem Si est: quae cum lateat in plerisque ob dolos, ideo incertum est, quodnam ex his experimentis sit verum, quidve falsum" (*Contradictiones* 2.2.7, *Opera* 6:480 [and similarly elsewhere in the same *quaestio*]). On the standard list of magical objects and effects, repeated since antiquity, see Copenhaver, "A Tale of Two Fishes."

70. "Unde advertendum, multa esse per se pauci momenti viriumque contemptarum, quae tamen ex modo applicandi mirabiles faciunt effectus: velut aqua auget dolores, et putrefacit vulnera: copiosa tamen dolores levat, et assidue permutata vulnera sanat, ut ex Celso in librum de Animi immortalitate deduximus: quamobrem hoc genus non ad praecantationem, sed ad artem medicam deduco" (*Contradictiones* 2.2.7, *Opera* 6:482).

71. *De subtilitate* 19, *Opera* 3:656–57. *De subtilitate* was first published in 1550; Cardano stated that the case had occurred the previous year.

72. "Respondeo, quod damnantur ea quae verbis fiunt, ut merito: nam si operantur naturaliter, verba nullam habent vim, igitur sunt haec cum fraude, igitur non debent admitti. Idem dico de notis: si dicas habere vim secundum legem, igitur per daemones, quare committitur cultus daemonum, igitur nullo modo possunt admitti. Quae autem absque verbis fiunt si pertinent ad sanitatem, ut dixi, sunt de consideratione medici: si ad alium finem, ut de remora, et magnete,

sunt de consideratione philosophi naturalis: quare nullam aliam necesse est scientiam ponere. Igitur magia nulla est, nisi ponas eam partem vel medicinae vel scientiae naturalis, et hoc modo intellecta [1548: non] magis est illicita, quam ars ipsa fabrilis" (*Contradictiones* 2.2.7, *Opera* 6:483). Cardano would not necessarily have interpreted a ban on verbal invocations as prohibiting use of figures and symbols. See Brian Copenhaver, "Figure, Number, and Meaning in the Magical Cosmos of Giovanni Pico della Mirandola" (forthcoming).

73. "conabimur vero solvere iuxta nostra principia ac Aristotelis" (ibid., p. 480).

"[Pomponatius] modo Aristotelem, modo sequatur Platonem" (ibid., p. 478); see Copenhaver, "Did Science Have a Renaissance?" p. 401.

74. RV 16.90, *Opera* 3:310–12. Cardano discussed demons in *De subtilitate* 19, *Opera* 3:655–61, and RV 16.93, *Opera* 3:317–36. For discussion of these passages, see Müller-Jahncke, *Astrologisch-magische Theorie*, pp. 110–13. A diligent seventeenth-century expurgator of a copy of the Basel, 1557, edition of RV now in the New York Public Library (*KB 1557 [Cardano, G.] 85–259) sliced the whole of bk. 16 out of the volume.

75. *De subtilitate* 20, *Opera* 3:662.

76. "Omnibus igitur ad trutinam diligenter redactis, censendum est rationibus difficile est tueri, daemonum ac mortuorum animos hicinde dispersos esse: quod tamen experimento, et ordini rerum, et naturali inclinationi convenit, est ut illos haud dubie esse credamus" (RV 16.93, *Opera* 3:329).

77. "Deus an singula quaeque cognoscat" (*Contradictiones* 3.6, *Opera* 6:657–59). Not published in Cardano's lifetime, though apparently intended for publication; see chap. 3, n. 96.

78. Agostino Nifo, *De intellectu libri sex. Eiusdem de demonibus libri tres* (Venice, 1527), fols. 69r–76v. The evidence of the Paduan inquisitor is found on fol. 71r.

79. *Contradictiones* 3.6, *Opera* 6:659. I have not succeeded in locating the reference to the Neapolitan alchemist in Nifo's treatise but may have missed it.

80. "Tertium et, quod dantur genii singulorum qui ad unquem tantum sciunt, quantum illi ut genius Averroes, quantum novit Averroes in vita: et Avicennae, quantum Avicenna seu Hasen: Et hoc est valde verisimile ob ea quae in ea invocatione habentur, et concordat ad unguem cum experimentis primis. Et quod narravimus de illis duobus disputantibus, credendum est quod fuerint genii Averrois, et Algazelis: Et quod genius Averrois fuit ille qui minor videbatur corpore, et colore subnigro: Et Algazel fuit maior et rubicundior et disputaverunt super quarta disputatione, sciliet de mundi causa efficiente" (ibid.).

81. *De subtilitate* 19, *Opera* 3:656.

82. RV 16.93, *Opera* 3:335–36.

83. "Dico quod vel sunt perpetui, vel sunt mentes hominum vehiculo aereo imbutae, aliter essent duo in nobis qui idem intelligerent, anima et genius. Praeterea id concordat ad unguem cum nostris principiis, qui volumus animam non esse in nobis, nec ullibi: sed corpus esse in ea, et in corpore esse vitam, et forsan animam nutricem quae alit illud. Sed sensus et mens idem sunt quod genius: et assistunt corpori. . . . Sed dices, anima mea seu genius cuius aetatis doctrinam habebit. Si enim infantiae nullam, si mortis nullam, si praesentem qua ra-

tione magis, quam alterius temporis. Et etiam quia nunc multa scio, quae iam annis viginti nesciebam: et rursus multorum sum oblitus quae iam bene noveram. Respondeo, quod omnia quae unquam novi, licet enim oblitus sim. . . . genii isti norunt facta nostra, et nos ipsos . . ." (*Contradictiones* 3.6, *Opera* 6:659). Regarding Cardano's concept of his, and Socrates', genius, see further Ingegno, pp. 160–61.

84. *Contradictiones* 10.53, "Morborum quot genera propria" (*Opera* 6:921–23); not published in his lifetime.

85. "Fernelius quoque in secundo de abditis rerum causis ostendere nititur in similibus partibus fieri tria morborum genera, ut universa sint quinque. Tria sunt quae possunt vitiari materia forma et temperamentum. . . . In forma quoque cum vel iuncta putredine vel absque ea corrumpitur substantia. . . . Ad Fernelii argumenta quamvis pulcherrima: Respondeo quod venenum et febris pestilens prout corruptio est in substantia sunt causae, et non morborum genera; quia non nocent operationibus nisi cum qualitate" (ibid.).

86. Cardano, *De venenis* 1.14, *Opera* 7:293.

87. "Cum igitur spiritus amoveatur a propria functione, imaginatio refrigerat locum, aut movendo sanguinem excalefacit; igitur in fascinatione, et amore, ac huiuscemodi morbus est intemperies: sed qui existimantur morbi sunt illorum causae" (*Contradictiones* 10.53, *Opera* 6:923).

88. "cum qui hanc magiam fatentur, Platonici sint, mirum in modum addicti daemonum confessioni" (Cardano, *De venenis* 1.17, *Opera* 7:298).

89. Francisco Sanches, *De divinatione per somnum, ad Aristotelem*, in his *Opera philosophica* (Coimbra, 1955), pp. 107–16. Sanches (1551–1623), whose critique was based on *De rerum varietate*, was among those who categorized Cardano as primarily credulous. As a young man, Sanches studied philosophy and medicine in Rome and may have encountered Cardano there. See Francisco Sanches, *That Nothing Is Known*, ed. Elaine Limbrick and Douglas F. S. Thomson (Cambridge, 1988), pp. 13–14.

90. Müller-Jahncke, *Astrologisch-magische Theorie*, p. 113.

91. CA, *Opera* 7:253–64. Regarding the different versions and editions of this work, see chap. 2, n. 2.

92. "Usum quoque multorum simplicium introduxi, sed et medicamentorum. Validioribus tamen uti non audent [alii medici], cum ego semper sine errore illis usus sim" (ibid., p. 264).

93. Cardano found the patient sitting up in bed, breathing unnaturally and with a swollen face. He deduced that he had difficulty breathing, could not sleep, and had swollen feet, all of which turned out to be true, and predicted to the patient's relatives that he would die six days later, which he did, perhaps of congestive heart failure. Ibid., *praedictio* 6, p. 262.

94. Ibid., *curatio* 21, p. 259.

95. RV 8.43, "Hominis mirabilia" (*Opera* 3:160–61), includes an account of Cardano's own trances, visions, prophetic dreams, and so on. With specific reference to his visions, he stated: "Credo causam esse, vim virtutis imaginatricis, visusque subtilitatem." Of all these gifts, he asserted: "Haec si quis observet, ut naturalia, nec fallitur, nec Deum offendit: imo gratias illi reddere videtur, nisi apud superstitiosos, aut imperitos. Si ut a daemonibus immissa, idololatriam

aperte commitit, atque insanus est et vanus." On Cardano's view of his own nature, see also chap. 3 and Ingegno, "Il perfetto e il furioso."

96. "Quod vero contingit de Gaspare Roulla ... adeo miraculo proximum visum est omnibus, ut multi ad hunc visendum accurrerent. Nam nulla vi humana sanari posse videbatur, antequam per nos sanatus sit. Sed libet narrare historiam. Iacebat iam per annum integrum contractus in lecto, sed supremis quinque illius anni mensibus totus immobilis, non pedem, non caput aut brachium movere poterat, neque aliud quicquam. Praeter dolorem enim ingentem, membra, ut lapis, rigida obduruerant. Et erat media hyems. Constat hunc a me intra quadraginta dies plene sanatum, non admiratione, sed stupore maximo eorum qui illum viderunt. Alii enim sideratum, alii perculsum divina ira, alii resolutum, alii daemone correptum dicebant, ita ut non deessent supplicationes et execrationes" (CA, *curatio* 18, *Opera* 7:258).

97. "ut dixi, ter misso sanguine, non solum ob morbi magnitudinem, sed etiam quod ex vitae ratione et ipso morbo coniectarer, totam sanguinis congeriem corruptum esse. Ne fefellit me ulla ex parte de hac re iudicium factum. Siquidem totus qui exiit sanguis, putridus erat" (ibid.).

98. A helpful analysis of Cardano's statements about miracles is provided by Céard, "La notion de 'miraculum'"; see also idem, *La nature et les prodiges*, pp. 229–51.

99. RV 15.81, "Miracula," *Opera* 3:294–97, remark quoted at pp. 296–97.

100. Ibid., p. 294; *De subtilitate* 12, *Opera* 3:559. Daston, "Marvelous Facts," pp. 95–96, points out (not with reference to Cardano) that such an attitude is more or less Augustine's own.

101. VP 44, "Quae in diversis disciplinis digna adinveni" (*Opera* 1:40) (see chap. 2, above); ibid. 42, "Praecognoscendi vis in arte [medica], et aliis" (*Opera* 1:36–37).

102. For the expression *miraculorum ratio*, see next note. Cf. "L'intervention de la *ratio* dans le travail sur les songes et dans l'objet travaillé est étroitement liée au caractère 'naturel' du songe" (Jacques Le Brun, "Jérôme Cardan et l'interprétation des songes," Kessler, p. 194).

103. "Atque haec de aegris insignioribus, qui ex morbis desperatis a nobis curati sunt: quamquam innumeros alios temporis longitudo et oblivio aboleverit. Neque enim nisi paucis abhinc annis huius modi miraculorum rationem habui. Hoc unum satis sit, me semper in artis operibus felicissimum fuisse, adeo ut no[n]nulli ad casum, alii ad daemonem referrent. Verum ut nemo felicior perpetuo successu in curando, ita nullus ab erroribus et casibus adversis tutior meipso fuit: adeo ut in tota vita vix ter aut quater sinistre res cesserint. Itaque si ad foelicitatem medendi respicio, haud piget fortunae meae: quandoquidem videam Galenum tam paucorum meminisse, quos ex deploratis morbis sanaverit" (CA, *curatio* 30, *Opera* 7:261).

CHAPTER 8
THE MEDICINE OF DREAMS

1. The Borromeo included as part of their coat of arms the image of a serpent swallowing a child, also famous as the emblem of the Visconti: "un biscione di azzurro, ingoiante un puttino di carnagione" (*Enciclopedia storico-nobiliare*

italiana [Milan, 1928–35], 2:144). The coat of arms appears as frontispiece in Ginex Palmiere, *San Carlo Borromeo.*

2. The account summarized here is from SS 4.4, *Opera* 5:723–24. See also VP 33, *Opera* 1:25, and LP 1557, *Opera* 1:65. Judging by the various disputes that recurred throughout his military and political career, Count Camillo Borromeo (ca. 1500–1549) did indeed have a combative and violent nature. See *Dizionario biografici degli Italiani* 13 (Rome, 1971), p. 29.

3. "Ob hocque solum somnium, hoc opus conscripsi" (SS 4.4, *Opera* 5:725). The first edition is Cardano, *Somniorum synesiorum omnis generis insomnia explicantes libri IIII* . . . (Basel, 1562; IA *132. 083). The work was reissued twice more during the sixteenth century (Basel, 1585; IA *132. 125; and Basel, ca. 1590; IA *132. 126). There are also two sixteenth-century editions of a German translation (Basel, 1563; IA *132. 085; and Basel, 1564; IA *132. 095). Valuable studies are Alice Browne, "Girolamo Cardano's *Somniorum synesiorum libri IIII*," *Bibliothèque d'humanisme et Renaissance* 40 (1979): 123–35, and Le Brun, "Jérôme Cardan et l'interpretation des songes"; also useful are the introductions to the recent Italian translations of SS: of bk. 1, Gerolamo Cardano, *Sul sonno e sul sognare*, ed. Mauro Mancia and Agnese Grieco (Venice, 1989), pp. 11–22; and of bks. 2–3 with selections from bk. 4, idem, *Sogni*, ed. Agnese Grieco and Mauro Mancia (Venice, 1993), pp. 9–23. Less helpful is Markus Fierz, *Girolamo Cardano, 1501–1576* (Boston, 1983), pp. 125–55.

4. See Pierre Brind'amour, *Nostradamus astrophile: Les astres et L'astrologie dans la vie et l'oeuvre de Nostradamus* (Ottawa, 1993), pt. 1, "La carrière prophétique de Nostradamus," pp. 21–167; Richard L. Kagan, *Lucrecia's Dreams: Politics and Prophecy in Sixteenth-Century Spain* (Berkeley, 1990); William L. Christian, *Apparitions in Late Medieval and Renaissance Spain* (Princeton, 1981); on popular prophecy in Italy, see Ottavia Niccoli, *Prophecy and People in Renaissance Italy* (Princeton, 1990); see also, on Paracelsus and prophecy, Charles Webster, *From Paracelsus to Newton* (Cambridge, 1982), pp. 15–27; on dreams and the medical profession, see Richard Cooper, "Deux médecins royaux onirocrites: Jehan Thibault et Auger Ferrier," in *Le songe à la Renaissance*, ed. Françoise Charpentier (St. Etienne, 1987), pp. 53–59, esp. p. 53.

5. See, for example, LP 1562, *Opera* 1:108, and RV 17.100, *Opera* 3:348.

6. Both the original horoscope and Cardano's subsequent reflections are printed in his *In Cl[audii] Ptolemaei Pelusiensis IIII de astrorum iudiciis . . . libros* [= *Tetrabiblos*] *commentaria . . . . Praeterea eiusdem Hier[onymi] Cardani Geniturarum XII . . . exempla* (Basel, 1554; IA *132. 063), pp. 403–13. The version in *Liber duodecim geniturarum*, *Opera* 5:503–8, contains Cardano's apologia together with a version of the horoscope from which some of the specifics about Edward's future have been omitted.

7. Compare LP 1562, *Opera* 1:101, and VP 37, *Opera* 1:29.

8. RV 8.43–44, *Opera* 3:164–66.

9. Céard, *La nature et les prodiges*, p. 251.

10. "Dico ergo quod nemo potest dissolvere hanc difficultatem nisi quid [1568: qui] calleat artem Hippocraticam Ptolemei" (comm. *Prognost.* 3.5 [bk. 4 of commentary], *Opera* 8:746). See chap. 6, above.

11. Comm. *Epid.*, *Opera* 10:195, and chap. 6, above.

12. "Est igitur haec disciplina [sc. cognitio somniorum] in genere coniecturalium, qualis est medicina, agricultura et ars navigandi" (SS 1.6, *Opera* 5:602).

13. "Ergo videndum, an sit aliqua ars? Et certe si ad totum genus somniorum res haec referatur, ars omnino nulla est: sed si ad evidentia et perfecta, quorum maxima pars sortitur effectum, erit de illis ars atque scientia: plurima enim horum vera sunt, taliumque aliqua notitia: veluti sanationum nulla est scientia: quoniam plurimi casu sanantur: sanationum autem quae a medicis fiunt, ars aliqua est, et certa ratio" (ibid., 4.1, *Opera* 5:704).

14. See Giulio Guidorizzi, ed., *Il sogno in Grecia* (Rome, 1988); Tullio Gregory, ed., *I sogni nel Medioevo* (Rome, 1985); "Pour le Colloque 'Le Songe à la Renaissance,'" *Bulletin de l'Association d'Etude sur l'Humanisme, la Réforme et la Renaissance* 12 (1986): 43–65; Jacques Le Goff, "Dreams in the Culture and Collective Psychology of the Medieval West," in his *Time, Work, and Culture in the Middle Ages* (Chicago, 1980), pp. 201–4; Charpentier, *Le songe à la Renaissance*; Jean-Marie Wagner, "De la nécessaire distinction entre 'somnium'-songe et 'insomnium'-rêve," in *Acta Conventus Neo-Latini Turonensis*, ed. Jean-Claude Margolin (Paris, 1980), pp. 709–20. Luciano Bonuzzi, "Qualche considerazione su sonno e sogno dal tramonto della cultura classica all'età del manierismo," *Acta medicae historiae patavina* 20 (1973–74): 57–102; Steven F. Kruger, *Dreaming in the Middle Ages* (Cambridge, 1992).

15. On the interest in dreams of the Jewish physician and cabalist Abraham Yagel, see David B. Ruderman, *Kabbalah, Magic, and Science: The Cultural Universe of a Sixteenth-Century Jewish Physician* (Cambridge, Mass., 1988), pp. 31–32. Yagel read some of Cardano's works and, as Ruderman shows, his and Cardano's approach to medicine had much in common (ibid., pp. 91–96, 28). Conceivably Cardano himself knew something of Jewish traditions about dreams; he could have gained some awareness from personal contacts with Jewish physicians or cabalists (something for which I have, however, found no specific evidence) even in the absence of translations of Hebrew dream books. However, his reference to writings on dreams ascribed to "Salomon Iudaeus, non ille rex, sed longe posterior" (SS 1.1, *Opera* 5:596) probably refers to a medieval Latin text, perhaps *Somnia Salomonis regis filii David* [Venice, 1501]; see Durling, *Catalogue*, no. 4237, in which it is described as one of many apocryphal works attributed to Solomon; Durling also notes that a mention of Avicenna in the text establishes that the work was compiled no earlier than the eleventh century. Lynn Thorndike, *A History of Magic and Experimental Science*, vol. 6 (New York, 1941), p. 475, notes another edition entitled *Somnia Salomonis David regis filii una cum Danielis propheta somniorum interpretatione* (Venice, 1516). I have not seen either of these editions.

16. "Artemidorus et Iudaeus multa utilia tradidere" (SS 1.1, *Opera* 5:596). "Iudaeus" is presumably the same work mentioned by Cardano earlier on the same page and referred to in n. 15, above.

17. I have consulted *Artemidori Daldiani philosophi excellentissimi De somniorum interpretatione libri quinque*, trans. Janus Cornarius (Basel, 1539). The standard modern edition of the Greek text is *Artemidori Daldiani Onirocriticon Libri V*, ed. Roger A. Pack (Leipzig, 1963). See also Giulio Guidorizzi, "L'in-

terpretazione dei sogni nel mondo tardoantico: Oralità e scrittura," in *I sogni nel Medioevo*, at pp. 155–57, and the very helpful article of S.R.F. Price, "The Future of Dreams: From Freud to Artemidorus," *Past and Present*, no. 113 (1986): 3–37.

18. On the place of Artemidorus among the sources of medieval dream books, see François Berriot, ed., *Exposicions et significacions des songes et Les songes Daniel* (Geneva, 1989), introduction, p. 53; also Steven M. Oberhelman, *The Oneirocriticon of Achmet: A Medieval Greek and Arabic Treatise on the Interpretation of Dreams* (Lubbock, Tex., 1991), pp. 16–19. For the sixteenth-century editions and translations see IA, pt. 1, A/7 (Orleans, 1965), *109. 109–27.

19. "Hui, inquient . . . 'Quid minus opportuit quam somnia fallacia, inania, mentes ludificantia, et explosas ab omnibus nugas nunc tandem latinis hominibus communicare, et ex autore qui ne suo quidem tempore gentium philosophis tolerabilis erat?' . . . Somniorum interpretationem artem esse utilem apprime in vita, et non ut gentilem et vanam contemnandam sed ut piam Christiani etiam suspiciendam ac expetendam. Atque primum omnium ne permittimus quidem ut de somnis iudicent nisi viris valde gravibus, prudentibusque ac sobriis" (Artemidorus, *De somniorum interpretatione*, trans. Cornarius, translator's "Epistola dedicatoria," pp. 3–6).

20. Rütten, "Melanchthon's Rede 'De Hippocrate,'" pp. 25–26 (relations of Luther and Melanchthon with Cornarius); Niccoli, *Prophecy and People*, passim, but esp. the summary of conclusions, pp. 188–96.

21. Aristotle, *On Dreams* 458a35–462b10; *On Divination in Sleep* 462b13–464b18; *Problems* 30.14, 956b38–957a35.

22. SS 1.3, *Opera* 5:597–98.

23. "Quae ergo a superiore causa contingunt, moventur ab influxu qui a corporibus contingit coelestibus. . . . Ut sint ergo tria, quae differentiae causa sint; constitutio coeli valida aut imbecillis, res repraesentanda vulgaris aut rara, et imaginum copia et forma apposita ad rem referendam in anima somniantis" (ibid., *Opera* 5:598–99); for discussion of this passage and for a comparison of Cardano's dream theory with that of Aristotle, see Browne, "Cardano's *Somniorum synesiorum libri*," pp. 125–29.

24. "Itaque hoc opus est animae quiescentis, quae non impedita, curis, sensibus aut motionibus, nec crapula levissima sensilia percipit. . . . Hoc autem quod relucet, aut in ipso fati ordine constitutum est, aut in ipsius hominis deliberatione, aut in serie facti, aut a daemone subministrante, vel coelo. Ex coelo autem verisimillimum est: est enim causa omnium, et astrologi multa praedicunt, et in quibusdam est, quibusdam non. Imprimit autem magnum aliquid: quoniam quod imprimit, tale est" (SS 4.1, *Opera* 5:705).

25. On the medieval antecedents, see Tullio Gregory, "I sogni e gli astri," in *I sogni nel Medioevo*, pp. 111–48; I have not noticed any evidence that Cardano cited medieval scholastic authors on the connection between meaningful dreams and the stars. Gaurico, *Super diebus decretoriis*, pp. 120–28, "Hyppocratis libellus de somnis aegrotantium"; the abbreviated text of *Dreams* is broken up into numbered aphorisms. On *Regimen* 4 and celestial influences see chap. 4, n. 20, and below. On Gaurico and the relation of prophecy and astrology see Paola Zambelli, "Many Ends for the World: Luca Gaurico, Instigator of the Debate in

Italy and Germany," in *"Astrologi hallucinati": Stars and the End of the World in Luther's Time*, ed. Paola Zambelli (Berlin, 1986), pp. 239–63.

26. See Niccoli, *Prophecy and People*, pp. 140–67.

27. *Synesius de somniis translatus a Marsili Ficino Florentino* in Marsilio Ficino, *Opera omnia* (Turin, 1959; facsimile reproduction of the edition of Basel, 1576), 2:1968–79. On Synesius and his doctrine in this work, see Jay Bregman, *Synesius of Cyrene* (Berkeley and Los Angeles, 1982), esp. pp. 145–54. On Ficino's use of Synesius, see Brian P. Copenhaver, "Iamblichus, Synesius and the Chaldaean Oracles in Marsilio Ficino's *De vita libri tres*: Hermetic Magic or Neoplatonic Magic," in *Supplementum Festivum: Studies in Honor of Paul Oskar Kristeller*, ed. James Hankins, John Monfasani, and Frederick Purnell (Binghamton, N.Y., 1987), pp. 441–55.

28. Ibid., esp. pp. 446–47.

29. "Non negaverim in quibusdam huiusmodi idola a Diis velut et in defectu artis medicae sanationes, immitti: quale illud: 'Surge, et tolle puerum, et vade in Aegyptum: sunt enim qui animam pueri quaerant.' Sed miracula sunt, et extra artis considerationem, sicut et sanationes illae, et reliqua huiusce generis" (SS 2.18, *Opera* 3:690). For Cardano's views on miracles, see Céard, "La notion de 'miraculum,' " and chap. 7, above.

30. SS *Opera* 5:593–595, esp. p. 594.

31. His silence on this score is also noted by Agnese Grieco; see Cardano, *Sogni*, introduction, p. 11.

32. Auger Ferrier, *Liber de somniis. Hippocratis de insomniis liber. Galeni liber de insomniis. Synesii liber de somnis* (Lyon, 1549), pp. 29–33. On Ferrier and his dream book, see Cooper, "Deux medécins royaux onirocrites," pp. 56–60; for his career at Toulouse, see Sanches, *That Nothing Is Known*, ed. Limbrick and Thomson, p. 23.

33. "Quippe Iosephus in Pharaone per vaccas pingues, non vaccas, sed annorum ubertatem interpretatus est. . . . Tum vero huiusmodi somnia neque a Deo, neque a daemonibus immitti, his argumentis perspicuum est: nam tam visionum quam idolorum illi causae essent: cur ergo opus illis esset ut occultarent quod docere vellent? praesertim tot ambagibus? An non possunt, cum volunt, huiusmodi, si libet, clare docere?" (SS 2.18, *Opera* 5:689).

34. Ibid. 4.3, *Opera* 5:711.

35. Cardano, *Dialogus Hieronymi Cardani et Facii Cardani ipsius patris*, *Opera* 1:637–40; this work was not published during Girolamo's lifetime. See also SS 4.4, *Opera* 5:719.

36. See Natalie Zemon Davis, "Ghosts, Kin, and Progeny: Some Features of Family Life in Early Modern France," *Daedalus* 106 (1977): 87–114, at p. 94.

37. VP 39, *Opera* 1:31.

38. "Quis locus somniis?" is part of the title of VP 33, *Opera* 1:24.

39. On the medieval medical sources, see Marta Fattori, "Sogni e temperamenti," in *I sogni nel Medioevo*, pp. 87–109. Between 1481 and the mid–sixteenth century, as well as appearing in independent editions, *Dreams* (*Regimen* 4) was published as part of the various editions of Hippocrates' *Opera*, included in one version of the *Articella*, and issued in several collections with various other treatises. See Littré 6:464–65, and nn. 25 and 32, above. See also chap. 3, nn. 103 and 105, and chap. 4, n. 20.

40. *Hippocratis Liber de somniis cum Iulii Caesaris Scaligeris commentariis* (Lyon, 1539).

41. Galen, *De dignotione ex insomniis libellus*, in *Opera*, ed. Kühn, 6:832–35. For the sixteenth-century publications of this work, see Durling, "Chronological Census," p. 284.

42. See n. 32, above. According to Cooper, "Deux médecins royaux onirocrites," an earlier, less complete, edition of this collection had appeared in 1540.

43. *Regimen IV or Dreams* 90, in *Hippocrates*, ed. and trans. W.H.S. Jones (Loeb), 4:438.

44. "Si quis in somnis incendium quidem videt, a flava bile vexatur; si fumum, vel caliginem, vel profundas tenebras, ab atra bile; imber vero frigidam humidatem abundare indicat; nix et glacies et grando pituitam frigidam" (Galen, *De dignotione ex insomniis libellus*, Kühn 6:832). Examples occur on pp. 833–34. For discussion and an English translation of the Greek text, see Steven M. Oberhelman, "Galen, *On Diagnosis from Dreams*," *Journal of the History of Medicine and Allied Sciences* 38 (1983): 36–47, and idem, "The Diagnostic Dream in Ancient Medical Theory and Practice," *Bulletin of the History of Medicine* 61 (1987): 47–60.

45. ". . . immittunt iucunda, quae dulcem sanguinem generant. . . . viridis autem intensus cum splendore somnos suavesque excitant. . . . Non parum est iucunde dormire" (RV 8.45, *Opera* 3:165–66).

46. Cardano, *De subtilitate* 18, *Opera* 3:639; RV 15.80, *Opera* 3:292. On the social stratification of foodstuffs, see Grieco, "Social Politics."

47. SS 1.2–3, 9, *Opera* 5:596–99, 604.

48. "Decimus de exemplis, estque hic liber aliis iucundior lectu" (referring to a longer version of his dream book that he subsequently compressed to produce the work that survives). LP 1557, *Opera* 1:66.

49. Apart from Cardano himself, Hippocrates, and Galen, the recipients of dreams concerning health, disease, and medicine in bk. 4 of SS, *Opera*, vol. 5, are: 4.2, p. 706, Eudemus, friend of Aristotle; p. 707, the widow of Georgius Stachinus, medicus, a friend of Cardano; 4.3, p. 711, Fazio Cardano; pp. 711–12, Chiara Micheri (Girolamo Cardano's mother); p. 712, a patient of Rinaldus Vilanova [?Arnald of Villanova, d. 1311]; p. 714, the procurator of the college of *medici*; p. 714, a patient of Giovanni Matteo Ferrari de Gradi (fl. 15c); Dominico Confalonerio, a priest known to Cardano.

50. See chap. 6, n. 46.

51. "Relinquitur solum dicendum de interrogationibus a medico facientis (*sic*; pacientis). . . . de somno, et quantus, et qualis, et qua hora, et an insomnia et qualia in genere, non speciatim ne oniropolis habearis, tum maxime quomodo a somno se habuerit sciscitatus" (comm. VA 1, *Opera* 10:171).

52. SS 4.3, *Opera* 5:710. The story comes from a supposed letter of Hippocrates to Philopoemon. Of Renaissance Latin editions, I have consulted Hippocrates, *Opera* (Basel, 1526), pp. 479–80. However, Cardano seems to have quoted from one of the other translations. The Greek text is edited in *Hippocrates: Pseudepigraphic Writings*, ed. and trans. Smith, letter 15.

53. "Medicatio namque et vaticinatio cognatae sunt inter sese, quandoquidem et harum duarum artium pater et auctor est Apollo, proavusque noster praesentes et futuros morbos praedicebat, et affectos et afficiendos curabat"

(Hippocrates, *Epistolae*, in his *Opera*, trans. Calvi [Basel, 1526], p. 480). This closing sentence was not quoted by Cardano in the passage of SS referred to in the preceding note.

54. "Galeni quoque somnia inter haec admiranda recensere opera pretium fuerit, praecipue autem tria fuere patris repetita, quibus admonebatur, ut filium medicinae traderet. Aliud, quo ut scriberet de videndi ratione, cuius meminit in libris de Usu partium: velut alterius in Methodo, et de librorum propriorum ordine. Tertium magis dignum miraculo, cum bis per somnum monitus ut arteriam secaret, quae inter pollicem et indicem est, idque agens liberatus fit a diuturno dolore, quo infestabatur ea in parte qua septo transverso iecur iungitur: idque in libri de Sectione venae fine testatus est. Magno certe exemplo, quod tantus vir in medicina eam adhibuerit somnio fidem, ut in seipso periculum vitae subierit, in arte propria. Deinde probitatem admiror, ut quod potuerit solertia ingenii sibi inventum ascribere, Deo cui debebatur, reddiderit. Dignus vel hoc solo vir immortalitate nominis et librorum suorum" (SS 4.2, *Opera* 5:706).

55. Synesius, *De somniis*, in Ficino, *Opera* 2:1968–70; at p. 1970: "Studendum vero huic maxime prae caeteris disciplinis, quoniam ex nobis haec est, et intrinsecus, et uniuscuiusque animae propria."

56. "Phantasia est perspicatior quam sensus exterior"; "Spiritus phantasticus est primum animae vehiculum" (ibid., pp. 1970, 1971).

57. SS 1. 6, *Opera* 5:601. Compare Synesius, *De somniis*, in Ficino, *Opera* 2:1974.

58. Ibid., pp. 1976–77.

59. "Tradunt Deum aliis quidem dedisse facultatem ad perdiscendam luminis innotionem, alios autem etiam in somniis divini fructus vigorisque effecisse particeps" (ibid., p. 1970).

60. "Caeteris quidem cura est aliorum, hoc autem adest omnibus bonus unicuique daemon, atque iis qui vigilantes meditati sunt artificiose aliquid invenire, praeceptor occurrit. Adeo sapiens res est anima ocium agens a sensuum colluvione forensium animae naturas, undique inferentium alienas. Anima namque quocunque species habet, et quotcunque accipere solet a mente facta, quandoque sola perspicuas exhibet ad interiora conversis et quae veniunt a divino traducit. Nam anima [*sic*] ita se habenti Deus quoque mundanus se prorsus adiungit, propterea quod animae ipsius natura ex eodem simul atque ille profluxit. Haec igitur genera somniorum diviniora censentur atque vel omnino vel quasi penitus integra sunt atque perspicua, minimeque artis indigens adminiculo. Sed haec quidem solis contingunt hominibus virtute viventibus . . ." (ibid., p. 1975).

61. "Nam et per hoc diis quoque nonnunque propinquamus monentibus. . . . Mitto equidem in praesentia divulgatas somnii dotes, quibus saepe ab insidiis liberantur, et quod hominibus somnus accedens medicus adversum expulit valetudinem" (ibid., p. 1970). "Mihi quidem saepe libros mecum una, mentem enim instruxit, orationem composuit, diem partim quidem describeret, partim etiam commutaret, quandoque vero et totam linguae dispositionem stolidam atque tumentem nominum novitate ob nimium atheae linguae antiquioris, duriorisque amorem vaticinium hoc per Deum corrigens, et partim quidem dictans, partim vero, quid sit ostendens, tumores quosdam ingenitos linguae deliniens levigavit, tumorem expulit, modumque adhibuit" (ibid., p. 1975).

62. Ibid., p. 1977. SS 1.7, *Opera* 5:602–3.

63. SS 4.4, *Opera* 5:716.

64. Ibid. On the use of analogy as a means of selecting interpretations of dream images in Greek medicine, see Oberhelman, "Diagnostic Dream," and idem, "The Interpretation of Prescriptive Dreams in Ancient Greek Medicine," *Journal of the History of Medicine and Allied Sciences* 36 (1981): 416–24.

65. "Cum anno MDLVII somniassem, me audire harmoniam suavissimam atque coelestem, adeo ut etiam illius memoria recrearer: experrectus, statim inveni principium illud: Cur homines ex febribus alii necessario moriantur, alii non; cui quaesito iam prope vigintiquinque annis inveniendo incubueram. Eo ergo invento, statim mane coepi conscribere librum illum pulcherrimum Artis parvae medendi, quem post quatuor annos, postquam eum plusquam vicies aut transcripsissem, aut transcribi curassem, absolvi: in quo tota prorsus medicina continetur. Sic ex harmonia divina sapientia portendebatur" (SS 4.4, *Opera* 5:726). The work referred to is ACP, on which see chap. 2.

66. See, for example, SS 4.4, *Opera* 5:715, dream of 1528.

67. "At ego cum indies res mea deterior fieret, eo recurri quo solitus eram, scilicet ad Deum; quem supplicibus verbis exoravi, ut me per somnum admoneret, quid facere oporteret. Quievi autem ad solemnia sacra templi, quod divo Michaeli, ad Clusiam vocant, sacrum, e regione domus meae positum est. Tum praeter morem ante diem tempestivius experrectus, nihil me per somnum vidisse animadverti, verum credidi ob horam insuetam illam, qua experrectus fueram, admoneri, ut mihi ipsi consulerem, quod et feci" (UC 2.2, *Opera* 2:46). In the edition of 1561 the wording of the passage is slightly different, but the sense is the same. Cardano also described the location of this house (and various other addresses he lived at in Milan and other cities) in VP 24, *Opera* 1:16. The church of S. Michele alla Chiusa (at the lock, so called from a nearby lock on one of the city's canals) stood in the district of Milan known as Porta Ticinense, near what was in the sixteenth century the edge of the city. The church was demolished in the course of urban reconstruction during the 1930s; see Carlo Ponzoni, *Le chiese di Milano* (Milan, 1930), p. 426. I am grateful to Evelyn Welch for this reference. Regarding the urban geography of Renaissance Milan, see Evelyn S. Welch, *Art and Authority in Renaissance Milan* (New Haven, 1995).

68. "Tantum enim abfuit ut laeto vultu haec exciperet, ut etiam adiecerit me insanire, esseque hoc unum ex meis figmentis, appellabatque haec suo more imaginationes, id et, falsas (ut, quod dicere vellet magis, quam quod diceret, exprimam) imagines. Nec eo contentus subieci, nihil referre, quomodo quis medeatur: artem enim nihil ad salutem aegrorum conferre, sed sive quis bene vel male morbum agnoscat, sive etiam curet recte aut perperam, vel unum pro alio, statutum esse, qui debeant mori aut sanari" (ibid.).

69. ". . . mecumque dicebam, quid miseris istis, qui artis sunt ignari continget, si me, quem se fallere non posse intelligunt, ita tractant?" (ibid., p. 47).

70. "In templo Aesculapii aegri vera somniare soliti erant" (RV 8.44, p. 166). He made a similar assertion in his *Encomium medicinae, Opera* 6:2 (first published in his *Quaedam opuscula* (Basel, 1559).

71. There is a reference to cures in the temple of Asclepius in the proem to Cardano's comm. *Prognost., Opera* 8:586, but it does not mention incubation or dreams.

72. "Idem fiebat in templo Aesculapii, a quo vera existamabant immittii somnia. Et Calabri Podalyriam Aesculapii filium consulturi, iuxta illius sepulcrum in agminis pellibus obdormiscebant. Sic nanque quae in somnis quisque vidisset, tanquam vera, et certa divinitate praedita mirabatur, ac notabat. Nostris temporibus vero licet huiusmodi ritus non amplius admittatur, non desunt tamen superstitiosi quidam homines, qui certum locum sibi deligunt, in quo post multas ac varias expiationes, post religiosas quasdam obsecrationes, de quibus negotiis scire cupiunt, dormientes, admonentur" (Ferrier, *De somniis*, pp. 64–65).

73. J. C. Scaliger, *Hippocratis Liber de somniis cum . . . commentariis*, p. 7.

74. *Orationes Aristidis* (Florence, 1517; IA *107. 621). The *hieroi logoi* occupy fols. 167v–83r.

75. *Aelii Aristidis Adrianensis oratoris clarissimi orationum tomi tres nunc primum latine versi a Guilielmo Cantero . . .* (Basel, 1566), with *Sacrorum sermones primus . . . sextus* at 1:154–208.

76. "Praesentiam quidem numinis mihi affuisse non dicam, sed tamen haud absurde forsan id mihi persuasi, quandoquidem primum monitus toties per somnium multa peregi, multaque declinavi: quae si evenissent, non hucusque pervenire potuissem" (LP 1562, *Opera* 1:129).

77. "Afferebant quoque nativitatum fasciculos ut de his pronunciarem tanquam ariolus et vates, non ut medicinae professor" (VP 33, *Opera* 1:25).

78. "Ergo iam videndum satis ostendisse, nullam esse de longinquis, remotisque per enthusiasmum, aut per somnum divinationem: imo nullam omnino esse, nisi quae in nobis, aut causis naturalibus fundamentum habet. Et quamvis concederemus esse aliquam, tamen inutilis esset omnimodo. Aut enim quae praesciuntur, vitari non possunt, aut possunt. Si non possunt, satis est nesciri, optima enim mors est, improvisa, dicebat Caesar. Si possunt, non ergo divinasti" (Sanches, *De divinatione per somnum*, p. 118). On this work, and Sanches in relation to Cardano, see also chap. 7, n. 89.

79. Ibid., pp. 122.

80. Ibid., pp. 120–21.

81. "Verum anno MDLVIII, quae aetatis nostrae fuit LVIII [*sic*] ab eo sensim destitui visus sum numine, quo impellebar: seu iam omnibus absolutis argumentis, et ferme etiam libris: seu intermittente se vi illa, non subducente: seu alia quacunque causa: certum est, cum alias nihil esset de quo per somnum non monerer: deinde annis iam decem abhinc illis cessantibus ardor ille accederet, quo nihil arduum mihi putarem: et hic maxima ex parte cessaverit, nec aetatis vitio, siquidem ad alia promptior factus sum: vim aliquam coelestem me deseruisse, quae diu antea dux mihi fuit ad obeunda negocia illa" (LP 1562, *Opera* 1:129).

CHAPTER 9
HISTORIA, NARRATIVE, AND MEDICINE

1. Gabriel Naudé, *Vita Cardani*, Cardano, *Opera* 1:i r–v.

2. The relation between Cardano's autobiography and autobiographical elements in his other writings is discussed in Gregori, "Rappresentazione e difesa."

3. For an interesting analysis of narrative in modern medicine, see Kathryn

Montgomery Hunter, *Doctors' Stories: The Narrative Structure of Medical Knowledge* (Princeton, 1991); for some comments on the status of patients' narratives in eighteenth-century medicine, see Roy Porter, "The Rise of Physical Examination," in *Medicine and the Five Senses*, ed. W. F. Bynum and Roy Porter (Cambridge, 1993), pp. 179–97; on narrative and scientific writing more generally, see Peter Dear, ed., *The Literary Structure of Scientific Argument: Historical Studies* (Philadelphia, 1991).

4. "Medicam artem antiquis temporibus maximo in pretio habitam fuisse historiae, et divina scriptura tradiderunt: cum tamen ab initio conditae artis, Gnidiae sententiae praevalerent, quas sapientissimus Hippocrates, libro de victus ratione in acutis inscribitur, reprobavit" (MM, *Opera* 7:199). See LP 1562, *Opera* 1:107, and similarly LP 1557, *Opera* 1:70 (n. 23 to chap. 6).

5. See, for example, *De optima secta ad Thrasybulum*, chap. 14, Kühn 1:142–49, where the misuse of *historia* by the Empiric sect is criticized. The "case histories" collected in the Hippocratic *Epidemics* are not termed histories in the text; see Hans-Josef Kühn and Ulrich Fleischer, *Index Hippocraticus* (Gottingen, 1986–89), 2:400.

6. Cardano, *Encomium Neronis* (also entitled *Neronis encomium*), *Opera* 1:179–220 (published with his *Somniorum synesiorum* [Basel, 1562; IA *132. 083]). The *Encomium* is discussed in Ingegno, pp. 184–208; on Cardano's views on Roman history, see also Alexander Demandt, *Der Fall Roms* (Munich, 1984), pp. 100–101.

7. *Discorsi*, preface to bk. 1. I owe this reference to Anthony Grafton.

8. See Arno Seifert, *Cognitio historica* (Berlin, 1976); on the influence of Roman historians and the idea of history as example in the fifteenth to seventeenth centuries, see also George H. Nadel, "Philosophy of History before Historicism," *History and Theory* 3 (1964): 291–315.

9. On Cardano's astrology see Ernst, " 'Veritatis amor dulcissimus,' " and Grafton, *Girolamo Cardano and the Tradition of Classical Astrology* (and the forthcoming studies by Grafton mentioned in n. 33 to chap. 1, above). For Cardano's commentary on *Airs Waters Places*, see chap. 6, above.

10. For ancient precedents, see Anthony Grafton and Noel M. Swerdlow, "Technical Chronology and Astrological History in Varro, Censorinus, and Others," *Classical Quarterly* 35 (1985): 454–65. Another ancient precedent for the collection of individual horoscopes and the associated life stories for subsequent analysis (for purposes of astrological, not historical, theory, however) was provided by Vettius Valens; see O. Neugebauer and H. B. Van Hoesen, *Greek Horoscopes* (Philadelphia, 1959), p. 176. On astrology and history in the Renaissance more generally, see Paola Zambelli, "Introduction: Astrologer's Theory of History," in *"Astrologi hallucinati": Stars and the End of the World in Luther's Time*, ed. Paola Zambelli (Berlin and New York, 1986), pp. 1–28, and Garin, *Lo zodiaco della vita*.

11. "Iuvat et hic liber ad cognoscendum praesentia et praeterita eadem ratione qua futura" (proem, comm. *Tetrabiblos*, *Opera* 5:93). The commentary extends to p. 368.

12. For example, "Maius est discrimen inter Ptolemaei praecepta, et omnium reliquorum qui eum secuti sunt, quam inter smaragdum et lutum" (Cardano,

Aphorismorum astronomicorum segmenta septem 1.101, *Opera* 5:35). A *Peroratio* concluding this work begins "Propositum nostri negocii in hoc libro fuit ut artem iam ad infamiam, vicio professorum redactam, ab iniuria vindicaremus . . ." (ibid. 5:90).

13. Cardano, *Liber de exemplis centum geniturarum, Opera* 5:458–502; Julius II is no. 48, p. 484 (Nuremberg, 1547; IA *132. 054).

14. Cardano, *De interrogationibus, quaesitum* 17, *Opera* 5:557–58. At p. 557: "Et ut huius rei exemplum rarissimum proponam (nam rarissima solum me propositurum sum testatus) subiungo bifariam exemplum imo trifarium admirabile. Primum quidem narranda est historia brevissime, deinde colligenda horum."

Cardano's remarks on Giovio occur in the *Encomium Neronis, Opera* 1:216, and are noted and discussed in Zimmerman, *Paolo Giovio*, p. 264, and n. 9, where a passage alluded to by Cardano is identified as found in Giovio's *Illustrium virorum vitae*, first published Florence, 1551 (for the date of publication, Zimmerman, *Paolo Giovio*, p. 373). Cardano's first reference to the composition of the *Encomium Neronis* appears to be in LP 1557, *Opera* 1:74; as noted previously, LP 1557 has the explicit 1554. On Giovio's family background, humanistic, philosophical, and medical education, and medical practice (and authorship), see Zimmerman, *Paolo Giovio*, pp. 1–19. For Cardano's comments on the empire and the expected results of the voyages, see VP 9 and 41, *Opera* 1:7 and 34–35.

15. "Est autem ars haec [sc. astrologia] philosophiae pars prognostica et praecognoscere docens, unde non vere scientia, sed ut ad [1554: quoad] medicinam se habet liber praedictionum Hippocratis aut Galeni, ita hic ad totam philosophiam" (Cardano, comm. *Tetrabiblos*, proem, *Opera* 5:93). See also Céard, *La nature et les prodiges*, pp. 229–51.

16. See Andrew Wear, "Explorations in Renaissance Writings on the Practice of Medicine," in *The Medical Renaissance of the Sixteenth Century*, ed. Andrew Wear, R. K. French and I. M. Lonie (Cambridge, 1985), pp. 118–45.

17. Vesalius, *Fabrica* 1.18 (Basel, 1555), p. 103.

18. Taddeo Alderotti, *Expositiones in arduum aphorismorum Ipocratis volumen, In divinum pronosticorum Ipocratis librum, In preclarum regiminis acutorum Ipocratis opus, In subtilissimum Joannitii Isagogarum libellum* (Venice, 1527), fols. 247v–50v; for discussion, Siraisi, *Taddeo Alderotti*, pp. 124–25.

19. Interesting comparisons are suggested by the analysis of narratives of personal history for a purpose in Natalie Z. Davis, *Fiction in the Archives: Pardon Tales and Their Tellers in Sixteenth-Century France* (Stanford, 1987).

20. For example, Vesalius denied the Galenic theory that special foramina in the sphenoid or the cribriform plate of the ethmoid bone were provided for the sake of purging phlegm from the brain, but then had to postulate the transmission of this substance through other, hypothetical channels (*Fabrica* 7.11 [Basel, 1543], pp. 640–42, translated with anatomical annotation in Charles Singer, *Vesalius on the Human Brain* [London, New York, Toronto, 1952], pp. 51–56).

21. *On Prognosis* was translated into Latin from Greek in Italy during the fourteenth century, perhaps by Niccolo da Reggio (fl. 1308–45); of the five

Latin manuscripts, only two antedate the mid–fifteenth century. See Galen, *On Prognosis*, ed. and trans. Vivian Nutton, *Corpus medicorum graecorum* V 8 1 (Berlin, 1979), pp. 26–34.

22. *Methodus medendi* occupies the whole of Kühn, vol. 10. There were three medieval translations. A paraphrase from the Arabic by Constantinus Africanus circulated under the title *Megategni*; a translation of the whole work by Gerard of Cremona was known as *De ingenio sanitatis*; Burgundio of Pisa's translation of bks. 7–14 with bk. 14 completed by Pietro d'Abano was known as *Terapeutica*. According to Pearl Kibre and R. J. Durling, "A List of Latin Manuscripts Containing Medieval Versions of the *Methodus medendi*," in *Galen's Method of Healing*, ed. Fridolf Kudlien and Richard J. Durling (Leiden, 1991), pp. 117–22, there are collectively over one hundred manuscripts. *De locis affectis* was known in an Arabo-Latin version under the title *De interioribus*. Galen's use of case histories in *Methodus medendi* is discussed in Vivian Nutton, "Style and Context in the *Method of Healing*," ibid., pp. 1–25, at pp. 9–11.

23. *Cyrurgia Guidonis de Cauliaco. Et Cyrurgia Bruni Theodorici Rogerii Rolandi Bertapalie Lanfranci* (Venice, 1498), fols. 177(176), 187(186).

24. For example, Guglielmo da Saliceto (fl. 1276), *Cyrurgia*, printed with his *Summa conservationis et curationis* (Venice, 1489), 2.15, sig. X4v; Rolando da Parma (fl. early thirteenth century), *Libellus de cyrurgia*, in *Cyrurgia Guidonis de Cauliaco* 3.25, fol. 157(156)r. On Guglielmo da Saliceto's use of stories, see Nancy G. Siraisi, "How to Write a Latin Book on Surgery: Organizing Principles and Authorial Devices in Guglielmo da Saliceto and Dino del Garbo," in *Practical Medicine from Salerno to the Black Death*, ed. Luis Garcia Ballester et al. (Cambridge, 1993), 88–109. Another well-known example is the list of patients cured of anal fistula provided by the fourteenth-century English surgeon John of Arderne; see Peter Murray Jones, "John of Arderne and the Mediterranean Tradition of Scholastic Surgery," ibid., 289–321.

25. Jacquart, "Theory, Everyday Practice," esp. p. 160.

26. For example, there are 304 in a collection of *consilia* by Bartolomeo da Montagnana (d. before 1452), printed in eleven editions between 1472 and 1673, often together with over 150 *consilia* by Antonio Cermisone (d. 1441). Manuscripts and editions are listed in Tiziana Pesenti, *Professori e promotori di medicina nello Studio di Padova dal 1405 al 1509: Repertorio bio-bibliografico* (Trieste and Padua, 1984), pp. 76–89, 143–54. On the development of the genre in the thirteenth to fifteenth centuries, see Agrimi and Crisciani, *Les consilia médicaux*, and Chiara Crisciani, "L' 'individuale' nella medicina tra medioevo e Rinascimento" (forthcoming in the proceedings of the colloquium *Umanesimo e medicina*, held at the Centro di Studi sul Classicismo, San Gimignano, June 3–4, 1994, ed. Roberto Cardini). For thirteenth- and early-fourteenth-century *consilia*, see also Siraisi, *Taddeo Alderotti*, chap. 9.

27. Cardano, *Consilia*, no. 6, *Opera* 9:55.

28. Noted in Bylebyl, "Teaching 'Methodus Medendi,'" p. 162.

29. For example, *Consilia Jo[hannis] Ma[tthaei] de Gradi .... secundam viam Avicen[nae]* (Venice, 1521).

30. For example, the sons of Baverio Baviera compiled his *consilia* into a col-

lection after his death and published them prefaced by a dedicatory epistle to an ecclesiastic who had been their father's patron (*Consilia Bavierii* [Pavia, 1521]; the work first appeared in 1489).

31. The work was edited for Borso d'Este by Pier Candido Decembrio and printed in the collection *De balneis omnia quae extant apud Graecos, Latinos, et Arabas* . . . (Venice, 1553), fols. 47r–57r.

32. Vivian Nutton, "Case Histories in the Early Renaissance," *Journal of the History of Medicine and Allied Sciences* (forthcoming).

33. See Ambroise Paré, *The Apologie and Treatise Containing the Voyages Made into Divers Places*, ed. Geoffrey Keynes (New York, 1968), pp. 33–37, 39–40; William Clowes, *A Profitable and Necessarie Booke of Observations, for all those that are burned with the flame of Gun powder, &c* . . . (London, 1596), facsimile with introduction by De Witt T. Starnes and Chauncey D. Leake (New York, 1945). Nutton, "Case Histories," discusses Clowes's similarly structured books on syphilis, surgery, and struma.

34. Da Monte, *In tertium primi Epidemiorum*. On Da Monte's *consilia*, see Bylebyl, "Teaching 'Methodus Medendi,' " pp. 183–85.

35. Giovanni Argenterio, *Tres in Artem medicam Galeni commentarii*, in his *Opera*, 3 vols. in 1 (Venice, 1592), 1:390; see Siraisi, "Giovanni Argenterio," pp. 171–72.

36. *Fabrica* (1543), 1.11, p. 46, and 5.17, p. 543.

37. Findlen, *Possessing Nature*, pp. 304–8.

38. Cunningham, "Fabricius and the 'Aristotle Project.' "

39. The fourteenth-century translation of *On Prognosis* was printed in the 1490 edition of Galen's *Opera* in Latin; the Greek text was edited in both the Aldine (1531) and Basel (1538) editions of Galen's works; six new Latin translations were made between the 1520s and 1560s (Galen, *On Prognosis*, ed. Nutton, pp. 34–42). Nutton, "Style and Context," pp. 9–11, and Bylebyl, "Teaching 'Methodus medendi.' "

40. Gabriele Falloppia, *Observationes anatomicae*, preface, in his *Opera omnia* (Venice, 1584), preface, fol. 221r–v.

41. On Baillou, see Lonie, "The Paris Hippocratics," pp. 169–74; Baillou's work, like Cardano's commentaries on the *Epidemics*, was not published until the seventeenth century. According to Vivian Nutton, "Pieter Van Foreest and the Plagues of Europe: Some Observations on the Observationes," in *Pieter Van Foreest: Een Hollands medicus in de zestiende eeuw*, ed. H. L. Houtzager (Amsterdam, 1989), pp. 25–39, Van Foreest's *Observationes et curationes medicinales* (1588) also makes use of the model of the *Epidemics* and contains observations of cases probably made many years before the work was published.

42. "Opusculum hoc Domine aggressus sum, ut non haec ipsa viginti duo Hippocratis solum exempla declararem: vel morborum et causarum historiam exindeque curationem docerem: aut etiam reliquorum viginti aegrorum quae ibidem ascripta sunt vel caeterorum qui in libris Epidemiorum quotquot supersint, sed ut quod latebat reconditi aperirem. Et ut quivis ex arte similibus observationibus illam augere valeret quod nostris temporibus tanto facilius fieri poterit et melius quanto aetas nostra arte dissecandi corpora humana illustrior evasit" (*Examen*, dedicatory proem, *Opera* 9:36). In the manuscript of Cardano's com-

mentary on *Epidemics* 1, the case histories are rendered more prominent than in the printed version in *Opera* 10 by headings that set off each case history with the rubric "languens" and number the lectures (Biblioteca Apostolica Vaticana, MS vat. lat. 5848, fols. 52r–74v, *lectio* 36–49, on *languens* 2–14), devoting a full lecture—and in one instance two—to each history.

43. Cardano, *Consilia*, no. 22, *Opera*, 9:123–52.

44. See Vivian Nutton, "Galen and Medical Autobiography," in his *From Democedes to Harvey: Studies in the History of Medicine* (London, 1988).

45. For example, *Liber de exemplis centum geniturarum* and SS, bk. 4, both in *Opera*, vol. 5.

46. I owe this suggestion to Vivian Nutton.

47. CA, *curatio* 12, *Opera* 7:255.

48. Ibid., *curatio* 30, *Opera* 7:261; VP 40, *Opera* 1:34.

49. CA, *curationes* 5, p. 254; 14, p. 256; 15, pp. 256–57.

50. "Vincentius Cospus Bononiensis, Senator, amicus meus, annos agens quinquaginta, procerae staturae, crassus corpore, cruribus gracilibus, pravi coloris, timidus praeter modum, fontem in brachio iam pluribus annis gerens, multum se exercens, et post quiescens: multi cibi, varii, crassi, mali, adeo ut castaneas, itria, legumina, et caseum uno prandio, tum alia etiam devoraret. Anno hoc pepones tres aut quatuor una die edebat. Ad XII calendas Novembris MDLXIX correptus est febre duplici tertiana; erat autem dies Veneris rigor, et in eo vomitus, et egestio fusca, non sudebat: febris finiebatur. In quinta circa vesperi vocatus, nullum praeter haec aliud symptomata agnovi, mane satis bene videbatur se habet: iam autem cibum sumpserat, panem coctum cum iure: sed et aquam bibit, imminebat enim accessio. Vesperi cum reversus essem, pulsu carere animadverti. Laetus decumbebat super latus sinistrum, ut exciperet (credo) venientes. Ubi saepius tetigisse nec invenissem, dubitaremque, ne id mihi causa mea contingeret, scilicet ob stuporem. Iterum aggressus sum tangere illum, animadverti me non esse deceptum, nam pulsam quidem inveni, sed languidissimum, parvum, celerem non multum, sed frequentiorem. Certus ergo de eius statu, admonito altero medico, in coena cum ferculo et luteo ovi, vini diluti parum dedi. Mane sequenti exhibuimus theriacen, et ventriculum absynthio fovimus, et cor etiam inunximus; successit febris sine vomitu atque deiectione. Pulsus satis robustus, et ut solet magnus, velox, frequens. Sudor successit copiosus, cum et praecedenti nocte sudasset. Cum transacta esset septima, verebamur circuitum; facta sunt auxilia praecedentis diei: cum advenissem circiter horam XVI (iam vero sumpserat cibum) inveni etiam febrire, cum nondum accessio supervenisset (exacerbabatur autem diebus paribus, et post ponebat) superveniente accessione ac rigore pauco vires collapsae, egessit autem non multa, ut in sexta: et nihil vomuit, ante solis occasum interit." Cardano, *Paralipomena*, bk. 3, *Opera* 10:501.

51. "Relinquitur solum dicendum de interrogationibus a medico facientis (*sic*; pacientis): hae sunt . . . circa res naturales, non naturales et praeter naturam. . . . iubeat autem illum circumvertere se, et tunc inspice caput, quam facile attollat, non interogare [*sic*] autem opportet, sed videre aut tangere pulsum, respirationem, feces, utinam, sputa, sudores. . . . tange ventrem, si tumet, si dolitat, si durus est aut tensus, cordis molestia, mentis vacillatio, quomodo circa viscera et

spirationem se habuerit. . . . Hoc autem Mediolani servatur, aliud Bononiae, ut singulorum dierum acta et insultus et casus scribantur. Nam per illa circuituum rationem coniectari licet" (comm. VA, *Opera* 10:171).

52. See chap. 6, n. 123.

53. "Dicam autem egregium exemplum, quod contigit, ut hodie viderem, dum haec scribo VII, scilicet Idus septembris anni MDLXVI et ut intelligant medici quantum fallantur in dignotione morborum interiorum membrorum, quod etiam testatur Hippocrates: et quantum profit sectio corporum illorum qui ex morbis obiere: quantumque prodesse possit optima cura. Aegrotabat iam mensibus fere medicus et artis eiusdem professor Ioann. Baptista Peregrinus Bononiensis, vir studiosissimus e probus admodum, aetatis annorum XLVIII, totus habitus melancholici, timidus, tardus, niger, macilentus, pauci cibi, et potus moderatus, uxorem habens forsan iuniorem, quam illius temperatura, et curae exposcerent, cum quinque filiis: res domestica tenuis, et difficultates multae. Igitur ab initio intamuit [*sic*; intumuit] venter, advocavit medicum celebrem, qui ratus esse, ut erat, ascitem, fomenta calida exterius multa applicuit. . . . Demum quasi sponte post menses, anno iam ad unguem exacto, scilicet VIII Idus [septembris] anni MDLXV (mortuus est enim heri) coepit deiecere humores crudos, et aquam multam per alvum per diesque multos, et ita detumuit venter: surrexit, et per hyemem ambulabat cum baculo tamen, et per domum tantum, durus tumor videbatur esse in dextro hypochondrio, et ipse non se erigere poterat, trahebatur deorsum, quasi vinculo intus, et difficulter spirabat. Vere autem et spiratio facta est deterior et tensio loci augebatur: sentiebatque dum se verteret, quasi pondus in praecordiis transferri ex dextra parte in sinistram, et febris intendebatur, rursus ergo coactus est decumbere, et auxilia illa calida, et unguenta emollienta experiri, atque ita per totam aestatem e malo in peius decidendo curabatur. . . . Fortefortuna cum, ut mutuo peterem, quaedam commentaria illum adiissem, inveni febricitantem continua febre, pulsum magnum velocem, et frequentem, modo durum, modo satis mollem: invadebat eum febris circa meridiem modo cum frigore alternis scilicet diebus, modo erat exacerbatio tantum, somni pene nulli, appetitus cibi constans, difficultas spirandi magna, praecordia palpitabant, et dextrum satis tensum erat. Medicus ille alter curabat illum ut hecticum. . . . hecticum autem non credebam esse, post quadraginta dies, et fuit circa mensis Augusti medium (nam ab hac sententia circiter viginti dies supervixit) dixi aperte, me morbum tenere non esse ullo pacto scirrhum in iecore, nec ullo membrorum naturalium, sed fore morbum totum ferme principaliterque in pulmone: esseque oedema, et suffocatum iri. Itaque curam aggressus, nihil profeci, sed paulo post ab ea strangulatus est." Comm. *Prognost.* 2.2–3, *Opera* 8:649. The description of the autopsy follows.

CHAPTER 10

THE PHYSICIAN AS PATIENT

1. Cardano included his own horoscope in two collections of examples of horoscopes, namely the *Liber de exemplis centum geniturarum* and the *Liber duodecim geniturarum*, the second of which went into three editions before being included in the *Opera*. The first horoscope is Cardano, *Libelli quinque* . . . . *V. de*

exemplis centum geniturarum (Nuremberg, 1547; IA *132. 054), no. 19 (*Opera* 5:468–72). The remark "pervenisset caput ad Lunam in 43 annis [of Cardano's life] iam, id est anno praeterito," gives the date of composition. Cardano's second horoscope, recast on different principles and accompanied by a greatly expanded narrative, is no. 8 in . . . . *Geniturarum XII . . . utilia exempla*, printed with his *In Cl. Ptolemaei Pelusiensis IIII de astrorum iudiciis aut ut vulgo vocant, quadripartititae constructionis libros commentaria* (Basel, 1554; IA *132.063), pp. 430–75 (an octavo edition was published in Lyon, 1555; IA *132.066). Cardano revised horoscope and narrative once more, presumably in or shortly after 1564, since he stated in the present tense, "Patior etiam in sinistro oculo lachrymam, quae eo anno coepit quo et podagra. Anno 64. Aprile 4" (*Opera* 5:523). This revision was presumably included in the third edition of the commentary on Ptolemy (Basel, 1578; IA *132. 112, of which I have not seen a copy) and appears, as *Liber duodecim geniturarum*, in *Opera* 5:517–41. VP 6, *De valetudine, Opera* 1:5–6. VP is dated by the statement "usque ad praesentem diem (finem scilicet Octobris, an. 1575)" (ibid., p. 3).

2. Cardano, *De exemplis centum geniturarum, Opera* 5:470. With reference to ages and or dates, one cannot always be sure whether Cardano meant, e.g., "when I was twenty" or "in my twentieth year," or even "in 1520."

3. "tandem evasi nutu divino, natura tamen robusta erat, quia Luna erat potens, et illustrata radiis Iovis et Martis . . ." (ibid.).

4. "et timui ne morerer, et non apparuit egritudo qua decumberem, sed sola copia urinae, quae excedebat generaliter XXX uncias singulas nocte, et cogebar quater surgere ad mingendum, et erat sine ardore, et ego intelligens causam auxiliatus sum cum calidis, et protinus cessavit multitudo, ut nullo modo cogar surgere de nocte, attamen remansit semper maior quantitas urinae quam prius solerem emittere, et quamvis propter trinum Veneris, qui succedit corpori Saturni, res cemper cesserit in melius, nunquam tamen ex toto liberabor, tum maxime quia pater meus mortu[u]s est cum urinae profluvio" (ibid.).

5. On Cardano's astrological techniques and their critics, see the forthcoming study by Anthony Grafton, *Cardano's Cosmos* (as in n. 33 to chap. 1, above).

6. Cardano, *Liber duodecim geniturarum* (Basel, 1554), pp. 443–45.

7. "Ab eo tempore cum nunquam vel unam diem valetudine firmus, et sine dolore duxerim, nihilominus per 44 annos sequentes vix toto triduo, et semel tantum in lecto morbo oppressus decubui" (ibid., p. 430).

8. Ibid., pp. 436, 441.

9. "Animadvertendum etiam, quod morbus octavi anni fuit adeo saevus, ut post illum relictus sit sudor perpetuus singulis noctibus universi corporis, usque ad 36 annum, et tunc mutatus est in urinae profluvium, ideo fuit quasi naturalis, et minori cum periculo, sed etiam difficilioris sanationis" (ibid., pp. 442–43).

10. "Quod etiam natus sim parentibus senibus, fui minus pulcher et validus. Mater enim cum me genuit 37 pater 56 annum agebant" (ibid., p. 443).

11. Ibid., pp. 444–45; *Opera* 5:521–23; "transmutabitur in ramices, aut calculum, quod et accidit iam" (ibid., p. 523; cf. *Liber duodecim geniturarum* [1554], p. 445: "a 61 ad 69 transmutabitur . . .).

12. Notably in *La carne impassibile* (Milan, 1983).

13. *Encomium medicinae, Opera* 6:5. The *Encomium*, first published in 1559 (see n. 70 to chap. 8), is an oration, probably delivered at the University of Pavia.

14. Gianbattista Da Monte, *Lectiones . . . in secundam fen primi Canonis Avicennae* (Venice, 1557), pp. 54–56. The passage is part of a long disquisition on accident, sign, symptom, and cause in disease that fills lectures 3–6 (pp. 27–79). For brief discussion, see Siraisi, *Avicenna*, pp. 346–48. On the Renaissance debates on disease, see further Nutton, "Seeds of Disease" and "Reception of Fracastoro's Theory."

15. VP 1, *Patria et maiores, Opera* 1:1–2; 2, *Nativitas nostra*, ibid., p. 2. ". . . destitutus corporeis viribus" (ibid.).

16. "Infirmo statu corporis plurifariam fui, natura, casu, symptomatibus" (ibid., p. 5).

17. "Inde anno MDXXXVI (quis credidisset?) correptus fluxu urinae, et magno etiam, cum annis pene XL laborem [*sic*] eodem, a LX unciis ad centum in singolos dies, vivo, nec contabesco (inditio annuli iidem) nec sitio: et multi eodem anno hoc malo correpti adiutore nullo, longe plus perdurarunt, quam qui medicorum opem quaesiere" (ibid.).

18. *Contradictiones* 2.6.14, *Opera* 6:636.

19. VP 6, *Opera* 1:5–6.

20. Giovanni Argenterio, *Varia opera de re medica* (Florence, 1550), reprinted in his *Opera* (Venice, 1592), vol. 2. The theme of Galen's inconsistency in defining disease, symptom, etc., recurs throughout Argenterio's treatises on disease; for examples, see *Opera* (Venice, 1592), 2:1–2, 91. For brief discussion, see Siraisi, "Giovanni Argenterio," pp. 170–72. The views of Da Monte (n. 14, above) and Argenterio on disease, its causes, means of transmission, and proper definition form part of the same body of debate.

21. UC 2.2, 4, 9, 10, 13, *Opera* 2:46–48, 50–51, 76, 76–77, 80.

22. "Nam et hoc incredibile malum mihi successit anno aetatis vigesimo primo. Quo nescio, quo casu abreptus peste pueris familiari, coepi primum cum iuvencula concumbere de more, iam satis, ut mihi videbar, ad venerem validus ac promptus. Verum aliter res cessit. Nam redire in patriam coactus, ab eo tempore usque at trigesimum primum annum exactum, hoc est, integro decennio, nusquam mihi licuit cum muliere concumbere. Etsi enim plures mecum dormitum ducerem maxime eo anno, quo Academiam Patavinam regere contigit, liber animo, viribus caetera validus, aetate florentissima, abstinentia ac ciborum delectu pari industria utens, omnes tamen siccas reliqui: ita ut cum saepius idem fecissem, taedio, pudore, desperatione, in totum ab hac experientia desistere decreverim: nempe aliquando tribus perpetuis noctibus apud me mulierculas habueram, nec quidquam profeceram. Fateor ingenue hoc unum mihi malorum fuisse gravissimum. Non servitus paterna, non paupertas, non morbi, non inimicitia, lites, iniuriae civium, repulsa medicorum, falsae calumniae, infinitaque illa malorum congeries me ad desperationem, vitae odium, voluptatum contemptum, tristitiamque perpetuam adigere potuerunt: hoc unum certe potuit. Deflebam calamitatem, ludibrium naturae; deflebam veritas nuptias et perpetuam orbitatem" (ibid., 2.10, *Opera* 2:76–77). In the first edition of *De utilitate ex*

adversis capienda (Basel, 1561; IA *132.082), pp. 280–81, the wording of the first two sentences of the passage quoted is slightly different, but the sense is the same.

23. "Ergo hac cura, tum etiam purgatione corporis in priore morbo, atque auxiliis ob eum adhibitis, sanus non solum vixi . . . sed quasi adverso flumine devectus, quamquam ingravescente indies aetate, prosperiore tamen valetudine sum usus" (ibid., 2.2, *Opera* 2:48).

24. VP 6, *Opera* 1:5.

<h2 style="text-align:center">EPILOGUE</h2>

1. Gliozzi, "Cardano, Gerolamo," pp. 760–61. The inquisitor's sentence and Cardano's written acceptance of it are edited in Alessandro Simili, *Gerolamo Cardano nella luce e nell'ombra del suo tempo*, Istituto di Storia della Medicina della R. Università di Bologna (Milan, 1941), pp. 14–15.

2. Biblioteca Apostolica Vaticana, MS reg. lat. 2023, fol. 66r (fol. 67v, "Supplica a sua s.ta. Alla Cong. dell' Ill.mo Card.le delle Indici di Hieronimo Cardano Med."). The letter is discussed and in part quoted in Di Rienzo, "Cardaniana," p. 106. It is undated, but in it Cardano refers to himself as seventy-three years old.

3. Maclean, "Cardano and His Publishers," p. 318. On Cardano's religious ideas and contacts, see also Di Rienzo, "La religione di Cardano."

4. I have consulted Biblioteca Apostolica Vaticana, MS ottobon. lat. 2173, 26 fols., H. Cardani in suorum librum castigationes Praefatio. Inc.: "Non solum decet (dicebat C. Caesar) Caesaris uxorem carere culpa. . . ." This is one of two manuscripts of this work in the Vatican Library; the other, in the fondo Ludovisi-Boncompagni, is described in Di Rienzo, "Cardaniana." The incipits and outline of the contents match, but I have not confronted the manuscripts themselves. The date of the version of the work in ottobon. lat. 2173 is established on fol. 8r: "Anno quoque praeterito silicet MDLXXII. . . ." On the early stages of the composition of the *Castigationes*, see Di Rienzo, "Cardaniana," pp. 105–6.

5. Comm. *Aliment*, 1574 (chap. 6, n. 32), ST (chap. 4, n. 2); *Examen*, 1574 or 1575 (chap. 6, n. 27). No doubt some of the other miscellaneous or fragmentary medical and nonmedical writings first published in vols. 9 and 10 of the *Opera* may also have been written or revised at Rome.

6. Maclean, "Cardano and His Publishers," p. 329.

7. "Vestrae enim sanctitatis pro sua humanitate Cardanum vivum dilexit, et mortui memoriam conservat, et auctoritate promotus, et ope sublevatus, multo celerius quam fecissem opus ipsum promulgavi" (Rodolfo Silvestri, dedicatory epistle to Gregory XIII, ST [Rome, 1580], a2r); see also chap. 4, n. 2, and Maclean, "Cardano and His Publishers," p. 327.

8. "Quanto al utile, el si vede chiaro che qua a Roma ho fatto tante cure maravigliose ch'io mai non feci la quarta parte nè a Pavia nè a Bologna, nè a Milano nè in Inghilterra, e tutto è statto causa l'haver l'animo sencero tutto rivolto

solo al medicar con diligentia" (Cardano to Annibale Osio, segretario del Reggimento, April 25, 1573, edited in Costa, "Gerolamo Cardano allo Studio di Bologna," pp. 432–33, at p. 433).

9. *Visitatio cadaverica oratoris Francorum*, March 7, 1575, document edited in Bertolotti, "I testamenti," appendix of documents, no. 7, pp. 647–48.

10. Biblioteca Apostolica Vaticana, MS vat. lat. 6535, fols. 9–11r, supposedly autograph, *consilium* by Cardano; vat. lat. 7250, 17c, fol. 33r, Ricordo del Cardano per il Conclave (presumably the one resulting in the election of Gregory XIII).

11. Rome, Archivio di Stato, Università, busta 48, Liber Decretorum, 1568–82, fol. 77r–v. Fols. 78r–97r include records of other meetings attended by Cardano or in which he was referred to. I am deeply grateful to Dr. Andrea Carlino for generously drawing my attention to this document and helping me to obtain photocopies.

12. Ibid., fols. 94v, 97r.

13. "Quaerit medicus, an morbi, an sanationes a Deo immitantur, quemadmodum facit Hippocrates. Sursumque mentem dirigens theologus evadit. Idem quid sit anima, an mortalis, an immortalis, idem quid astra possint, et eodem modo an ab illis morbi sanationesque pendeant: ab iisdem enim utrumque fieri, a quo alterum eorum fiat verisimile est. Ita motus siderum, et exortus considerans atque occasus, tempora quoque geniturarum reditus non mediocrem astrologiae partem tractat. Inde ad ventos, anni constitutiones, pluvias, serenitatem aut nubes siccas, frigora caloresque metheorologicum dicetis exquisitissimum. Rursus cum domorum considerat structuram commodaque, architectum peritissimum. Quibus ventis exponendae fenestrae, porticus, atrium: quibus lignis constare debeant aedes: quae cubicula aut coenacula et quomodo construenda, ut hyemali sole tepeant, aestiva aura refrigerentur. Mitto coquorum artem, quam penitissime oportet ut norit, totque alia quae nunc enumerando potius ad ostentationem protrahi oratio forsan videri posset, quam necessitatis causa recitari: haec solum adiiciam, quae ad medicum tantum pertinent, eique sunt propria: quorum scientia adeo admirabilis est, ut unus medicus plura scire videatur, quam universi alii artifices aut philosophi. Quid enim maius dici apud mortales aut excogitare potest, quam hominem unum non solum noscere plantas omnes ac fructus tum lapides, metalla, pisces, aves, serpentes, quadrupedia membraque illorum universa: sed generationem tum illorum, tum etiam eorum animalium quae insecta dicuntur? Sed formam et regiones ubi nascantur, quaeque optima pessimave sint? et quod maximum est, vires, secretasque potentias ac miracula? Ut si haec in parte medicus philosopho conferatur, videatur sane philosophus parvulus, viro comparatus. Nonne medicus herbas, arbores, fructus, semina, flores, solus depingit? solus quid possint novit? atque idem in omnibus quae terra producit facit? Quid dicam postmodum de dissectione illa admirabili corporum nostrorum, deque notitia usus uniuscuiusque partis? Ille solus vim etiam elementorum novit: ille morum perturbationes etiam sanare docet: nonne haec (ingenue fateamur, quae manifestissima sunt) prope ad divinitatem accedunt. Quid subtilissima illa pulsuum atque urinarum cognitio, ac adeo admirabilis, ut multi eam esse negent, in qua cum natura ipsa cum ipso rerum opifice (sed tamen id me-

mentote, omnem humanam scientiam umbram quandam esse, cum ad divinam immensitatem comparatur) contendere velle videtur? Quid dicam de divinis medici periti oraculis in praedicendo, cum et mortem et salutem, et tempora et qualitatem adeo norit, ut nullus vates, nulla deorum responsa mereantur illis conferri?" (*Encomium medicinae, Opera* 6:6–7).

BIBLIOGRAPHY

PRIMARY SOURCES

Works of Girolamo Cardano

MANUSCRIPTS

Rome, Biblioteca Nazionale Centrale

S. Francesca a Ripa 1, 16c, pp. 1–285, Cardano, *Proptuarium, seu manuarium.*

S. Francesca a Ripa 2, 16c, 95 fols., Cardano, *Experimenta.*

S. Francesca a Ripa 4, 16c, 99 fols., many blank. Cardano, [*Experimenta*].

S. Francesca a Ripa 11, 125 fols. Fol. 1r, heading: "Hieronimi Cardani Mediolensis medici civisque Bononiensis professoris supraordinarii publice profitentis in libro de victu in acutis commentaria anni 1569."

Vatican City, Biblioteca Apostolica Vaticana

Chigi E. V. 171, *Hieronymi Cardani dialogus cui nomen Carcer.* 17c copy, fols. 7r–68v, bound with 16c original, fols. 70r–98r.

Ottobon. lat. 2173, 16c, fols. 1–26. *H. Cardani in suorum librorum castigatio.*

Reg. lat. 2023, 16c, fols. 66r–67v. Letter from Cardano.

Vat. lat. 5848, fols. 1r–106v, Cardano, comm. *Epidemics*, 71 numbered lectures. Fol. 1r, heading: Hieronymi Cardani Mediolanensis civisque Bononiensis professoris supra ordinarii medicinae in expositione primorum librorum Epidemiorum praefatio anni MCDLXIII.

Vat. lat. 6535, miscellany, fols. 9r–10v, undated, *consilium* by Cardano.

Vat. lat. 7250, 17c, fol. 33r, *Ricordo del Cardano per il Conclave.*

PRINTED BOOKS

In the case of works consulted both in independent editions published during Cardano's lifetime or within five years of his death and in the *Opera omnia*, the location in the *Opera* is given immediately following the reference to the sixteenth-century edition.

Anathomiae Mundini cum expositione. Opera 10:129–67.

Ars curandi parva quae est absolutissimus medendi methodos et alia nunc prima aedita opera. 2 vols. Basel, 1564, 1566. (Vol. 1 = *Opera* 7:143–99.)

The Book of My Life (De vita propria liber). Translated by Jean Stoner. New York, 1930, 1962.

Commentaria in libros Hippocratis de victu in acutis. Opera 10:168–92.

Commentaria in quatuor primas Principis primae sectionis docrinas [sic], seu Floridorum libri duo. Opera 9:453–567 (= *In primam primi Hasen* = Avicenna, *Canon* 1.1.1–4).

Commentarii in Hippocratis de aere, aquis, et locis opus. Basel, 1570. (*Opera* 8:1–212.)

Commentarii tres in primum Epidemiorum Hippocratis librum. Commentarii duo in secundum Hippocratis [Epidemiorum] librum. Opera 10:168–387.

Consilia medica ad varios partium morbos spectantia. Opera 9:47–246.

Contradicentium medicorum liber continens contradictiones centum octo. Venice, 1545.

Contradicentium medicorum liber primus [-secundus] continens contradictiones centum et octo. Lyon, 1548. (*Opera* 6:295–654.)

De causis, signis, ac locis morborum, liber unus. Bologna, 1569. (*Opera* 7:65–108).

De malo recentiorum medicorum medendi usu libellus ad illustrem virum D. Philippum Archintum. . . . Eiusdem libellus de simplicium medicinarum noxa. Venice, 1536.

De malo recentiorum medicorum medendi usu libellus, centum errores illorum continens. Eiusdem libellus de simplicium medicinarum noxa. Venice, 1545. (= *De methodo medendi sectiones tres*, secs. 1 and 2, *Opera* 7:199–252.)

De methodo medendi sectiones quatuor. Paris, 1565. (Secs. 1–3 = *Opera* 7:199–264.)

De oxymelitis usu in pleuritide. Ad Thaddaeum Dunum epistola. Opera 7:271–74. Also in Duno's letter collection; see under Duno, Taddeo, below.

De propria vita liber. Opera 1:1–54.

De radice cina, De sarzaparilia. In Auger Ferrier, *De pudendagra lue hispanica libri duo. Adiecimus De radice cina, et Sarzaparilia Hieronymi Cardani medici.* Antwerp, 1564. (*Opera* 7:265–66, 271.)

De rerum varietate libri XVII. Basel, 1557.

De sapientia libri quinque. . . . Eiusdem de libris propriis, liber unus. Nuremberg, 1544. (*Opera* 1:492–582, 55–59.)

De subtilitate libri XXI. Lyon, 1550.

De subtilitate libri XXI. Basel, 1560. (*Opera* 3:357–672.)

De urinis liber. Opera 7:109–42.

De usu ciborum liber. Opera 7:1–64.

De utilitate ex adversis capienda libri IIII. Basel, 1561. (*Opera* 2:1–282.)

Della mia vita. Translated into Italian, with introduction and notes, by Alfonso Ingegno. Milan, 1982.

Dialogus Hieronymi Cardani et Facii Cardani ipsius patris. Opera 1:637–40.

Encomia medicinae Johannis Beverovicii, Desiderii Erasmi Roterodami, Hieronymi Cardani, necnon Philippi Melancthonii. Rotterdam, 1665.

"Ex Hieronymi Gardani [*sic*] Contradictionibus, Contradictione III. Articulari morbo, an balneum competat [= *Contradictiones* 1.4.3]." In *De balneis omnia quae extant apud Graecos, Latinos, et Arabas, tam medicos quam quoscunque caeterarum artium probatos scriptores,* fol. 226v. Venice 1553.

Examen XX aegrorum Hippocratis [from *Epidemics* 1 and 3]. *Opera* 9:36–46.

The First Book of Jerome Cardan's De Subtilitate. Edited and translated by Myrtle Marguerite Cass. Williamsport, Pa., 1934.

In Cl[audii] Ptolemaei Pelusiensis IIII de astrorum iudiciis aut ut vulgo vocant quadripartitae constructionis libros [= *Tetrabiblos*] *commentaria. . . . Praeterea eiusdem Hier[onymi] Cardani Geniturarum XII ... utilia exempla.* Basel, 1554.

In Hippocratis Coi prognostica, opus divinum. . . . Atque etiam in Galeni prognosticorum expositionem, commentarii absolutissimi. Item in libros Hippocratis de septimestri et octomestri partu, et simul in eorum Galeni commentaria, Cardani commentarii. Basel, 1568. In fact, no commentary on *De octimestri partu* is included. (*Opera* 8:581–806; 9: 1–36.)

In librum Hippocratis de alimento commentaria praelecta dum profiteretur supraordinariam medicinae, Bononiae anno MDLXVIII. Rome, 1574. (*Opera* 7:356–515.)

In septem Aphorismorum Hippocratis particulas commentaria. . . . Eiusdem de venenorum differentiis, viribus et adversus ea remediorum praesidiis ac praesertim De pestis generibus omnibus praeservatione et cura libri III. Basel, 1564. (*Opera* 8:213–580; 7:275–355.)

Lettura della fronte: Metoposcopia. Edited by Alberto Arecchi. Milan, 1994.

Libelli quinque. . . . V. de exemplis centum geniturarum. . . . Nuremberg, 1547. (*Opera* 5:458–502.)

Liber de libris propriis, eorumque ordine et usu, ac de mirabilibus operibus in arte medica per ipsum factis. Lyon, 1557. (*Opera* 1:60–95.)

Opera omnia. Edited by C. Spon. 10 vols. Lyon, 1663. Facsimile edition, New York and London, 1967.

Opus novum cunctis de sanitate tuenda ac vita producenda studiosis apprime necessarium: in quatuor libros digestum. A Rodulpho Sylvestrio Bononiensi Medico, recens in lucem editum. Rome, 1580. (*Opera* 6:8–294.)

Opuscula medica senilia (*De dentibus, De rationali curandi ratione, De facultatibus medicamentorum, De morbo regio*). Lyon 1638. (*Opera* 9:247–452, where *De morbis articularibus* is added.)

Quaedam opuscula, artem medicam exercentibus utilissima, ut sunt, de aqua et aethere, de cyna radice. . . . Medicinae encomium. . . . Basel, 1559. (*Opera* 2:570–614; 7:266–70; 6:1–7.)

Sogni. Edited by Agnese Grieco and Mauro Mancia. Venice, 1993. (Italian translation of *Somniorum synesiorum libri,* bks. 2 and 3 and selections from bk. 4.)

Somniorum synesiorum omnis generis insomnia explicantes libri IIII. . . . Quibus accedunt eiusdem haec etiam: De libris propriis. De curationibus et praedictionibus admirandis. Neronis encomium. . . . Basel 1562. (*Opera* 5:593–727; 1:96–150; 7:252–64; 1:179–220.)

Sul sonno e sul sognare. Edited by Mauro Mancia and Agnese Grieco. Venice, 1989. (Italian translation of *Somniorum synesiorum libri,* bk. 1.)

Theonoston. Opera 2:299–454.

Other Primary Sources

MANUSCRIPT

Rome, Archivio di Stato, Università, busta 48, Liber Decretorum, 1568–82, fols. 77r–97r. Minutes of meetings of the College of Physicians (*Collegium physicorum*) of Rome, 1574–76.

PRINTED BOOKS

Alderotti, Taddeo. *Expositiones in arduum aphorismorum Ipocratis volumen, In divinum pronosticorum Ipocratis librum, In preclarum regiminis acutorum Ipocratis opus, In subtilissimum Joannitii Isagogarum libellum.* Venice, 1527.

Alemanus. See L'Alemant.

Argenterio, Giovanni. *Tres in Artem medicam Galeni commentarii.* In his *Opera,* vol. 1. 3 vols. in 1. Venice, 1592.

————. *Varia opera de re medica.* Florence, 1550.

Aristides, Aelius. *Orationum tomi tres nunc primum latine versi a Guilielmo Cantero. . . .* Basel, 1566. *Sacrorum sermones primus . . . sextus* at 1:154–208.

Artemidorus Daldianus. *De somniorum interpretatione libri quinque.* Translated by Janus Cornarius. Basel, 1539.

Articella nuperrime impressa. Lyon, 1515.

Avicenna latinus. Liber de anima seu sextus de naturalibus IV–V. Edited by S. Van Riet with introduction by G. Verbeke. Louvain, 1968.

Baveria, Baverio. *Consilia Bavierii.* Pavia, 1521.

Belon, Pierre. *L'histoire naturelle des estranges poissons marins. . . .* Paris, 1551.

Benedetti, Alessandro. *Historia corporis humani sive Anatomice.* Venice, 1502.

Benivieni, Antonio. *De abditis non nullis ac mirandis morborum et sanationum causis.* Edited in A. Costa and G. Weber, *L'inizio dell'anatomia patologica nel Quattrocento fiorentino, sui testi di Antonio Benivieni, Bernardo Torni, Leonardo da Vinci. Archivio "De Vecchi" per l'Anatomia Patologica,* vol. 39, fasc. 2, pp. 429–821. Florence, 1963 (recently reissued, with revised and abbreviated introductory material, as Benivieni, Antonio. *De abditis nonnullis ac mirandis morborum et sanationum causis.* Edited by Giorgio Weber. Florence, 1994).

————. *De abditis nonnullis ac mirandis morborum et sanationum causis.* Facsimile of edition of Florence, 1507, with English translation by Charles Singer and introduction by Esmond R. Long. Springfield, Ill., 1954.

————. *Encomion Cosmi ad Laurentiam Medicem. Riproduzione dell'autografo con proemio e trascrizione.* Edited by Renato Piattoli. Florence, 1949.

Berengario da Carpi, Jacopo. *Isagoge breves perlucide ac uberime [sic] in Anatomiam.* Venice, 1535.

————. *A Short Introduction to Anatomy (Isagoge Breves).* Translated by L. R. Lind. Chicago, 1959.

Berriot, François, ed. *Exposicions et significacions des songes et Les songes Daniel.* Geneva, 1989.

Brain, Peter. *Galen on Bloodletting: A Study of the Origins, Development and Validity of His Opinions, with a Translation of Three Works.* Cambridge, 1986.

Brasavola, Antonio Musa. *In octo libros Aphorismorum Hippocratis et Galeni commentaria et annotationes.* Basel, 1546.

Camuzio, Andrea. *Disputationes, quibus Hieronymi Cardani magni nominis viri conclusiones infirmantur, Galenus ab eiusdem iniuria vindicatur, Hippocratis praeterea aliquot loca diligentius multo, quam unquam alias, explicantur. . . .* Pavia, 1563.

Carcano Leone, Gianbattista. *Exenterationis cadaveris illustrissimi Cardinalis*

Borrhomaei Mediolani Archiepiscopi . . . verissima, atque elegantissima enarratio. Milan, 1584.

Cattani, Andrea. *Opus de intellectu et de causis mirabilium effectuum.* N.p., n.d., but thought to be Florence, ca. 1502.

Clowes, William. *A Profitable and Necessarie Booke of Observations, for all those that are burned with the flame of Gun powder, &c.* Facsimile of the edition of London, 1596, with introduction by De Witt T. Starnes and Chauncey D. Leake. New York, 1945.

Cogliati Arano, Luisa, ed. *The Medieval Health Handbook: Tacuinum sanitatis.* New York, 1976.

Cornaro, Alvise. *Scritti sulla vita sobria, elogio e lettere.* Edited by Marisa Milani. Venice, 1983.

Corti, Matteo. *In Mundini Anatomen commentarius.* Lyon, 1551.

Costeo, Giovanni. *Disquisitionum physiologicarum . . . in primam primi Canonis Avicennae sectionem libri sex. . . .* Bologna, 1589.

Cyrurgia Guidonis de Cauliaco. Et Cyrurgia Bruni Theodorici Rogerii Rolandi Bertapalie Lanfranci. Venice, 1498.

Dallari, Umberto, ed. *I rotuli dei lettori legisti e artisti dello Studio bolognese dal 1384 al 1799,* vol. 2. 2 vols. Bologna, 1889.

Da Monte, Gianbattista (Montanus). *In tertium primi Epidemiorum sectionem explanationes.* Venice, 1554.

———. *Lectiones . . . in secundam fen primi Canonis Avicennae.* Venice, 1557.

Daza Chacon, Dionisio. *Practica y teorica de Cirugia.* 2 vols. Madrid, 1678.

Dubois, Jacques (Sylvius). *Ordo et ordinis ratio in legendis Hippocratis et Galeni libris.* Paris, 1548.

Duno, Taddeo. *Thaddaei Duni Locarniensis medici et Francisci Cigalini, Ioannisque Pauli Turriani medicorum Novocomensium clarissimorum, item Hieronymi Cardani medici et philosophi celeberrimi disputationum per epistolas liber unus.* Zurich, n.d. (preface dated 1555).

Estienne, Charles. *De dissectione partium corporis humani libri tres.* Paris, 1545.

Falloppia, Gabriele. *Observationes anatomicae.* Venice, 1561.

Fernel, Jean. *Universa medicina tribus et viginti libris absoluta. Ab ipso quidem authore ante obitum diligenter recognita, et quatuor libris nunquam ante editis, ad praxim tamen perquam necessariis, aucta.* Lyon, 1581.

Ferrier, Auger. *Liber de somniis. Hippocratis de insomniis liber. Galeni liber de insomniis. Synesii liber de somnis.* Lyon, 1549.

Ficino, Marsilio. *Three Books on Life.* Edited and translated by Carol V. Kaske and John R. Clark. Binghamton, N.Y., 1989.

Fuchs, Leonhart. *Errata recentiorum medicorum LX numero, adiectis eorundem confutationibus.* Hagenau, 1530.

———. *Hippocratis Coi medicorum omnium sine controversia principis Aphorismorum sectiones septem recens e Graeco in Latinum sermonem conversae, et luculentissimis, iisdemque breviss. commentariis illustratae et expositae.* Paris, 1545.

———. *Hippocratis medicorum omnium longe principis Epidemiorum Liber Sextus. . . . Addita est luculenta universi eius libri expositio.* Hagenau, 1532.

Galen. *Galeni in primum Hippocratis de morbis vulgaribus librum commentarius primus Hermanno Cruserio Campensi interprete.* Paris, 1534 [title page missing in the New York Academy of Medicine copy].

———. *In Hippocratis Epidemiarum libros I et II.* Edited by Ernst Wenkebach and Franz Pfaff. *Corpus Medicorum Graecorum* V 10, 1. Berlin, 1934.

———. *On Prognosis.* Edited and translated by Vivian Nutton. *Corpus Medicorum Graecorum* V 8, 1. Berlin, 1979.

———. *On the Usefulness of the Parts of the Body.* Translated by Margaret T. May. 2 vols. Ithaca, 1968.

———. *Opera omnia.* Edited by C. G. Kühn. 20 vols. Leipzig, 1821–33.

Gaurico, Luca. *Super diebus decretoriis (quos etiam criticos vocitant) axiomata, sive aphorismi grandes utique sententiae brevi oratione compraehensae. Enucleavit item pleraque Hippocratis, et Galeni theoremata, quae medici rerum coelestium expertes vix olfecerunt. Isagogicus astrologiae Tractatus medicis admodum oportunus. . . .* Rome, 1546.

Gesner, Conrad. *Historiae animalium liber IIII, qui est de Piscium et Aquatilium animantium natura.* Zurich, 1558.

Giovio, Paolo. *De piscibus.* In his *Opera* 9:11–64. Edited by Ernesto Travi and Mariagrazia Penco. Rome, 1984.

Gradi, Giovanni Matteo Ferrari de. *Consilia . . . secundam viam Avicen[nae].* Venice, 1521.

Guglielmo da Saliceto. *Cyrurgia.* Printed with his *Summa conservationis et curationis.* Venice, 1489.

———. *Summa conservationis et curationis.* Venice, 1489.

Hansen, Bert. *Nicole Oresme and the Marvels of Nature: A Study of His "De causis mirabilium" with Critical Edition, Translation, and Commentary.* Toronto, 1985.

Heseler, Baldasar. *Andreas Vesalius' First Public Anatomy at Bologna 1540: An Eyewitness Report.* Edited by Ruben Eriksson. Uppsala, 1959.

Hippocrates. *De l'Aliment.* In *Hippocrate,* vol. 6, pt. 2. Edited and translated into French by Robert Joly. Paris, 1972.

———. *Epidemie libro sesto.* Edited and translated into Italian by Daniela Manetti and Amneris Roselli. Florence, 1982.

———. *Octoginta volumina . . . per M. Fabium Calvum Latinitate donata. . . .* Rome, 1525.

———. *Oeuvres complètes d'Hippocrate.* Edited and translated by E. Littré. 10 vols. Paris, 1839–61.

———. *Opera . . . nunc tandem per M. Fabium Rhavennatem, Guilielmum Copum Basiliensem, Nicolaum Leonicenum, et Andream Brentium, viros doctissimos Latinitate donata.* Basel, 1526.

———. *Opera quae ad nos extant omnia. Per Ianum Cornarium medicum physicum latina lingua conscripta.* Basel, 1546.

———. Loeb Classical Library. 7 vols. Cambridge, Mass., 1972–94.

Incisa Della Rochetta, G., et al., eds. *Il primo processo per San Filippo Neri.* 4 vols. Vatican City, 1957–63.

L'Alemant, Adrien (Alemanus). *Hippocratis medicorum omnium principis, de aere, aquis, et locis, Liber olim mancus nunc integer . . . commentariis quatuor illustratus.* Paris, 1557.

Legio, Leonardo. *Practice ordinarie ibidem interpretis fabrica regiminis sanitatis.* Milan, 1522.

Lind, L. R. *Studies in Pre-Vesalian Anatomy: Biography, Translations, Documents.* Philadelphia, 1975.

Liuzzi, Mondino de'. *Anothomia.* Edited by Piero P. Giorgi and Gian Franco Pasini. Bologna, 1992.

Massa, Niccolò. *Anatomiae liber introductorius.* Venice, 1559.

Matal (Metellus), Jean. Letter to George Cassandre, April 15, 1565, printed in J.-P. Nicéron, *Mémoires pour servir à l'histoire des hommes illustrés dans la république des lettres,* 10:153–54. Paris, 1731.

Memorie e documenti per la storia dell'Università di Pavia e degli uomini più illustri che v'insegnavano. Pavia, 1875.

Mercuriale, Girolamo. *De morbis puerorum. Item de venenis et morbis venenosis. Quibus adiuncta est Censura Hippocratis.* Basel, 1584.

Mercurio, Girolamo (fra' Scipione). *La commare o riccoglitrice.* Excerpts edited in Maria Luisa Altieri Biagi et al., *Medicina per le donne nel Cinquecento: Testi di Giovanni Marinello e di Girolamo Mercurio.* Turin, 1992.

Montanus. See Da Monte.

Nardi, G. M. "Antonio Benivieni ed un suo scritto inedito sulla peste." *Atti e memorie dell'Accademia di Storia d'Arte Sanitaria* 4 (1938): 124–33, 190–97.

Nifo, Agostino. *De intellectu libri sex. Eiusdem de demonibus libri tres.* Venice, 1527.

Paré, Ambroise. *The Apologie and Treatise Containing the Voyages Made into Divers Places.* Edited by Geoffrey Keynes. New York, 1968.

Parodi, Giacomo. *Elenchus privilegiorum, et actuum publice Ticinensis Studii a seculo nono ad nostra tempora.* Pavia, 1753.

Pico, Gianfrancesco. *Examen vanitatis doctrinae gentium et veritatis Christianae disciplinae.* Mirandola, 1520.

Pico della Mirandola, Giovanni. *Disputationes adversus astrologiam divinatricem.* Edited by Eugenio Garin. 2 vols. Florence, 1946.

Pietro d'Abano. *Conciliator: Ristampa fotomeccanica dell'edizione Venetiis apud Iuntas 1565.* Edited by Ezio Riondato and Luigi Olivieri. Padua, 1985.

Platina, Bartolomeo. *De honesta voluptate et valetudine. . . .* Venice, 1475.

Pomponazzi, Pietro. *De naturalium effectuum admirandorum causis et de incantationibus liber.* In his *Opera.* Basel, 1567.

Rangone, Tommaso. *Iulio Tertio Sanctissimo. Thomae Philologi Ravenna De vita homini ultra CXX annos protrahenda.* Venice, 1553.

Rondelet, Guillaume. *Libri de piscibus marinis.* Lyon, 1554.

Salviani, Ippolito. *Aquatilium animantium historia liber primus.* Rome, 1554 [1558].

Sanches, Francisco. *De divinatione per somnum, ad Aristotelem.* In his *Opera philosophica.* Coimbra, 1955.

———. *That Nothing Is Known.* Edited by Elaine Limbrick and Douglas F. S. Thomson. Cambridge, 1988.

Savonarola, Michele. *Libreto de tute le cosse che se manzano.* Edited by Jane Nystedt. Stockholm, 1982.

Scaliger, Julius Caesar. *Exotericarum exercitationes libri XV de subtilitate ad Hieronymum Cardanum.* Frankfurt, 1592.

———. *Hippocratis Liber de somniis cum Iulii Caesaris Scaligeris commentariis.* Lyon, 1539.

Scappi, Bartolomeo. *Opera di M. Bartolomeo Scappi cuoco secreto di Papa Pio Quinto.* Florence, 1570.

Smith, Wesley D., ed. and trans. *Hippocrates: Pseudepigraphic Writings.* Leiden, 1990.

Statuti e ordinamenti per l'Università di Pavia dall'anno 1361 al 1859. Pavia, 1925.

Synesius of Cyrene. *Synesius de somniis translatus a Marsili Ficino Florentino.* In Marsilio Ficino, *Opera omnia* 2:1968–79. Turin, 1959; facsimile reproduction of the edition of Basel, 1576.

Torrigiani, Pietro. *Turisani monaci plusquam commentum in microtegni Galieni. Cum questione eiusdem de Ypostasi.* Venice, 1512.

Valles, Francisco. *Controversiarum medicarum et philosophicarum . . . libri decem. . . .* Frankfurt, 1590.

Verde, Armando F. *Lo studio fiorentino 1473–1503: Ricerche e documenti.* Vol. 2, *Docenti-dottorati.* Florence, 1973.

Vesalius, Andreas. *Anatomicarum Gabrielis Falloppii observationum examen. . . .* Venice, 1564.

———. *The Bloodletting Letter of 1539.* Translated by J. B. de C. M. Saunders and C. D. O'Malley. New York, n.d.

———. *De humani corporis fabrica libri septem.* Basel, 1543.

Zerbi, Gabriele. *Gerontocomia, On the Care of the Aged,* and Maximianus, *Elegies on Old Age and Love.* Translated by L. R. Lind. Memoirs of the American Philosophical Society, vol. 182. Philadelphia, 1988.

Secondary Studies and Reference Works

Agrimi, Jole, and Chiara Crisciani. *Les consilia médicaux.* Typologie des sources du Moyen Age Occidental, fasc. 69. Turnhout, 1994.

———. *Edocere medicos.* Naples, 1988.

———. "Medicina e logica in maestri bolognesi tra Due e Trecento: Problemi e temi di ricerca." In *L'insegnamento della logica a Bologna nel XIV secolo,* edited by Dino Buzzetti et al., pp. 187–239. Bologna, 1992.

Albini, Giuliana. *Guerra, fame, peste: Crisi di mortalità e sistema sanitario nella Lombardia tardomedioevale.* Bologna, 1982.

Appleby, Andrew W. "Diet in Sixteenth-Century England: Sources, Problems, Possibilities." In *Health, Medicine and Mortality in the Sixteenth Century,* edited by Charles Webster, pp. 97–116. Cambridge, 1979.

Ashworth, William B. "Natural History and the Emblematic World View." In *Reappraisals of the Scientific Revolution,* edited by David C. Lindberg and Robert Westman, pp. 304–32. Cambridge, 1990.

Barton, Tamsyn S. *Power and Knowledge: Astrology, Physiognomics, and Medicine under the Roman Empire.* Ann Arbor, Mich., 1994.

Bellagarda, G. "G. Cardano e la scoperta dell'infezione focale." *Minerva stomatologica* 15 (1966): 563–66.

———. "Quattro studi su G. Cardano. II. Il 'De dentibus' di G. Cardano." *Minerva stomatologica* 14 (1965): 563–67.

———. "Quattro studi su G. Cardano. IV. G. Cardano e l'odontoiatria." *Minerva stomatologica* 15 (1966): 695–99.

Belloni, Luigi. "L'aneurisma di S. Filippo Neri nella relazione di Antonio Porto." *Rendiconti dell'Istituto Lombardo di Scienze e Lettere. Classe di scienze* 83 (1950): 665–80.

Benson, Pamela Joseph. *The Invention of the Renaissance Woman: The Challenge of Female Independence in the Literature and Thought of Italy and England.* University Park, Pa., 1992.

Bertolotti, A. "I testamenti di Girolamo Cardano, medico, filosofo e matematico nel secolo XVI." *Archivio storico lombardo* 9 (1882): 615–60.

Biagioli, Mario. "The Social Status of Italian Mathematicians, 1450–1600." *History of Science* 27 (1989): 41–95.

Bianchi, Massimo Luigi. "Scholastische Motive im ersten und zweiten Buch des *De subtilitate* Girolamo Cardanos." In *Girolamo Cardano: Philosoph, Naturforscher, Arzt*, edited by Eckhard Kessler, pp. 115–30. Wiesbaden, 1994.

Bilancioni, Guglielmo. "Leonardo e Cardano." *Rivista di storia delle scienze mediche e naturali* 12 (1930): 302–29.

Blair, Ann. "Humanist Methods in Natural Philosophy: The Commonplace Book." *Journal of the History of Ideas* 53 (1992): 541–51.

———. *The Theater of Nature: Jean Bodin and Renaissance Science.* Princeton: Princeton University Press, forthcoming, 1997.

Blok, Josine. *The Early Amazons: Modern and Ancient Perspectives on a Persistent Myth.* Leiden, 1995.

Bono, James J. "Medical Spirits and the Medieval Language of Life." *Traditio* 40 (1984): 91–130.

———. *The Word of God and the Languages of Man: Interpreting Nature in Early Modern Science and Medicine.* Vol. 1, *Ficino to Descartes.* Madison, 1995.

Bonuzzi, Luciano. "Qualche considerazione su sonno e sogno dal tramonto della cultura classica all'età del manierismo." *Acta medicae historiae patavina* 20 (1973–74): 57–102.

Bottero, A. "I più antichi statuti del collegio dei medici di Milano." *Archivio storico lombardo*, n.s., 8 (1943): 72–112.

Braudel, Fernand. *The Mediterranean and the Mediterranean World in the Age of Philip II.* 2 vols. New York, 1972.

Bregman, Jay. *Synesius of Cyrene.* Berkeley and Los Angeles, 1982.

Brind'amour, Pierre. *Nostradamus astrophile: Les astres et L'astrologie dans la vie et l'oeuvre de Nostradamus.* Ottawa, 1993.

Browne, Alice. "Girolamo Cardano's *Somniorum synesiorum libri IIII*." *Bibliothèque d'humanisme et Renaissance* 40 (1979): 123–35.

Burrow, J. A. *The Ages of Man: A Study in Medieval Writing and Thought.* Oxford, 1986.

Bylebyl, Jerome J. "The School of Padua: Humanistic Medicine in the Sixteenth Century." In *Health, Medicine and Mortality in the Sixteenth Century*, edited by Charles Webster, pp. 335–70. Cambridge, 1979.

————. "Teaching *Methodus medendi* in the Renaissance." In *Galen's Method of Healing*, edited by Fridolf Kudlien and Richard J. Durling, pp. 157–89. Leiden, 1991.

Calvi, Giulia. *Histories of a Plague Year: The Social and the Imaginary in Baroque Florence*. Berkeley, 1989.

Campana, Augusto. "Manente Leontini Fiorentino, medico e traduttore di medici greci." *La Rinascita* 4 (1961): 499–15.

Camporesi, Piero. *Bread of Dreams: Food and Fantasy in Early Modern Europe*. Cambridge, 1989. Originally published as *La carne impassibile*. Milan, 1983.

Carlino, Andrea. *La fabbrica del corpo: Libri e dissezione nel Rinascimento*. Turin, 1994.

————. "'Knowe thyself': Anatomical Figures in Early Modern Europe." *Res* 27, *Anthropology and Aesthetics* (Spring 1995): 52–69.

Carmichael, Ann. "Diseases of the Renaissance and Early Modern Europe." In *The Cambridge World History of Human Disease*, edited by Kenneth R. Kiple, pp. 279–87. Cambridge, 1993.

————. "The Health Status of Florentines in the Fifteenth Century." In *Life and Death in Fifteenth-Century Florence*, edited by Marcel Tetel, Ronald G. Witt, and Rona Goffen, pp. 28–45. Durham, N.C., 1989.

Carugo, Adriano. "Giuseppe Moleto: Mathematics and the Aristotelian Theory of Science at Padua in the Second Half of the Sixteenth Century." In *Aristotelismo veneto e scienza moderna*, pp. 509–16. Padua, 1983.

Cavagna, Anna Giulia. *Libri e tipografi a Pavia nel Cinquecento: Note per la storia dell'Università e della cultura*. Milan, 1981.

Céard, Jean. "La diététique dans la médecine de la Renaissance." In *Pratiques et discours alimentaires à la Renaissance*, edited by Jean-Claude Margolin and Robert Sauzet, pp. 21–36. Paris, 1982.

————. *La nature et les prodiges: L'insolite au XVIe siècle en France*. Paris, 1977.

————. "La notion de 'miraculum' dans la pensée de Cardan." In *Acta conventus neo-latini turonensis*, edited by Jean-Claude Margolin, 2:924–37. 2 vols. Paris, 1976.

Christian, William L. *Apparitions in Late Medieval and Renaissance Spain*. Princeton, 1981.

Cipolla, Carlo. *Public Health and the Medical Profession in the Renaissance*. Cambridge, 1976.

Clarke, John R. "Roger Bacon and the Composition of Marsilio Ficino's *De Vita longa* (*De vita*, Book II)." *Journal of the Warburg and Courtauld Institutes* 49 (1986): 230–33.

Connors, Joseph. "*Ars tornandi*: Baroque Architecture and the Lathe." *Journal of the Warburg and Courtauld Institutes* 53 (1990): 217–36.

Cooper, Richard. "Deux médecins royaux onirocrites: Jehan Thibault et Auger Ferrier." In *Le songe à la Renaissance*, edited by Françoise Charpentier, pp. 53–59. St. Etienne, 1987.

Copenhaver, Brian. "Did Science Have a Renaissance?" *Isis* 83 (1992): 387–407.

————. "Iamblichus, Synesius and the Chaldean Oracles in Marsilio Ficino's *De vita libri tres*: Hermetic Magic or Neoplatonic Magic." In *Supplementum Festivum: Studies in Honor of Paul Oskar Kristeller*, edited by James Hankins, John Monfasani, and Frederick Purnell, pp. 441–55. Binghamton, N.Y., 1987.

————. "Renaissance Magic and Neoplatonic Philosophy: 'Ennead' 4. 3–5 in Ficino's 'De vita coelitus comparanda.'" In *Marsilio Ficino e il ritorno di Platone: Studi e documenti*, edited by Gian Carlo Garfagnini, 2:451–69. 2 vols. Florence, 1986.

————. *Symphorien Champier and the Reception of the Occultist Tradition in Renaissance France*. The Hague, 1978.

————. "A Tale of Two Fishes: Magical Objects in Natural History from Antiquity through the Scientific Revolution." *Journal of the History of Ideas* 52 (1991): 373–98.

Costa, Emilio. "Gerolamo Cardano allo Studio di Bologna." *Archivio storico italiano*, 5th ser., 35 (1905): 425–36.

Coturri, Enrico. "L'inizio di una 'Practica' lasciata incompiuta e ancora inedita di Antonio Benivieni." *Episteme: Rivista critica di storia delle scienze mediche e biologiche* 8 (1974): 3–25.

Crisciani, Chiara. "History, Novelty, and Progress in Scholastic Medicine." *Osiris* 6 (1990): 118–39.

Crummer, Leroy. "Early Anatomical Fugitive Sheets." *Annals of Medical History* 5 (1923): 189–209.

Cunningham, Andrew. "Fabricius and the 'Aristotle Project' in Anatomical Teaching and Research at Padua." In *The Medical Renaissance of the Sixteenth Century*, edited by Andrew Wear, Roger French, and I. M. Lonie, pp. 195–22. Cambridge, 1985.

Cushing, Harvey. *A Bio-Bibliography of Andreas Vesalius*. New York, 1943.

Dall'Osso, Eugenio. "Aranzio, Giulio Cesare." *Dictionary of Scientific Biography*, 1:204. New York, 1970.

Daston, Lorraine. "Marvelous Facts and Miraculous Evidence in Early Modern Europe." *Critical Inquiry* 18 (1991): 93–124.

Davis, Natalie Zemon. *Fiction in the Archives: Pardon Tales and Their Tellers in Sixteenth-Century France*. Stanford, 1987.

————. "Ghosts, Kin, and Progeny: Some Features of Family Life in Early Modern France." *Daedalus* 106 (1977): 87–114.

De Ferrari, A. "Corti (Curti, Curzio, de Curte, de Corte), Matteo." *Dizionario biografico degli italiani*, 29:795–97. Rome, 1983.

De Vecchi, Bindo. "I libri di un medico umanista fiorentino del sec. XV dai 'Ricordi' di maestro Antonio Benivieni." *La bibliofilia* 34 (1932): 293–301.

Dear, Peter, ed. *The Literary Structure of Scientific Argument: Historical Studies*. Philadelphia, 1991.

Demaitre, Luke, "The Care and Extension of Old Age in Medieval Medicine." In *Aging and the Aged in Medieval Europe*, edited by Michael M. Sheehan, pp. 3–22. Toronto, 1990.

————. "The Care of Health in Old Age: The Development of Gerocomy in the Renaissance." In *Aging and the Life Cycle in the Renaissance: The Interaction between Representation and Experience*, edited by Adele Seefe and Edward Ansello. University of Delaware Press, forthcoming.

Demandt, Alexander. *Der Fall Roms*. Munich, 1984.

Di Rienzo, Eugenio. "Cardaniana: Su alcuni manoscritti inediti di Cardano conservati alla Biblioteca Vaticana." *Rivista di storia e letteratura religiosa* 25 (1989): 102–10.

———. "La religione di Cardano." In *Girolamo Cardano: Philosoph, Naturforscher, Arzt*, edited by Eckhard Kessler, pp. 49–76. Wiesbaden, 1994.

Durling, Richard J. *A Catalogue of Sixteenth Century Printed Books in the National Library of Medicine*. Bethesda, 1967.

———. "A Chronological Census of Renaissance Editions and Translations of Galen." *Journal of the Warburg and Courtauld Institutes* 24 (1961): 230–305.

———. "An Early Manual for the Medical Student and the Newly-Fledged Practitioner: Martin Stainpeis' *Liber de modo studendi seu legendi in medicina* ([Vienna] 1520)." *Clio Medica* 3 (1970): 5–33.

Eamon, William. *Science and the Secrets of Nature: Books of Secrets in Medieval and Early Modern Culture*. Princeton, 1994.

Eckman, James. *Jerome Cardan. Supplements to the Bulletin of the History of Medicine*, no. 7. Baltimore, 1946.

Ernst, Germana. "'Veritatis amor dulcissimus': Aspetti dell'astrologia in Cardano." In *Girolamo Cardano: Philosoph, Naturforscher, Arzt*, edited by Eckhard Kessler, pp. 158–54. Wiesbaden, 1994.

Faccioli, Emilio. "La cucina dal Platina allo Scappi." In *Trattati scientifici nel Veneto fra XV e XVI secolo*, edited by Ezio Riondati. Vicenza, 1985.

Fattori, Marta. "Sogni e temperamenti." In *I sogni nel Medioevo*, edited by Tullio Gregory, pp. 87–109. Rome, 1985.

Ferrari, Giovanna. "Public Anatomy Lessons and the Carnival: The Anatomy Theatre of Bologna." *Past and Present* 117 (1987): 51–106.

Ferrary, Jean-Louis. *Correspondance de Lelio Torelli avec Antonio Agustín et Jean Matal (1542–53)*. Como, 1993.

Fierz, Markus. *Girolamo Cardano, 1501–1576*. Boston, 1983.

Findlen, Paula. *Possessing Nature: Museums, Collecting, and Scientific Culture in Early Modern Italy*. Berkeley and Los Angeles, 1994.

Firpo, Massimo. *Inquisizione romana e Controriforma: Studi sul cardinale Giovanni Morone e il suo processo d'eresia*. Bologna, 1992.

———, ed. *Il processo inquisitoriale del cardinale Giovanni Morone*. Vols. 1–6. Rome, 1981–95.

Folena, Gianfranco. "Per la storia della ittionimia volgare: Tra cucina e scienza naturale." *Bollettino dell'Atlante Linguistico Mediterraneo* 5–6 (1963–64): 61–137.

Frame, Donald. *Montaigne's Essais: A Study*. Englewood Cliffs, N.J., 1969.

French, Roger. "Berengario da Carpi and the Use of Commentary in Anatomical Teaching." In *The Medical Renaissance of the Sixteenth Century*, edited by Andrew Wear, Roger French, and I. M. Lonie, pp. 42–74. Cambridge, 1985.

———. *William Harvey's Natural Philosophy*. Cambridge, 1994.

Friedman, John B. *The Monstrous Races in Medieval Art and Thought*. Cambridge, Mass., 1981.

Garin, Eugenio. *Medioevo e Rinascimento*. Bari, 1961.

———. *Lo zodiaco della vita*. Bari and Rome, 1976.

Gil Sotres, Pedro. "Le regole della salute." In *Storia del pensiero medico occidentale*. Vol. 1, *Antichità e Medioevo*, edited by Mirko D. Grmek, pp. 399–438. Rome and Bari, 1993.

Ginex Palmiere, Ede. *San Carlo Borromeo: L'uomo e la sua epoca*. Milan, 1984.

Glacken, Clarence J. *Traces on the Rhodian Shore: Nature and Culture in Western Thought from Ancient Times to the End of the Eighteenth Century*. Berkeley, 1967.

Gliozzi, G. "Cardano, Gerolamo." *Dizionario biografico degli italiani*, 19:758–63. Rome, 1976.

Gourevitch, Danielle. *Le triangle hippocratique dans le monde gréco-romain: Le malade, sa maladie et son médecin*. Rome, 1984.

Grafton, Anthony. *Cardano's Cosmos: The Three Worlds of a Renaissance Magus*. Cambridge: Harvard University Press, forthcoming, 1997.

———. *Defenders of the Text: The Traditions of Scholarship in an Age of Science, 1450–1800*. Cambridge, Mass., 1991.

———. *Forgers and Critics: Creativity and Duplicity in Western Scholarship*. Princeton, 1990.

———. "From Apotheosis to Analysis: Some Late Renaissance Histories of Classical Astronomy." In *History and the Disciplines*, edited by Donald E. Kelley. Rochester, N.Y.: Rochester University Press, forthcoming, 1997.

———. *Girolamo Cardano and the Tradition of Classical Astrology*. Rothschild Lecture, 1995, Department of the History of Science, Harvard University. Cambridge, 1996.

———. "Humanism, Magic, and Science." In *The Impact of Humanism on Western Europe*, edited by Anthony Goodman and Angus MacKay, pp. 99–117. London and New York, 1990.

———. *Joseph Scaliger: A Study in the History of Classical Scholarship*. Vol. 1, *Textual Criticism and Exegesis*. Oxford, 1983.

———. *New Worlds, Ancient Texts*. Cambridge, Mass., 1992.

———. "On the Scholarship of Politian and Its Context." *Journal of the Warburg and Courtauld Institutes* 40 (1977): 150–88.

———. "L'umanista come lettore." In *Storia della lettura nel mondo occidentale*, edited by Guglielmo Cavallo and Roger Chartier, pp. 199–242. Rome and Bari, 1995.

Grafton, Anthony, and Noel M. Swerdlow. "Technical Chronology and Astrological History in Varro, Censorinus, and Others." *Classical Quarterly* 35 (1985): 454–65.

Grant, Edward. "Medieval and Renaissance Scholastic Conceptions of the Influence of the Celestial Regions on the Terrestrial." *Journal of Medieval and Renaissance Studies* 17 (1987): 1–23.

Gregori, Carlo. "L'elogio del silenzio e la simulazione come modelli di comportamento in Gerolamo Cardano." In *Sapere e/è potere. Discipline, dispute e professioni nell'università medievale e moderna. Il caso bolognese a confronto.* Vol. 3, *Dalle discipline ai ruoli sociali,* edited by Angela De Benedictis, pp. 73–84. Bologna, 1990.

Gregori, Carlo. "Rappresentazione e difesa: Osservazioni sul *De vita propria* di Gerolamo Cardano." *Quaderni storici* 73 (1990): 225–34.

Gregory, Tullio. "I sogni e gli astri." In *I sogni nel Medioevo,* edited by Tullio Gregory, pp. 111–48. Rome, 1985.

———, ed. *I sogni nel Medioevo.* Rome, 1985.

Grieco, Allen J. "Les plantes, les régimes végétariens et la mélancholie à la fin du Moyen Age et au début de la Renaissance italien." In *Le monde végétal (XIIe–XVIIe siècles): Savoirs et usages sociaux,* edited by Allen J. Grieco et al., pp. 11–29. Saint-Denis, 1993.

———. "The Social Politics of Pre-Linnean Botanical Classification." *I Tatti Studies: Essays in the Renaissance* 4 (1991): 131–49.

Gruman, Gerald J. *A History of Ideas about the Prolongation of Life: The Evolution of Prolongevity Hypotheses to 1800. Transactions of the American Philosophical Society,* n.s., 56, pt. 9. Philadelphia, 1966.

Guidorizzi, Giulio. "L'interpretazione dei sogni nel mondo tardantico: Oralità e scrittura." In *I sogni nel Medioevo,* edited by Tullio Gregory. Rome, 1985.

———, ed. *Il sogno in Grecia.* Rome, 1988.

Hall, Thomas S. "Life, Death and the Radical Moisture." *Clio medica* 6 (1971): 3–23.

Harcourt, Glen. "Andreas Vesalius and the Anatomy of Antique Sculpture." *Representations,* no. 17 (1987): 28–61.

Harvey, Barbara. *Living and Dying in England 1100–1540: The Monastic Experience.* Oxford, 1993.

Haviland, Thomas N., and Lawrence C. Parish. "A Brief Account of the Use of Wax Models in the Study of Medicine." *Journal of the History of Medicine and Allied Sciences* 25 (1970): 52–75.

Henderson, John. *Piety and Charity in Late Medieval Florence.* Oxford, 1994.

Herrlinger, Robert. *Volcher Coiter.* Nuremberg, 1952.

Hodgen, Margaret. *Early Anthropology in the Sixteenth and Seventeenth Centuries.* Philadelphia, 1964, 1971.

Hunter, Kathryn Montgomery. *Doctors' Stories: The Narrative Structure of Medical Knowledge.* Princeton, 1991.

Ilberg, Johann. "Zur Ueberlierferung des hippokratischen Corpus." *Rheinisches Museum für Philologie* 21 (1887): 436–61.

Index aureliensis: Catalogus librorum sedicimo saeculo impressorum. Pt. 1, vol. 6. Orleans, 1976.

Ingegno, Alfonso. "Cardano e Bruno. Altri spunti per una storia dell''uomo perfetto.'" In *Girolamo Cardano: Philosoph, Naturforscher, Arzt,* edited by Eckhard Kessler, pp. 77–90. Wiesbaden, 1994.

———. "Il perfetto e il furioso." *Il piccolo Hans: Rivista di analisi materialistica* 75/76 (Autumn–Winter 1992–93): 11–31.

———. *Saggi sulla filosofia di Cardano.* Florence, 1980.

Jacquart, Danielle. "La question disputée dans les facultés de médecine." In Bernardo C. Bàzan, John F. Wippel, Gérard Fransen, and Danielle Jacquart,

Les questions disputées et les questions quodlibétiques dans les facultés de théologie, de droit et de médecine, fasc. 44–45, pp. 281–313. Typologie des sources du Moyen Age occidental. Turnhout, 1983.

———. "Theory, Everyday Practice, and Three Fifteenth-Century Physicians." *Osiris* 6 (1990): 161–80.

Jensen, Kristian. "Cardanus and His Readers in the Sixteenth Century." In *Girolamo Cardano: Philosoph, Naturforscher, Arzt,* edited by Eckhard Kessler, pp. 265–308. Wiesbaden, 1994.

Jones, Peter Murray. "John of Arderne and the Mediterranean Tradition of Scholastic Surgery." In *Practical Medicine from Salerno to the Black Death,* edited by Luis Garcia-Ballester et al., pp. 289–321. Cambridge, 1991.

———. "Thomas Lorkyn's Dissections." *Transactions of the Cambridge Bibliographical Society* 9 (1988): 209–30.

Julia, Dominique, Jacques Revel, and Roger Chartier, eds. *Les universités européennes du XVIe au XVIIIe siècle: Histoire sociale des populations étudiantes.* Vol. 1. Paris, 1986.

Kagan, Richard L. *Lucrecia's Dreams: Politics and Prophecy in Sixteenth-Century Spain.* Berkeley, 1990.

———. "Universities in Italy 1500–1700." In *Les universités européennes du XVIe au XVIIIe siècle: Histoire sociale des populations étudiantes,* vol. 1, edited by Dominique Julia, Jacques Revel, and Roger Chartier, pp. 153–86. Paris, 1986.

Keil, Gundolf, ed. *Der Humanismus und die oberen Facultäten.* Weinheim, 1987.

Kemp, Martin. "From 'Mimesis' to 'Fantasia': The Quattrocento Vocabulary of Creation, Inspiration, and Genius in the Visual Arts." *Viator* 8 (1977): 347–99.

Kessler, Eckhard. "*Alles ist Eines wie der Mensch und das Pferd.* Zu Cardano's Naturbegriff." In *Girolamo Cardano: Philosoph, Naturforscher, Arzt,* edited by Eckhard Kessler, pp. 91–114. Wiesbaden, 1994.

———, ed. *Girolamo Cardano: Philosoph, Naturforscher, Arzt.* Wiesbaden, 1994.

Kibre, Pearl. *Hippocrates latinus.* New York, 1985.

Kibre, Pearl, and R. J. Durling. "A List of Latin Manuscripts Containing Medieval Versions of the *Methodus medendi.*" In *Galen's Method of Healing,* edited by Fridolf Kudlien and Richard J. Durling, pp. 117–22. Leiden, 1991.

King, Margaret L. *The Death of the Child Valerio Marcello.* Chicago, 1994.

Kleinbaum, Abby Wettan. *The War against the Amazons.* New York, 1983.

Kristeller, Paul Oskar. "Bartolomeo, Musandino, Mauro di Salerno e altri antichi commentatori dell''Articella,' con un elenco di testi e di manoscritti." In his *Studi sulla scuola medica salernitana,* pp. 97–151. Naples, 1986.

Krivatsky, Peter. *A Catalogue of Seventeenth Century Printed Books in the National Library of Medicine.* Bethesda, 1989.

Kruger, Steven F. *Dreaming in the Middle Ages.* Cambridge, 1992.

Kümmel, Werner Friedrich. "Der Homo litteratus und die Kunst, gesund zu leben. Zur Entfaltung eines Zweiges der Diätetik im Humanismus." In *Humanismus und Medizin,* edited by Rudolf Schmitz and Gundolf Keil, pp. 67–85. Bonn, 1984.

Kusukawa, Sachiko. *The Transformation of Natural Philosophy: The Case of Philip Melanchthon.* Cambridge, 1995.

La Ca' Granda: Cinque secoli di storia e d'arte dell'Ospedale Maggiore di Milano. Milan, 1981.

Lawn, Brian. *The Rise and Decline of the Scholastic "Quaestio Disputata" with Special Emphasis on Its Use in the Teaching of Medicine and Science.* Leiden, 1993.

———. *The Salernitan Questions: An Introduction to the History of Medieval and Renaissance Problem Literature.* Oxford, 1963.

Le Brun, Jacques. "Jérôme Cardan et l'interpretation des songes." In *Girolamo Cardano: Philosoph, Naturforscher, Arzt*, edited by Eckhard Kessler, pp. 185–206. Wiesbaden, 1994.

Le Goff, Jacques. "Dreams in the Culture and Collective Psychology of the Medieval West." In his *Time, Work, and Culture in the Middle Ages*, pp. 201–4. Chicago, 1980.

Lehoux, Françoise. *Le cadre de vie des médecins parisiens aux XVIe et XVIIe siècles.* Paris, 1976.

Lloyd, G.E.R. "Galen on Hellenistics and Hippocratics: Contemporary Battles and Past Authorities." In his *Methods and Problems in Greek Science*, pp. 398–416. Cambridge, 1991.

Lohr, Charles H. *Latin Aristotle Commentaries.* Vol. 2, *Renaissance Authors.* Florence, 1988. Vol. 3, *Index initiorum—Index finium.* Florence, 1995.

Long, Esmond R. "Jean Fernel's Conception of Tuberculosis." In *Science, Medicine and History*, edited by E. Ashworth Underwood, 1:401–7. 2 vols. Oxford, 1953.

Lonie, Iain M. "Cos versus Cnidus and the Historians: Part 1." *History of Science* 16 (1978): 42–75.

———. "The Paris Hippocratics." In *The Medical Renaissance of the Sixteenth Century*, edited by Andrew Wear, R. K. French, and I. M. Lonie, pp. 155–74. Cambridge, 1985.

Lopez Piñero, José Maria. *Los temas polémicos de la medicina renacentista: Las Controversias (1556), de Francisco Valles.* Madrid, 1988.

Lubkin, Gregory. *A Renaissance Court: Milan under Galeazzo Maria Sforza.* Berkeley and Los Angeles, 1994.

Maclean, Ian. "Cardano and His Publishers, 1534–1663." In *Girolamo Cardano: Philosoph, Naturforscher, Arzt*, edited by Eckhard Kessler, pp. 309–38. Wiesbaden, 1994.

———. "The Interpretation of Natural Signs: Cardano's *De subtilitate* versus Scaliger's *Exercitationes*." In *Occult and Scientific Mentalities in the Renaissance*, edited by Brian Vickers, pp. 231–52. Cambridge, 1984.

———. "Montaigne, Cardano: The Reading of Subtlety / the Subtlety of Reading." *French Studies* 37 (1983): 143–56.

———. *The Renaissance Notion of Woman: A Study in the Fortunes of Scholasticism and Medical Science in European Intellectual Life.* Cambridge, 1980.

Maloney, G., and R. Savoie. *Cinq cent ans de bibliographie hippocratique, 1483–1982.* St.-Jean-Chrysostome, Québec, 1982.

Margolin, Jean-Claude. "Analogie et causalité chez Jérome Cardan." In *Sciences de la Renaissance. VIIIe Congrès International de Tours*, pp. 67–81. Paris, 1973.

———. "Cardan, interprête d'Aristote." In *Platon et Aristote à la Renaissance. XVIe Colloque International de Tours*, pp. 307–33. Paris, 1976.

Martinoli Santini, Livia. "Le traduzioni dal Greco." In *Un pontificato ed una città: Sisto IV (19471–1484). Atti del Convegno, Roma 3–7 Dicembre, 1984*, edited by Massimo Miglio et al., pp. 81–101. Rome, 1986.

Martinotti, Giovanni. "L'insegnamento dell'anatomia in Bologna prima del secolo XIX." *Studi e memorie per la storia dell'Università di Bologna* 2 (1911): 3–146.

Mazzini, Innocenzo. "Manente Leontini, Übersetzer der hippokratischen Epidemien (cod. Laurent. 73, 12): Bemerkungen zu seiner Übersetzung von Epidemien Buch 6." In *Die hippokratischen Epidemien: Theorie—Praxis—Tradition*, edited by Gerhard Baader and Rolf Winau, pp. 312–28. *Sudhoffs Archiv*, Beiheft 27. Stuttgart, 1989.

McNair, Philip. "Poliziano's Horoscope." In *Cultural Aspects of the Italian Renaissance: Essays in Honour of Paul Oskar Kristeller*, pp. 262–75. Manchester and New York, 1976.

McVaugh, Michael R. "The Nature and Limits of Medical Certitude at Early Fourteenth-Century Montpellier." *Osiris* 6 (1990): 62–84.

McVaugh, Michael, and Nancy G. Siraisi, eds. *Renaissance Medical Learning: Evolution of a Tradition. Osiris* 6 (1990).

Mercati, Giovanni. "Altre notizie di M. Fabio Calvo." *Bessarione* 25 (1919): 159–63.

———. "Su Francesco Calvo da Menaggio primo stampatore e Marco Fabio Calvo da Ravenna primo traduttore latino del corpo ippocratico." *Notizie varie di antica letteratura medica e di bibliografia. Studi e testi* 31 (Rome, 1917): 47–71.

Minois, George. *History of Old Age from Antiquity to the Renaissance*. Cambridge, 1989.

Montanari, Massimo. *The Culture of Food*. Oxford, 1994. Originally published as *La fame e l'abbondanza: Storia dell'alimentazione in Europa*. Rome and Bari, 1991.

Mugnai Carrara, Daniela. *La biblioteca di Nicolò Leoniceno*. Florence, 1991.

Müller-Jahncke, Wolf-Dieter. *Astrologisch-magische Theorie und Praxis in der Heilkunde der frühen Neuzeit. Sudhoffs Archiv*, Beiheft 25. Stuttgart, 1985.

Münster, Ladislao. "La medicina legale in Bologna dai suoi albori fino alla fine del secolo XIV." *Bollettino dell'Accademia Medica Pistoiese Filippo Pacini* 26 (1955): 257–71.

Nada Patrone, Anna Maria. *Il cibo del ricco ed il cibo del povero. Contributo alla storia qualitativa dell'alimentazione: L'area pedemontana negli ultimi secoli del Medio Evo*. Turin, 1981.

Nadel, George H. "Philosophy of History before Historicism." *History and Theory* 3 (1964): 291–315.

Niccoli, Ottavia. *Prophecy and People in Renaissance Italy*. Princeton, 1990.

North, J. D. "Astrology and the Fortunes of Churches." *Centaurus* 24 (1980): 181–211.

Nutton, Vivian. "The Changing Languages of Medicine, 1450–1550." In *Vo-*

cabulary of Teaching and Research between Middle Ages and Renaissance, edited by Olga Weijers, pp. 183–98. Turnhout, 1995.

Nutton, Vivian. "Galen and Medical Autobiography." In his *From Democedes to Harvey: Studies in the History of Medicine*. London, 1988.

———. "Hippocrates in the Renaissance." In *Die hippokratischen Epidemien: Theorie-Praxis-Tradition*, edited by Gerhard Baader and Rolf Winau, pp. 420–39. *Sudhoffs Archiv*, Beiheft 27. Stuttgart, 1989.

———. *John Caius and the Manuscripts of Galen*. Supplementary vol. no. 13, Cambridge Philological Society, 1987.

———. "Pieter Van Foreest and the Plagues of Europe: Some Observations on the *Observationes*." In *Pieter Van Foreest: Een Hollands medicus in de zestiende eeuw*, edited by H. L. Houtzager, pp. 25–39. Amsterdam, 1989.

———. "'Qui magni Galeni doctrinam in re medica primus revocavit': Matteo Corti und der Galenismus im medizinischen Unterricht der Renaissance." In *Der Humanismus und die oberen Facultäten*, edited by Gundolf Keil, pp. 173–84. Weinheim, 1987.

———. "The Reception of Fracastoro's Theory of Contagion: The Seed That Fell among Thorns." *Osiris* 6 (1990): 196–234.

———. "The Seeds of Disease: An Explanation of Contagion and Infection from the Greeks to the Renaissance." *Medical History* 27 (1983): 1–34.

———. "Style and Context in the *Method of Healing*." In *Galen's Method of Healing*, edited by Fridolf Kudlien and Richard J. Durling, pp. 1–25. Leiden, 1991.

———. "Wittenberg Anatomy." In *Medicine and the Reformation*, edited by Ole Peter Grell and Andrew Cunningham, pp. 11–32. London, 1993.

———, ed. *Medicine at the Courts of Europe*. London, 1990.

Oberhelman, Steven M. "The Diagnostic Dream in Ancient Medical Theory and Practice." *Bulletin of the History of Medicine* 61 (1987): 47–60.

———. "Galen, *On Diagnosis from Dreams*." *Journal of the History of Medicine and Allied Sciences* 38 (1983): 36–47.

———. "The Interpretation of Prescriptive Dreams in Ancient Greek Medicine." *Journal of the History of Medicine and Allied Sciences* 36 (1981): 416–24.

———. *The Oneirocriticon of Achmet: A Medieval Greek and Arabic Treatise on the Interpretation of Dreams*. Lubbock, Tex., 1991.

Olmi, Giuseppe. *L'inventario del mondo: Catalogazione della natura e luoghi del sapere nella prima età moderna*. Bologna, 1992.

O'Malley, Charles D. *Andreas Vesalius of Brussels, 1514–1564*. Berkeley and Los Angeles, 1964.

———. "Varolio, Costanzo." *Dictionary of Scientific Biography*, 13:587–88. New York, 1976.

O'Malley, C. D., and J. B. de C. M. Saunders. *Leonardo da Vinci on the Human Body: The Anatomical, Physiological, and Embryological Drawings of Leonardo da Vinci*. New York, 1952, 1982.

Ongaro, Giuseppe. "Girolamo Cardano e Andrea Vesalio." *Rivista di storia della medicina* 13 (1969): 51–61.

Ore, Oystein. *Cardano, the Gambling Scholar*. Princeton, 1953.

Ottosson, Per-Gunnar. *Scholastic Medicine and Philosophy.* Naples, 1984.

Palmer, Richard. "Medicine at the Papal Court in the Sixteenth Century." In *Medicine at the Courts of Europe,* edited by Vivian Nutton, pp. 49–78. London, 1990.

Panofsky, Erwin. *Meaning in the Visual Arts.* Garden City, N.Y., 1955.

Paravicini Bagliani, Agostino. "Ruggero Bacone, Bonifacio VIII e la teoria della prolongatio vitae." In his *Medicina e scienza della natura alla corte dei papi del Duecento.* Spoleto, 1991.

Park, Katharine. "The Criminal and the Saintly Body: Autopsy and Dissection in Renaissance Italy." *Renaissance Quarterly* 47 (1994): 1–33.

Park, Katharine, and Lorraine J. Daston. "Unnatural Conceptions: The Study of Monsters in Sixteenth- and Seventeenth-Century France and England." *Past and Present* 92 (1981): 20–54.

———. *Wonders and the Order of Nature, 1150–1750.* New York: Zone Press, forthcoming, 1997.

Pélicier, Yves. "Les nourritures à la Renaissance: Essai de typologie." In *Pratiques et discours alimentaires à la Renaissance,* edited by Jean-Claude Margolin and Robert Sauzet, pp. 15–20. Paris, 1982.

Pereira, Michela. "Un tesoro inestimabile: Elixir e 'prolongatio vitae' nell'alchimia del '300." *Micrologus* 1 (1993): 161–87.

Perosa, A. "Codici di Galeno postillati da Poliziano." In *Umanesimo e Rinascimento: Studi offerti a Paul Oskar Kristeller,* edited by Vittore Branca et al., pp. 80–87. Florence, 1980.

Pesenti, Tiziana. "Le 'articelle' di Daniele di Marsilio Santasofia (d. 1410), professore di medicina." *Studi petrarcheschi* 7 (1990): 50–92.

———. "Michele Savonarola a Padova: L'ambiente, le opere, la cultura medica." *Quaderni per la storia dell'Università di Padova* 9/10 (1977): 45–101.

———. "Le origini dell'insegnamento medico a Pavia." In *Storia di Pavia,* vol. 3, pt. 2, pp. 454–74. Milan, 1990.

———. *Professori e promotori di medicina nello Studio di Padova dal 1405 al 1509: Repertorio bio-bibliografico.* Trieste and Padua, 1984.

Peyronal Rambaldi, Susanna. *Speranza e crisi nel Cinquecento modenese: Tensioni religiose e vita cittadina ai tempi di Giovanni Morone.* Milan, 1979.

Pigeaud, Jackie. "Formes et normes dans le *De fabrica* de Vésale." In *Le corps à la Renaissance. Actes du XXXe Colloque de Tours 1987,* edited by Jean Céard, Marie Madeleine Fontaine, and Jean-Claude Margolin, pp. 399–421. Paris, 1990.

———. "L'Hippocratisme de Cardan: Etude sur le Commentaire d'AEL par Cardan." *Res publica litterarum* 8 (1975): 219–29.

———. "Homo quadratus: Variations sur la beauté et la santé dans la médecine antique." *Gesnerus* 42 (1985): 337–52.

———. "Les problèmes de la création chez Galien." In *Galen und das hellenistische Erbe,* edited by Jutta Kollesch and Diethard Nickel, pp. 87–103. Sudhoffs Archiv, Beiheft 32. Stuttgart, 1993.

Pinault, Jody Rubin. *Hippocratic Lives and Legends.* Leiden, 1992.

Polizzotto, Lorenzo. *The Elect Nation: The Savonarolan Movement in Florence, 1494–1545.* Oxford, 1994.

Pomata, Gianna. *La promessa di guarigione: Malati e curatori in antico regime: Bologna XVI–XVIII secolo.* Rome, 1994.

Porter, Roy. "The Rise of Physical Examination." In *Medicine and the Five Senses,* edited by W. F. Bynum and Roy Porter, pp. 179–97. Cambridge, 1993.

"Pour le Colloque 'Le Songe à la Renaissance.'" *Bulletin de l'Association d'Etude sur l'Humanisme, la Réforme et la Renaissance* 12 (1986): 43–65.

Price, S.R.F. "The Future of Dreams: From Freud to Artemidorus." *Past and Present,* no. 112 (1986): 3–37.

Reeds, Karen. *Botany in Medieval and Renaissance Universities.* New York, 1991.

Richardson, Linda Deer. "The Generation of Disease: Occult Causes and Disease of the Total Substance." In *The Medical Renaissance of the Sixteenth Century,* edited by Andrew Wear, R. K. French, and I. M. Lonie, pp. 175–94. Cambridge, 1985.

Ridder-Symoens, Hilde de, ed. *A History of the University in Europe.* Vol. 1, *Universities in the Middle Ages.* Cambridge, 1992.

Rivier, André. *Recherches sur la tradition manuscrite du traité hippocratique "De morbo sacro."* Bern, 1962.

Rizzo, Silvia. *Il lessico filologico degli umanisti.* Rome, 1984.

Roger, Jacques. *Jean Fernel et les problèmes de la médecine de la Renaissance.* Les Conférences du Palais de la Découverte, ser. D, no. 70. Paris, 1960.

Rossi, Paolo. *Immagini della scienza.* Rome, 1977.

————. *Philosophy, Technology, and the Arts in the Early Modern Era.* New York, 1970. (Originally published as *I filosofi e le macchine.* Milan, 1962.)

Ruderman, David B. *Kabbalah, Magic, and Science: The Cultural Universe of a Sixteenth-Century Jewish Physician.* Cambridge, Mass., 1988.

Rütten, Thomas. *Demokrit lachender Philosoph und sanguinischer Melancholiker: Eine pseudohippkratische Geschichte.* Leiden, 1992.

Rütten, Thomas, and Ulrich Rütten. "Melanchthon's Rede 'De Hippocrate.'" In *Melanchthon und die Naturwissenschaften seiner Zeit.* Sigmaringen, 1996.

Sanders-Goebel, Pamela. "Crisis and Controversy: Historical Patterns in Breast Cancer Surgery." *Canadian Bulletin of Medical History* 8 (1991): 77–90.

Saunders, J. B. de C. M., and Charles D. O'Malley. *The Illustrations from the Works of Andreas Vesalius of Brussels.* Cleveland, 1950; New York, 1973.

Schmidt, Paul Gerhardt. "Kritische Philologie und pseudoantike Literatur." In *Die Antike-Rezeption in der Wissenschaften während der Renaissance,* pp. 117–27. Weinberg, 1983.

Schmitt, Charles B. *Aristotle and the Renaissance.* Cambridge, Mass., 1983.

————. *Studies in Renaissance Philosophy and Science.* London, 1981.

Schmitt, Charles B., et al., eds. *The Cambridge History of Renaissance Philosophy.* Cambridge, 1988.

Schullian, Dorothy M. "Coiter, Volcher." *Dictionary of Scientific Biography,* 3:342–43. New York, 1971.

Schultz, John B. *Art and Anatomy in Renaissance Italy*. Ann Arbor, 1985.

Schupbach, William. *The Paradox of Rembrandt's "Anatomy of Dr. Tulp."* *Medical History*, supplement no. 2. London, 1982.

Sclavi, Susanna. "La biblioteca di Antonio Benivieni." *Physis* 17 (1975): 255–68.

Scully, Terence. "The Sickdish in Early French Recipe Collections." In *Health, Disease, and Healing in Medieval Culture*, edited by Sheila Campbell, Bert Hall, and David Klausner, pp. 132–40. New York, 1992.

Sears, Elizabeth. *The Ages of Man: Medieval Interpretations of the Life Cycle*. Princeton, 1986.

Seifert, Arno. *Cognitio historica*. Berlin, 1976.

Serrai, Alfredo. *Conrad Gesner*. Edited by Maria Cocchetti. Rome, 1990.

Sherrington, Charles. *The Endeavor of Jean Fernel*. London, 1946. Reprint, Folkestone and London, 1974.

Simili, Alessandro. "Gerolamo Cardano, lettore e medico a Bologna: Nota I. La condotta di G. Cardano." *Atti e memorie dell'Accademia di Storia dell'Arte Sanitaria* 39 (1940): 1–62.

———. "Gerolamo Cardano, lettore e medico a Bologna: Nota II. Il soggiorno e gli insegnamenti." *Archiginnasio: Bollettino della Biblioteca Comunale di Bologna* 61 (1966): 384–507.

———. "Gerolamo Cardano, lettore e medico a Bologna: Nota III. Le accuse e la partenza." *Atti e memorie dell'Accademia di Storia dell'Arte Sanitaria*, 2d ser., 32 (1966): 1–7.

———. *Gerolamo Cardano nella luce e nell'ombra del suo tempo*. Istituto di Storia della Medicina della R. Università di Bologna. Milan, 1941.

Siraisi, Nancy G. *Avicenna in Renaissance Italy*. Princeton, 1987.

———. "The Faculty of Medicine." In *A History of the University in Europe*, vol. 1, *Universities in the Middle Ages*, edited by Hilde de Ridder-Symoens, pp. 360–87. Cambridge, 1992.

———. "Giovanni Argenterio and Sixteenth-Century Medical Innovation: Between Princely Patronage and Academic Controversy." *Osiris* 6 (1990): 161–80.

———. "How to Write a Latin Book on Surgery: Organizing Principles and Authorial Devices in Guglielmo da Saliceto and Dino del Garbo." In *Practical Medicine from Salerno to the Black Death*, edited by Luis Garcia Ballester et al., pp. 88–109. Cambridge, 1993.

———. "Medicine, Physiology, and Anatomy in Early Sixteenth-Century Critiques of the Arts and Sciences." In *New Perspectives on Renaissance Thought*, edited by John Henry and Sarah Hutton, pp. 214–29. London, 1990.

———. "The Physician's Task: Medical Reputations in Humanist Collective Biographies." In *The Rational Arts of Living*, edited by A. C. Crombie and Nancy G. Siraisi, pp. 105–33. Smith College Studies in History, vol. 50. Northampton, Mass., 1987.

———. *Taddeo Alderotti and His Pupils*. Princeton, 1981.

———. "Vesalius on Human Diversity." *Journal of the Warburg and Courtauld Institutes* 57 (1994): 60–88.

Smith, Wesley D. *The Hippocratic Tradition*. Ithaca and London, 1979.

Spinelli, Salvatore. *La Ca' Granda, 1456–1956*. Milan, 1956.

Stefanutti, U. "Benivieni, Antonio." *Dizionario biografici degli italiani*, 8:543–45. Rome, 1966.

Storia di Milano. Vols. 8, 9, 10. Milan, 1957.

Taufer, Alison. "The Only Good Amazon Is a Converted Amazon: The Woman Warrior and Christianity in the *Amadis Cycle*." In *Playing with Gender: A Renaissance Pursuit*, edited by Jean R. Brink, Maryanne C. Horowitz, and Allison P. Coudert, pp. 35–51. Urbana, 1991.

Temkin, Owsei. *Galenism*. Ithaca, 1973.

———. *Hippocrates in a World of Pagans and Christians*. Baltimore, 1991.

Thorndike, Lynn. *A History of Magic and Experimental Science*. Vol. 5. New York, 1941.

Thorndike, Lynn, and Pearl Kibre. *A Catalogue of Incipits of Mediaeval Scientific Writings in Latin*. 2d ed. Cambridge, Mass., 1963.

Tooley, Marian J. "Bodin and the Medieval Theory of Climate." *Speculum* 28 (1953): 64–83.

Truman, Ron. "Jean Matal and His Relations with Antonio Agustín, Jerónimo Osório da Fonseca and Pedro Ximenes." In *Antonio Agustín between Renaissance and Counter-Reform*, edited by M. H. Crawford, pp. 247–63. Warburg Institute Surveys and Texts 24. London, 1993.

Vaccari, Pietro. *Storia della Università di Pavia*. 2d ed. Pavia, 1957.

Vickers, Brian, ed. *Occult and Scientific Mentalities in the Renaissance*. Cambridge, 1984.

Von Staden, Heinrich. "Anatomy as Rhetoric: Galen on Dissection and Persuasion." *Journal of the History of Medicine and Allied Sciences* 50 (1995): 47–66.

Wagner, Jean-Marie. "De la nécessaire distinction entre 'somnium'-songe et 'insomnium'-rêve." In *Acta Conventus Neo-Latini Turonensis*, edited by Jean-Claude Margolin, pp. 709–20. Paris, 1980.

Walker, D. P. *Spiritual and Demonic Magic from Ficino to Campanella*. London, 1958.

Wear, Andrew. "Explorations in Renaissance Writings on the Practice of Medicine." In *The Medical Renaissance of the Sixteenth Century*, edited by Andrew Wear, R. K. French, and I. M. Lonie. Cambridge, 1985.

Wear, Andrew, R. K. French, and I. M. Lonie, eds. *The Medical Renaissance of the Sixteenth Century*. Cambridge, 1985.

Webster, Charles. *From Paracelsus to Newton*. Cambridge, 1982.

———, ed. *Health, Medicine and Mortality in the Sixteenth Century*. Cambridge, 1979.

Webster, Charles, and Margaret Pelling. "Medical Practitioners." In *Health, Medicine and Mortality in the Sixteenth Century*, edited by Charles Webster, pp. 165–235. Cambridge, 1979.

Welch, Evelyn S. *Art and Authority in Renaissance Milan*. New Haven, 1995.

Wenskus, Otta. *Astronomische Zeitangaben von Homer bis Theophrast. Hermes: Zeitschrift für klassische Philologie*, Einzelschriften 55. Stuttgart, 1990.

Yates, Frances. *The Art of Memory*. Chicago, 1966.

———. *Giordano Bruno and the Hermetic Tradition*. London, 1964.

Zambelli, Paola. *L'ambigua natura della magia*. Milan, 1991.

―――. "Introduction: Astrologer's Theory of History." In *"Astrologi hallucinati": Stars and the End of the World in Luther's Time*, edited by Paola Zambelli, pp. 1–28. Berlin and New York, 1986.

―――. "Many Ends for the World: Luca Gaurico, Instigator of the Debate in Italy and Germany." In *"Astrologi hallucinati": Stars and the End of the World in Luther's Time*, edited by Paola Zambelli, pp. 239–63. Berlin and New York, 1986.

Zanetti, Dante. "La morte a Milano nei secoli XVI–XVIII: Appunti per una ricerca." *Rivista storica italiana* 88 (1976): 803–51.

Zanier, Giancarlo. "Cardano e la critica delle religioni." *Giornale critico della filosofia italiana* 54 (1979): 89–98.

―――. *Medicina e filosofia tra '500 e '600*. Milan, 1983.

―――. *Ricerche sulla diffusione e fortuna del "De incantationibus" di Pomponazzi*. Florence, 1975.

Zimmerman, T. C. Price. *Paolo Giovio: The Historian and the Crisis of Sixteenth-Century Italy*. Princeton, 1995.

Zöllner, F. *Vitruvs Proportionsfigur: Quellenkritische Studien zur Kunstliteratur im 15. und 16. Jahrhundert*. Worms, 1987.

INDEX

Frequently occurring names (e.g., Hippocrates, Galen) are indexed very selectively; titles of works by Girolamo Cardano analyzed in the text are not indexed.

About the Author

NANCY G. SIRAISI is Professor of History at Hunter College and the Graduate School of the City University of New York. Her books include *Avicenna in Renaissance Italy* and *Taddeo Alderotti and His Pupils*, both published by Princeton University Press, and *Medieval and Early Renaissance Medicine* (Chicago).